NURSING SCHOOL ENTRANCE EXAMS PREP

TENTH EDITION

ALSO FROM KAPLAN NURSING

Books

NCLEX-RN® Prep

NCLEX-RN® Content Review Guide

NCLEX-PN® Prep

NCLEX-PN® Content Review Guide

The Basics: A Comprehensive Outline of Nursing School Content

NCLEX® Medication Review

Dosage Calculation Workbook

Talk Like a Nurse

Online

Kaplan NCLEX-RN® Qbank

Kaplan NCLEX-PN® Qbank

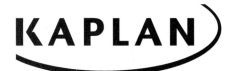

NURSING SCHOOL ENTRANCE EXAMS

PREP

TENTH EDITION

Our 80 years' expertise = Your competitive advantage

YOUR ALL-IN-ONE GUIDE TO THE KAPLAN AND HESI® EXAMS

© 2023 by Kaplan North America, LLC

Published by Kaplan North America, LLC dba Kaplan Publishing
1515 West Cypress Creek Road
Fort Lauderdale, Florida 33309

10 9 8 7 6 5 4 3 2

ISBN: 978-1-5062-9036-2

Kaplan North America, LLC print books are available at special quantity discounts to use for sales promotions, employee premiums, or educational purposes. For more information or to purchase books, please call the Simon & Schuster special sales department at 866-506-1949.

Contents

KAPLAN

How to Use This Book

Congratulations! You've taken the first step to prepare yourself for the two most popular nursing school entrance exams: Kaplan Nursing Admission Test and the HESI A2. This book contains the information you want and need to do your best on both exams and get into the school of your choice. Use the icons beside each topic head to tailor your studies to the exam you are taking: **K** for the Kaplan and **H** for the HESI.

To get you started, Part One provides important information about each test and offers practical tips for handling Test Day stress.

Chapter One includes test-taking strategies that will boost your confidence on this or any test you take. The tips in this chapter show you how to increase your score. It also includes tips to minimize your stress on Test Day. Learn the habits that will help you keep cool under any testing conditions.

Before you start your review, find out exactly what your strengths and weaknesses are. The 60-question diagnostic quiz in Chapter Two will help you focus your studies so you don't waste time reviewing topics you have already mastered.

Parts Three through Five of this book offer you targeted lessons, strategies, and review questions. These sections are tailored to the content tested on the most popular nursing exams: verbal and language content (in Chapters Three through Five), mathematics (Chapter Six), and Science (Chapters Seven through Nine). In short, the lessons and practice in these sections will prepare you for success.

Once you have learned about the test and reviewed the subjects covered, you are ready for more practice. Part Six includes two practice tests modeled on the content of the Kaplan exam and two practice tests modeled on the content of the HESI A2 exam. Each practice test comes complete with answer keys and detailed answer explanations. By taking these practice tests, you will be able to apply the test-taking strategies you have learned, as well as identify areas in which you have improved and areas that still require further study.

KAPLAN

Finally, the Learning Resources found in Part Seven will serve as a quick reference for useful information. Look here to quickly find frequently used math formulas, commonly misspelled words, and other key study resources. In addition, you will find a directory of State Boards of Nursing.

By using Kaplan's *Nursing School Entrance Exams Prep*, you are taking an important step in getting the score you need to start a successful nursing career. Good luck!

kaptest.com/retail-book-corrections-and-updates

The material in this book is up-to-date at the time of publication. However, changes may have been instituted in the tests after this book was published.

If there are any important late-breaking developments—or changes or corrections to the Kaplan test preparation materials in this book—we will post that information online at kaptest.com/publishing. Check to see if there is any information posted there regarding this book.

About the Tests

INTRODUCTION

Congratulations! You have chosen to read a book that could very well change your life. When you take the nursing school entrance exam, you will feel confident, and you will be prepared to excel. You won't face unwanted surprises.

In the eyes of the schools you want to be admitted to, your successful test results demonstrate your real potential for learning. The schools need to know that you possess basic math, science, and verbal skills. It's a win-win situation for both you and the schools.

Nursing schools across the country use several different tests to determine who is admitted to their programs. Although these exams have different names and different formats, they all ask you to verify the same skills. In short, nursing schools want to know that you have basic knowledge in 3 main subjects: Verbal and Language, Mathematics, and Science.

The two most popular nursing school entrance exams, the Kaplan Nursing Admission Test and the HESI A2 exam (short for Health Education Systems, Inc., Admissions Assessment), cover many of the same areas but have different emphases. For example, both tests include questions that assess reading and writing skills; however, the HESI A2 exam has a section devoted specifically to the topic of vocabulary, while the Kaplan exam does not. Does this mean you should skip material related to vocabulary if you are taking the Kaplan exam? No. But knowing which areas are highlighted on each test can help you concentrate your studies more effectively. This book uses icons to help you identify at a glance which exam each topic appears on: (K) for the Kaplan and (H) for the HESI.

Here's how the Kaplan exam breaks down, complete with the number of questions and the amount of testing time allotted to complete each section:

Section	# of Questions	# of Minutes to Complete
Reading Comprehension	22	45
Writing	21	45
Math	28	45
Science	20	30
Totals	**91**	**165 (2 hours 45 minutes)**

KAPLAN)

Here's how the HESI exam breaks down, complete with the number of questions and the amount of testing time allotted to each section:

Section	# of Questions	# of Minutes to Complete
Reading Comprehension	47	60
Vocabulary	50	50
Grammar	50	50
Mathematics	50	50
Biology	25	25
Chemistry	25	25
Anatomy and Physiology	25	25
Totals	272	285 (4 hours 45 minutes)

The HESI also includes unscored questions to assess the test taker's learning style and personality profile. These are meant to help you identify your personal best strategies for success in a nursing program.

As you can see, the HESI exam is a much larger test, with less time allotted per question. But don't assume that the Kaplan exam is therefore "easier."

ABOUT THE READING COMPREHENSION SECTION

In this section, you will read several passages and answer the questions that follow each of them. All of the questions are multiple-choice, with 4 answer choices (A–D).

The Passages
The passages in this section range from fairly long (up to 650 words), to medium (around 400 words) and short (around 100 words). The passage topics vary, but many of them have a science- or nature-based theme.

The Questions
There are 5 main question types:

- Main Idea
- Author purpose
- Detail
- Inference
- Vocabulary-in-Context

To learn more about these question types, refer to Chapter Three, Reading Comprehension Review.

ABOUT THE VOCABULARY, SPELLING, AND GRAMMAR SECTION

All of the questions in this section are multiple-choice, with 4 answer choices (A–D).

Vocabulary Questions

These questions test your ability to understand how to use specific vocabulary terms. In some cases, you will be asked to choose the best definition for a specific word; you might even get to see the word being used in a sentence, which can provide context clues to the word's meaning. In other cases, you will be asked to choose the best word to complete a sentence. Whatever nursing exam you take, you are likely to encounter an emphasis on words that are likely to be used in a professional medical environment.

Spelling Questions

These questions test your ability to recognize a misspelled word. The good thing about the spelling questions is that you don't have to know the correct spelling of a word to answer correctly; you only have to recognize an *incorrect* spelling of a word. There are two types of spelling questions, and 10 of each type appear in this section:

- The first type offers you *four words*, one of which is misspelled. You must choose the word that is misspelled.
- The second type offers you *three sentences*. One of the sentences may have a misspelled word in it, or instead, there may be no spelling mistake in any of the sentences. If there is a misspelled word, you should select that sentence. If there are no spelling mistakes in any of the three answer choices, you should select choice (D), no mistake.

Grammar Questions

These questions assess your ability to find and correct grammatical errors in sentences. Some questions will ask you to identify the sentence with a grammatical error or identify the incorrect word within a sentence. Other questions will ask you to choose the correct answer option to complete the sentence. Still other questions will ask you to identify specific parts of speech.

ABOUT THE WRITING SECTION

All of the questions in this section are multiple-choice format with four answer choices (A–D). These questions test your ability to identify and evaluate the logic and structure of a written passage. Some questions will ask you to identify unnecessary sentences or to place new sentences in the best location within an already written passage. Some questions will ask you to identify the main idea of a paragraph or to choose the best summary of a passage. You might also be asked about the purpose or function of words or phrases.

To learn more about the questions you will find in this section, turn to Chapter Five, Writing Review.

ABOUT THE MATHEMATICS SECTION

This section of the test covers math topics including basic operations, fractions, percentages, conversions, ratios, algebra, and word problems.

About the Questions

The Math questions are generally of 2 types:

- Equations
- Word Problems

Equations are straightforward questions that you must solve using basic operations. Word problems are slightly different. You are using the same math skills; however, the question appears in the form of a story.

To learn more about solving each type of math question, turn to Chapter Six, Mathematics Review.

ABOUT THE SCIENCE SECTION

Although the Kaplan exam combines science questions under a single section called Science, the HESI exam breaks these areas down into several topics. As in previous sections, all Science questions are multiple-choice, with four answer choices (A–D).

Biology Questions

These questions assess your knowledge of basic biological principles, including the structure of cells, cellular respiration, metabolism, photosynthesis, and genetics.

To learn more about these questions, turn to Chapter Seven, Biology Review.

Anatomy and Physiology Questions

These questions assess your knowledge of the various parts of the body, in particular its organ systems. Questions can range from the very basic (naming specific parts of the body) to the very complex (evaluating the specific medical condition suggested by a set of symptoms).

To learn more about these questions, turn to Chapter Eight, Anatomy and Physiology Review.

Physical Science Questions

These questions assess your knowledge of basic physical science areas, including chemistry and physics. You will encounter questions that demand knowledge of basic terms. You will also be required to complete mathematical calculations to answer physics-related questions.

To learn more about these questions, turn to Chapter Nine, Physical Science Review.

An Important Difference

It is important to realize that unlike other sections of the exam in which you can come to a conclusion about the answer quite reasonably, even with limited prior knowledge, the Science section is primarily a test of your knowledge. Although you can make educated guesses on this section, a large part of your success depends upon your knowledge of scientific concepts.

THE NEXT STEP

Now that you know more about it, you are ready to learn about the ways to succeed on the test. If you want to learn about test-taking and Test Day strategies, turn to Chapter One.

| PART ONE |

Strategies

- Test-Taking and Test Day Strategies

Chapter One: **Test-Taking and Test Day Strategies**

The tips in this chapter are designed to help you on your nursing school entrance exam, as well as other tests you may encounter during your career. In addition, you will find a schedule for counting down to Test Day, whether you have several months or just a few weeks.

HOW NURSING SCHOOL ENTRANCE EXAMS ARE ADMINISTERED

Your test will be administered either as a paper-based or a computer-based test. You will be told which format your test uses when you apply to take the test.

If Your Test Is Paper Based

In a paper-based test you can jump around within a section, answering the easy questions first and going back to the more difficult ones. You have to keep track of time yourself on a paper-based test, so wear a watch to be sure you're on schedule during each section. If you finish a test section before the time is up, you must wait until directed by the proctor to start the next section. Use this time to give your answers a second look.

Mark Your Booklet

You can usually write in your test booklet, so use this to your advantage: Circle each answer choice you've selected, and cross out any answer choice you've ruled out. Also circle each question you need to go back to. Do your math calculations beside the question.

Grid 5 or More Answers at Once

It sounds simple, but it's extremely important: Don't make mistakes filling out your answer grid. Use this strategy to ensure that you mark your grid correctly: Circle the answers in your test booklet, and transfer your answers after every five questions or at the end of each reading passage. Marking your booklet with answer selections and skipped questions makes it easy to check your answer grid later, to ensure your answers are beside the right question numbers.

KAPLAN

If Your Test Is Computer Based

On some computer-based tests, such as the TEAS, you can also jump around in a section answering the easy questions first. At the end of the PAX-RN you are shown which questions are still unanswered so you may go back. In the HESI, however, you must answer the questions in the order in which they are presented.

There is usually a timer on the screen, so you'll always know if you are on schedule. On most computer-based tests, if you complete a section before the time is up, you can move on to the next section.

Take Notes on Scrap Paper

Even though your test is on the screen, be sure to have scrap paper and pencils handy. You'll need them to write quick notes about the reading passages, to list questions you need to return to, and to record answer choices that you've eliminated while narrowing down your answer selection.

STRATEGIES FOR ALMOST ANY TEST

When you are faced with so much information to learn in preparation for a test, it can be helpful to know that there are some techniques you can use for any test you are taking. Here are some tips for you to learn and apply on Test Day. They may seem obvious, but they are easy to forget, so don't let that happen to you.

Guessing Advantage

Since most tests don't have a scoring penalty for guessing, you should try to answer every question. If you can determine that one or more answers are definitely wrong, then you should guess from the remaining choices. Even if you aren't sure which one of them is absolutely correct, you've at least increased your chances of success by paring the selection down.

Pace Yourself

Time limits on standardized exams are firm. If you spend too much time on items in the earlier part of the examination, you will likely leave some easier questions further along unanswered. This approach will really hurt your test score.

So you must consciously ration your time. For instance, if the test section has 50 questions and there is a 50-minute time limit, spend no more than 1 minute on each question. When half the allowed time has elapsed, you should be about halfway through the test.

Don't waste time on any question. If you don't know the answer, skip it and move on. Make a note to yourself, either by circling the unanswered question in your test booklet (if your test is paper based) or recording it by number on scrap paper (if your test is computer based). When you've tried every question at least once, return to your unanswered questions. Start at your first skipped question and make your best choice, then move on methodically to your next skipped question.

If your test doesn't allow you to skip and return to unanswered questions later, *don't leave any question blank*. Select an answer now by guessing strategically: Make a note of any answer choices you have ruled out. Then take your best guess from the remaining answer choices and move on. By eliminating answer choices, you'll improve your odds of guessing correctly. By moving on, you'll leave more time to spend on potentially easier questions later in the test.

Keep Track of Time

When you are coming to the end of a test section, you need to be careful about keeping track of how much time you have left to complete everything. You don't want to have your answers in the test booklet and not be able to transfer them to your answer grid because you have run out of time. If it gets down to the wire, and you still have a few questions left, it would be a good idea to start transferring your answers one by one to ensure that every question you answered earns credit.

Read the Question Carefully Before You Look at the Answers

There is a name for answer choices that look right but aren't: distracters. They are easy to choose if you haven't read the question carefully. If you choose an answer without being sure what you're looking for, you're much more likely to pick a distracter than a correct answer. Be especially careful of questions that include the word NOT or EXCEPT. If you misread the question and miss these words, you may end up falling into a wrong-answer trap. If you are taking a paper test, put a box around the word NOT or EXCEPT. Then when you look at the answer choices, cross out the answers that are true.

SELF-CARE AND DEALING WITH STRESS

Test taking can be stressful, but it doesn't have to be. An important part of taking any exam is having a cool, calm, and collected brain when you are prepping and on the day you take the test. On Test Day, few things can hurt your score more than being:

- Sleep deprived or burned out from studying
- In denial over your lack of preparation
- Clueless as to what to expect from the test
- Unaware of what to expect of yourself

This chapter teaches you:

- How to relax
- How to visualize success
- How to build your physical and mental strength

Dealing with Test Stress

Your nursing school entrance exam, like all tests, can be scary because it is the *unknown*. You don't know the exact questions that are going to be on it. You don't know how you are going to do. You don't know how your score will stand up at your school of choice. Humans are scared of the unknown. Let this book begin to ease that fear. Let's keep goals attainable. Let's focus on minimizing your unknowns so you can focus on one single thing—doing your best on your nursing school entrance exam.

The main point of this book is to help you exert control over your test experience. You can learn to control your anxiety the same way you can control how to approach a multiple-choice question—by knowing what to expect beforehand and developing strategies to deal with it. We will show you how to relieve stress and mentally prepare for the exam in five specific ways:

1. Identifying sources of stress
2. Visualizing success
3. Exercising away anxiety
4. Eating right
5. Doing isometric exercises

Sources of Test Stress

Grab a pencil. (Not a pen.) In the space provided, write down your sources of test-related stress. Take 5–10 minutes. The idea is to pin down your sources of anxiety so you can deal with them one by one.

First, read through these common examples. Feel free to use any that apply to you, along with the ones you think up on your own.

- I always freeze up on tests.
- I'm nervous about the math section (or the science section, or the reading section, etc.).
- I need a good/great score to get into my first-choice school.
- I'm afraid of losing my focus and concentration.
- I'm afraid I'm not spending enough time preparing.
- I study like crazy, but nothing seems to stick in my mind.
- I always run out of time and get panicky.

My Sources of Test Stress

_____

_____

_____

_____

_____

_____

_____

Great. Now read through the list. Take another few minutes. Cross out things or add things. Now rewrite the list in order of most bothersome to least bothersome.

My Sources of Test Stress, in Order

_____

_____

_____

_____

_____

_____

_____

What was your number-one source of stress? Chances are, the top of the list is a fairly accurate description of exactly what you need to tackle. Taking care of the top two or three items on the list should go a long way toward relieving your overall test anxiety. So write down your top three below.

My Top Three Sources of Test Stress

_____

_____

_____

The rest of this chapter will help you eliminate them.

Relaxation and Visualization

Now put away your pencil. Sit in a comfortable chair in a quiet setting. If you wear glasses, take them off. Close your eyes and breathe in a deep, satisfying breath of air. Really fill your lungs—to the point where your rib cage is fully expanded and you can't take in any more air. Now exhale the air slowly and completely. Imagine you're blowing out a candle with your last little puff of air. Do this two or three more times, filling your lungs to their maximum capacity and then emptying them totally. Keep your eyes closed, comfortably but not tightly. Let your body sink deeper into the chair as you become even more comfortable.

With your eyes shut and your body in a more relaxed state, you should begin to notice something very interesting. You're no longer dealing with the external worries of the world. Instead, you can concentrate on what happens inside. The more you recognize your own physical reactions to stress and anxiety, the more you can do about them. You may not realize it, but you've begun to regain the ability to stay in control.

Keeping your eyes closed, attempt to visualize TV or movie screens on the back of your eyelids; let relaxing images begin to form on those screens. Allow the images to come easily and naturally; don't force them. The images might be of a special place you've visited before or one you've read about. It can be a fictional location that you create in your imagination, but a real-life memory of a place or situation you know is usually better. Make it as detailed as possible, and notice as much about your surroundings as you can. Stay focused on the images as you sink further into your chair. Breathe easily and naturally. Try to feel the stress and tension drain from your muscles and begin to flow downward, toward your feet and then away from you. Do this for five minutes or so. Start now.

When you are done, slowly open your eyes. Take a moment to check how you're feeling. Notice how comfortable you've become.

Imagine how much easier it would be if you could take the test feeling this relaxed and in this state of ease. You've coupled the images of your special place with sensations of comfort and relaxation.

You've also found a way to become relaxed simply by visualizing your own safe, special place.

Visualize Success

This next part reinforces your *strengths* list and takes visualization one step further. Close your eyes and remember a real-life situation in which you did well on a test. If you can't come up with one, remember a situation in which you did something that you were really proud of—a genuine accomplishment.

Make the memory as detailed as possible. Think about the sights, sounds, smells, and even the tastes associated with this remembered experience. Remember how confident you felt as you accomplished your goal.

Now start thinking about the nursing school entrance exam as an extension of that successful feeling.

Keep your thoughts and feelings in line with that previous, successful experience. Don't make comparisons between them. Just imagine taking the test with the same feelings of confidence and relaxed control.

This exercise is a great way to bring the test down to earth. Any feelings of dread you may have associated with the test will be replaced by feelings of accomplishment. Practice your general relaxation technique and this success-oriented relaxation technique together at least three times a week, especially when you feel burned out on test prep. The more you practice relaxation and visualization, the more effective the exercise will be for you.

Exercise Away Your Anxiety

To be completely prepared for Test Day, you've got to be in shape—or get in shape—to do your best. Lots of people get out of the habit of regular exercise when they're prepping for an exam. But physical exercise is a very effective way to stimulate both your mind and body, as well as improve your ability to think and concentrate. Along with a good diet and adequate sleep, exercise is an important part of keeping yourself in fighting shape and thinking clearly.

Hop Like a Frog

Studying uses a lot of energy, but it's all mental. It's important to remember the importance of using up your physical energy too. When you take a study break, do something active. Take a 5–10 minute exercise break for every 50 or 60 minutes you study. Walk down the block. Do 20 sit-ups. Hop around like a frog. Whatever. The physical exertion helps keep your mind and body in sync. This way, when you finish studying for the night and go to bed, you won't lie there unable to sleep because your brain is exhausted while your body wants to run a marathon.

Oxygenate Your Brain

Exercise develops your mental stamina and increases the transfer of oxygen to your brain. The brain needs a strong, uninterrupted supply of oxygen to function at its best. Sedentary people have less oxygen in their blood than active people, so their brains receive less oxygen. Your ability to watch TV might not be affected by your brain receiving a little less oxygen, but your ability to think will be.

Happy Synapses

Exercise also releases your brain's endorphins. Endorphins have no side effects, and they're free! It just takes some exercise to release them. Running, bicycling, swimming, aerobics, and power walking all release endorphins that will occupy the happy spots in your brain's neural synapses.

Don't Run to Bed

One warning about exercise: It's not a good idea to exercise vigorously right before you go to bed. This could easily cause sleep-onset problems. For the same reason, it's not a good idea to study right up to bedtime. Make time for a buffer period before you go to bed. Take 30 to 60 minutes for yourself and watch some TV, take a long, hot shower, or meditate. Remember our relaxation and visualization tips? This is a good time to do them.

Squeeze Your Body

Here's a fast, natural route to relaxation and invigoration. You can do it whenever you get stressed out, including during the test. The idea is that by making your body as tense as possible and relaxing, you are releasing the tension from your body. The entire process takes five minutes from start to finish (maybe a couple of minutes during the test).

- Breathe slowly and easily.
- Close your eyes tightly.
- Squeeze your nose and mouth together so that your whole face is scrunched up. (If it makes you self-conscious to do this in the test room, skip this step.)
- Pull your chin into your chest, and pull your shoulders together.
- Tighten your arms to your body, then clench your fists.
- Pull in your stomach. Squeeze your thighs together, and tighten your calves.
- Stretch your feet, then curl your toes. (Watch out for cramping during this part.)

At this point, every muscle in your body should be tightened. Now, relax your body, one part at a time, in reverse order, starting with your toes. Let the tension drop out of each muscle. This clenching and unclenching exercise will feel silly at first, but it will leave you feeling very relaxed.

Say No to Drugs, Yes to Eating Right

Using drugs of any kind to prepare for a big test is not a good idea. Mild stimulants, such as coffee, cola, or over-the-counter caffeine pills can help you study longer because they keep you awake, but they can also lead to agitation, restlessness, and insomnia. To reduce stress, eat fruits and vegetables (raw, lightly steamed, or quickly nuked are best); low-fat sources of protein such as fish, skinless poultry, and legumes (lentils, beans, and nuts); and whole grains such as brown rice, whole wheat bread, and pasta (no bleached flour).

Don't eat sweet, high-fat snacks. Simple carbohydrates like sugar make stress worse, and fatty foods lower your immunity. Don't eat salty foods either. They can deplete potassium, which you need for nerve function.

Good Stress

We haven't said this yet, but it bears mentioning. A little anxiety is a good thing. You want to be relaxed when you take and prepare for the test, but some stress is healthy. The adrenaline that stress pumps into your bloodstream helps you stay alert and think more clearly. And that's a good thing.

STUDY TIMELINE FOR THE KAPLAN NURSING SCHOOL ADMISSION TEST

We've already covered some of the best strategies for taking any test. Now here are suggested timelines for organizing your study time if you have 6 months, 3 months, or 1 month to prepare for your nursing school entrance exam. This timeline is tailored to those taking the Kaplan exam; if you are taking the HESI exam, check out that timeline later in this chapter. This book provides practice tests for both the Kaplan and HESI exams. Although the two tests are quite different in some ways, the content they cover has considerable overlap. If you are taking the Kaplan exam, feel free to check out the HESI Practice Tests (Practice Tests Three and Four) as a way to review the information from a different angle, but remember that Practice Tests One and Two will better reflect the actual test you will be taking.

If You Have 6 Months

6 months before the test:

- Take the diagnostic quiz and assess which section is your weakest.
- Devote your study time this month to reviewing that chapter and any related materials in Part Seven, Learning Resources. Repeat that section of the diagnostic quiz.
- Study the answer explanations, review the chapter, and repeat the test as necessary.
- Supplement your study with textbooks and other study guides on the subject.

5 months before the test:

- Study Chapter Three, Reading Comprehension Review.
- Supplement with healthcare journal articles, picking out main ideas and looking up unfamiliar words.
- Read Chapter Seven, Biology Review, applying the skills you learned in Chapter Three.
- Take the Reading Comprehension section of Practice Test One and study the answer explanations.
- Review Chapter Three and repeat the practice test section as necessary.

4 months before the test: Study Chapter Seven, Biology Review, and Chapter Eight, Anatomy and Physiology Review. These are two very dense chapters filled with technical information. Understanding this material is key to performing well. The Kaplan exam is especially heavy on physiology content, so emphasize these concepts in your preparation.

3 months before the test:

- Take the Science section of Practice Test One and study the answer explanations.
- Review the Science chapters and repeat the practice test section as necessary.

2 months before the test:

- Study Chapter Six, Mathematics Review.
- Study "Math in a Nutshell" in Part Seven, Learning Resources.
- Take the Mathematics section of Practice Test One and study the answer explanations.
- Review the chapter and Learning Resources and repeat the practice test section as necessary.

4 weeks before the test:

- Study Chapter Four, Vocabulary, Spelling, and Grammar Review, and Chapter Five, Writing Review.
- Study the first three topics in Part Seven, Learning Resources: "Common Word Roots and Prefixes," "Frequently Misspelled Words," and "Words Commonly Confused for One Another."
- Take the Writing section of Practice Test One and study the answer explanations.
- Review the chapters and Learning Resources sections, and repeat the practice test section as necessary.

If You Have 3 Months

3 months before the test:

- Take the diagnostic quiz and assess your strengths and weaknesses.
- Study Chapter Three, Reading Comprehension Review; Chapter Four, Vocabulary, Spelling, and Grammar Review; and Chapter Five, Writing Review.
- Read the first three topics of Part Seven, Learning Resources: "Common Word Roots and Prefixes," "Frequently Misspelled Words," and "Words Commonly Confused for One Another."
- Take the Reading Comprehension and Writing sections of Practice Test One and study the answer explanations.
- Read Chapter Seven, Biology Review, applying the skills you learned in Chapter Three.
- Review the chapters and repeat the practice test sections as necessary.

2 months before the test:

- Study Chapter Seven, Biology Review, and Chapter Eight, Anatomy and Physiology Review. (Note that the Kaplan exam is especially heavy on physiology content, so emphasize these concepts in your preparation.)
- Take the Science section of Practice Test One and study the answer explanations.
- Review the chapters and repeat the practice test section as necessary.

4 weeks before the test:

- Study Chapter Six, Mathematics Review.
- Read "Math in a Nutshell" in Part Seven, Learning Resources.
- Take the Mathematics section of Practice Test One and study the answer explanations.
- Review the chapter and repeat the practice test section as necessary.

If You Have 1 Month

4 weeks before the test:

- Take the diagnostic quiz and assess your strengths and weaknesses.
- Study Chapter Three, Reading Comprehension Review; Chapter Four, Vocabulary, Spelling, and Grammar Review; and Chapter Five, Writing Review.
- Read the first three topics of Part Seven, Learning Resources: "Common Word Roots and Prefixes," "Frequently Misspelled Words," and "Words Commonly Confused for One Another."
- Take the Reading Comprehension and Writing sections of Practice Test One and study the answer explanations.
- Review the chapters and repeat the practice test sections as necessary.

3 weeks before the test:

- Study Chapter Seven, Biology Review, and Chapter Eight, Anatomy and Physiology Review. (Note that the Kaplan exam is especially heavy on physiology content, so emphasize these concepts in your preparation.)
- Take the Science section of Practice Test One and study the answer explanations.
- Review the chapters and repeat the practice test section as necessary.

2 weeks before the test:

- Study Chapter Six, Mathematics Review.
- Study "Math in a Nutshell" in Part Seven, Learning Resources.
- Take the Mathematics section of Practice Test One and study the answer explanations.
- Review Chapter Six, Mathematics Review, and "Math in a Nutshell," and repeat the practice test section as necessary.

STUDY TIMELINE FOR THE HESI A2 EXAM

Here are suggested timelines for organizing your study time if you have 6 months, 3 months, or 1 month to prepare for your HESI exam. This book provides practice tests for both the Kaplan and HESI exams. Although the two tests are quite different in some ways, the content they cover has considerable overlap. If you are taking the HESI exam, feel free to check out the Kaplan Practice Tests (Practice Tests One and Two) to review the information from a different angle, but remember that Practice Tests Three and Four will better reflect the actual test you will be taking.

If You Have 6 Months

6 months before the test:

- Take the diagnostic quiz and assess which section is your weakest.
- Devote your study time this month to reviewing that chapter and any related materials in Part Seven, Learning Resources. Repeat that section of the diagnostic quiz.
- Study the answer explanations, review the chapter, and repeat the test as necessary.
- Supplement your study with textbooks and other study guides on the subject.

5 months before the test:

- Study Chapter Three, Reading Comprehension Review, and Chapter Five, Writing Review. **Note:** Although the HESI exam does not have a Writing section, Chapter Five can help you better understand the "nuts and bolts" of a written passage.
- Supplement with healthcare journal articles, picking out main ideas and looking up unfamiliar words.
- Read Chapter Seven, Biology Review, applying the skills you learned in Chapter Three.
- Take the Reading Comprehension section of Practice Test Three and study the answer explanations.
- Review Chapter Three and repeat the practice test section as necessary.

4 months before the test: Study Chapter Seven, Biology Review; Chapter Eight, Anatomy and Physiology Review; and Chapter Nine, Physical Science Review. These are three very dense chapters filled with technical information. Understanding this material is key to performing well on any nursing school entrance exam.

3 months before the test:

- Take the Biology, Anatomy and Physiology, Chemistry, and Physics sections of Practice Test Three and study the answer explanations.
- Review the Science chapters and repeat the practice test sections as necessary.

2 months before the test:

- Study Chapter Six, Mathematics Review.
- Study "Math in a Nutshell" in Part Seven, Learning Resources.

- Take the Mathematics section of Practice Test Three and study the answer explanations.
- Review the chapter and Learning Resources and repeat the practice test section as necessary.

4 weeks before the test:

- Study Chapter Four, Vocabulary, Spelling, and Grammar Review.
- Study the first three topics in Part Seven, Learning Resources: "Common Word Roots and Prefixes," "Frequently Misspelled Words," and "Words Commonly Confused for One Another."
- Take the Vocabulary and Grammar sections of Practice Test Three and study the answer explanations.
- Review the chapter and Learning Resources sections, and repeat the practice test sections as necessary.

If You Have 3 Months

3 months before the test:

- Take the diagnostic quiz and assess your strengths and weaknesses.
- Study Chapter Three, Reading Comprehension Review; Chapter Four, Vocabulary, Spelling, and Grammar Review; and Chapter Five, Writing Review. Although the HESI exam does not have a Writing section, Chapter Five can help you better understand the "nuts and bolts" of a written passage.
- Read the first three topics of Part Seven, Learning Resources: "Common Word Roots and Prefixes," "Frequently Misspelled Words," and "Words Commonly Confused for One Another."
- Take the Reading Comprehension, Vocabulary, and Grammar sections of Practice Test Three and study the answer explanations.
- Read Chapter Seven, Biology Review, applying the skills you learned in Chapter Three.
- Review the chapters and repeat the practice test sections as necessary.

2 months before the test:

- Study Chapter Seven, Biology Review; Chapter Eight, Anatomy and Physiology Review; and Chapter Nine, Physical Science Review.
- Take the Biology, Anatomy and Physiology, Chemistry, and Physics sections of Practice Test Three and study the answer explanations.
- Review the chapters and repeat the practice test sections as necessary.

4 weeks before the test:

- Study Chapter Six, Mathematics Review.
- Read "Math in a Nutshell" in Part Seven, Learning Resources.
- Take the Mathematics section of Practice Test Three and study the answer explanations.
- Review the chapter and repeat the practice test section as necessary.

KAPLAN

If You Have 1 Month

4 weeks before the test:

- Take the diagnostic quiz and assess your strengths and weaknesses.
- Study Chapter Three, Reading Comprehension Review; Chapter Four, Vocabulary, Spelling, and Grammar Review; and Chapter Five, Writing Review. Although the HESI exam does not have a Writing section, Chapter Five can help you better understand the "nuts and bolts" of a written passage.
- Read the first three topics of Part Seven, Learning Resources: "Common Word Roots and Prefixes," "Frequently Misspelled Words," and "Words Commonly Confused for One Another."
- Take the Reading Comprehension, Vocabulary, and Grammar sections of Practice Test Three and study the answer explanations.
- Review the chapters and repeat the practice test sections as necessary.

3 weeks before the test:

- Study Chapter Seven, Biology Review; Chapter Eight, Anatomy and Physiology Review; and Chapter Nine, Physical Science Review.
- Take the Biology, Anatomy and Physiology, Chemistry, and Physics sections of Practice Test Three and study the answer explanations.
- Review the chapters and repeat the practice test sections as necessary.

2 weeks before the test:

- Study Chapter Six, Mathematics Review.
- Read "Math in a Nutshell" in Part Seven, Learning Resources.
- Take the Mathematics section of Practice Test Three and study the answer explanations.
- Review the chapter and repeat the practice test section as necessary.

COUNTDOWN TO TEST DAY

You've considered how to structure your study weeks or months before the test. Now here's a countdown schedule to prepare for Test Day.

3 to 10 Days Before the Test

Take Practice Test Two (to prepare for the Kaplan exam) or Practice Test Four (to prepare for the HESI exam). Use the techniques and strategies you've learned in this book. Approach the test strategically, actively, and confidently. We don't recommend taking a full practice test if you have less than 48 hours left before exam day. Doing so will probably exhaust you and hurt your score on the actual test.

2 Days Before the Test

Go over the results of your practice tests. Don't worry too much about your scores or whether you got a specific question right or wrong. The practice tests don't count. But do examine your performance on specific types of questions with an eye on how you might get through each one faster and with more ease on the test to come.

The Day Before the Test

Our advice is to not do any studying on this day. Instead, organize the things you may need to take to the test:

- A calculator with fresh batteries (Be sure to check with the test administrators to find out if you are allowed to use a calculator on your test.)
- A watch
- A few No. 2 pencils (Pencils with slightly dull points fill the ovals better.)
- Erasers
- Photo ID card
- Facial tissues
- A snack (There may be a break during the exam and you might be hungry.)

It is also important to know exactly where the test center is located, how you're getting there, and how long it takes to get there. If you can, it's a good idea to visit your test center sometime before the day of the test so you know what to expect—where to park, what the rooms are like, how the desks are set up, where the restrooms are, and so on. Relax the night before the test. Read a good book, take a long, hot shower, or watch something on TV. Go to bed early and get a good night's sleep. Finally, make sure to leave yourself extra time in the morning.

The Morning of the Test
After you wake up:

- Eat breakfast. Make it something substantial, but not anything too heavy or greasy.
- Don't drink a lot of coffee if you're not used to it. Bathroom breaks cut into your time, and too much caffeine may make you jittery.
- Dress in layers so that you can adjust to the temperature of the testing room.
- Read something. Warm up your brain with a newspaper or a magazine. You shouldn't let the test material be the first thing you read that day.
- Be sure to get there early. Allow yourself extra time for traffic, mass transit delays, or detours.

During the Test

If you find your confidence slipping, remind yourself how well you've prepared. If something goes really wrong, don't panic. If the test booklet is defective—two pages are stuck together or the ink has run—raise your hand, and tell the proctor you need new materials. If you accidentally misgrid your answer page or put your answers in the wrong section, raise your hand and tell the proctor. He or she might be able to arrange for you to regrid your test after it's over—when it won't cost you any time.

After the Test
Congratulate yourself.

Now, you might walk out of the exam thinking you blew it. This is a normal reaction. People tend to remember the questions that stumped them, not the ones they knew. However, we're positive you will perform well and score your best on the exam because you read Kaplan's *Nursing School Entrance Exams Prep*. Be confident that you will be prepared and do well, so you can celebrate when the test is a distant memory.

PART TWO

Diagnostic Quiz

- Nursing School Entrance Exams Diagnostic Quiz

Chapter Two: **Nursing School Entrance Exams Diagnostic Quiz**

Imagine if you were taking an exam that was testing your knowledge of colors and rare flowering plants of South America. Do you think you would spend much time reviewing color swatches and practicing to recognize the differences between green and purple? Or do you think you would spend more time reviewing content on the flowering plants of South America? Chances are, you are probably familiar enough with colors to do well on that part of the test, so you would concentrate on reviewing what you don't know.

That's how this diagnostic test is meant to work. You should take this 60-question test before you review any study materials. This way, your results on this test will give you important information about your strengths and weaknesses. For example, if you ace all the vocabulary and spelling questions on this test, you can limit the amount of time you spend reviewing Chapter Four. On the other hand, if you struggle with all of the science questions, you should spend more of your time reviewing Chapter Seven, Chapter Eight, and Chapter Nine. Please note that this diagnostic quiz covers knowledge areas of both the HESI and Kaplan exams. (Use the (H) and (K) icons provided in Chapters Three through Nine to see if the material covered by the question is actually relevant to the test you are taking. Be sure to focus your studies on the knowledge areas covered by the test you are taking.)

Having an understanding of what you know and what you don't know is an important first step in preparing for a major test. Allow 2 hours to take this diagnostic quiz; then be sure to review the answer explanations found at the end. Good luck!

KAPLAN

Nursing School Entrance Exams
Diagnostic Quiz
Answer Sheet

Reading Comprehension

1. Ⓐ Ⓑ Ⓒ Ⓓ	4. Ⓐ Ⓑ Ⓒ Ⓓ	7. Ⓐ Ⓑ Ⓒ Ⓓ	10. Ⓐ Ⓑ Ⓒ Ⓓ
2. Ⓐ Ⓑ Ⓒ Ⓓ	5. Ⓐ Ⓑ Ⓒ Ⓓ	8. Ⓐ Ⓑ Ⓒ Ⓓ	11. Ⓐ Ⓑ Ⓒ Ⓓ
3. Ⓐ Ⓑ Ⓒ Ⓓ	6. Ⓐ Ⓑ Ⓒ Ⓓ	9. Ⓐ Ⓑ Ⓒ Ⓓ	

Vocabulary and Spelling

1. Ⓐ Ⓑ Ⓒ Ⓓ	5. Ⓐ Ⓑ Ⓒ Ⓓ	9. Ⓐ Ⓑ Ⓒ Ⓓ	13. Ⓐ Ⓑ Ⓒ Ⓓ
2. Ⓐ Ⓑ Ⓒ Ⓓ	6. Ⓐ Ⓑ Ⓒ Ⓓ	10. Ⓐ Ⓑ Ⓒ Ⓓ	14. Ⓐ Ⓑ Ⓒ Ⓓ
3. Ⓐ Ⓑ Ⓒ Ⓓ	7. Ⓐ Ⓑ Ⓒ Ⓓ	11. Ⓐ Ⓑ Ⓒ Ⓓ	15. Ⓐ Ⓑ Ⓒ Ⓓ
4. Ⓐ Ⓑ Ⓒ Ⓓ	8. Ⓐ Ⓑ Ⓒ Ⓓ	12. Ⓐ Ⓑ Ⓒ Ⓓ	16. Ⓐ Ⓑ Ⓒ Ⓓ

Mathematics

1. Ⓐ Ⓑ Ⓒ Ⓓ	5. Ⓐ Ⓑ Ⓒ Ⓓ	9. Ⓐ Ⓑ Ⓒ Ⓓ	13. Ⓐ Ⓑ Ⓒ Ⓓ	17. Ⓐ Ⓑ Ⓒ Ⓓ
2. Ⓐ Ⓑ Ⓒ Ⓓ	6. Ⓐ Ⓑ Ⓒ Ⓓ	10. Ⓐ Ⓑ Ⓒ Ⓓ	14. Ⓐ Ⓑ Ⓒ Ⓓ	
3. Ⓐ Ⓑ Ⓒ Ⓓ	7. Ⓐ Ⓑ Ⓒ Ⓓ	11. Ⓐ Ⓑ Ⓒ Ⓓ	15. Ⓐ Ⓑ Ⓒ Ⓓ	
4. Ⓐ Ⓑ Ⓒ Ⓓ	8. Ⓐ Ⓑ Ⓒ Ⓓ	12. Ⓐ Ⓑ Ⓒ Ⓓ	16. Ⓐ Ⓑ Ⓒ Ⓓ	

Science

1. Ⓐ Ⓑ Ⓒ Ⓓ	5. Ⓐ Ⓑ Ⓒ Ⓓ	9. Ⓐ Ⓑ Ⓒ Ⓓ	13. Ⓐ Ⓑ Ⓒ Ⓓ
2. Ⓐ Ⓑ Ⓒ Ⓓ	6. Ⓐ Ⓑ Ⓒ Ⓓ	10. Ⓐ Ⓑ Ⓒ Ⓓ	14. Ⓐ Ⓑ Ⓒ Ⓓ
3. Ⓐ Ⓑ Ⓒ Ⓓ	7. Ⓐ Ⓑ Ⓒ Ⓓ	11. Ⓐ Ⓑ Ⓒ Ⓓ	15. Ⓐ Ⓑ Ⓒ Ⓓ
4. Ⓐ Ⓑ Ⓒ Ⓓ	8. Ⓐ Ⓑ Ⓒ Ⓓ	12. Ⓐ Ⓑ Ⓒ Ⓓ	16. Ⓐ Ⓑ Ⓒ Ⓓ

Section 1: Reading Comprehension

Questions 1–2 are based on the following passage.

The rarely sighted three-toed sloth, long mistaken for a species of monkey, is one of the most unusual animals on earth. In fact, many characteristics of this tree-dwelling mammal seem to run counter to the instincts displayed by almost all wild animals. First, sloths are incredibly slow, tending to move no faster than six feet per minute, even when confronted by a predator. As a result, most sloths spend years in a single tree, making their way from branch to branch almost imperceptibly. Second, sloths spend almost their entire lives hanging upside down, even when eating, sleeping, mating, and—perhaps most remarkably—giving birth.

1. The author's reference to sloths moving "almost imperceptibly" is meant to show that these animals:

   (A) Move in ways that can be difficult to detect.
   (B) Intentionally hide their movements.
   (C) Are essentially impossible to observe.
   (D) Are physically unable to move with any speed.

2. According to the passage, the three-toed sloth's lack of speed and tendency to hang upside down are:

   (A) Entirely unique evolutionary traits.
   (B) Characteristics shared by some monkeys.
   (C) Apparently contrary to the usual behavior of most wild animals.
   (D) Detrimental to their eating, sleeping, and mating habits.

Questions 3–4 are based on the following passage.

Ecologists apply the term *biome* to the major divisions of ecosystem types, largely based on the structure of their most prevalent vegetation. The tundra biome, for example, found in the Arctic and high in the mountains of all latitudes, is characterized by low-growing perennial plants that can survive in soil that remains frozen for most of the year. The temperate grassland biome, on the other hand, is found in those areas of the world that remain relatively dry throughout the year and is distinguished by the structurally simple grasses and scrub brush that dominate the landscape.

3. Judging from the passage, *dominate* most probably means:

   (A) Control.
   (B) Rule over.
   (C) Overwhelm.
   (D) Overshadow.

4. According to the last sentence, the grasses and scrub brush:

   (A) Live only in the temperate grassland biome.
   (B) Can thrive only in dry climates.
   (C) Require relatively little water to survive.
   (D) Are, by definition, structurally simple.

GO ON TO THE NEXT PAGE

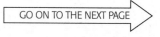

Questions 5–7 are based on the following passage.

   Although the brain comprises only 2 percent of the human body's average weight, the billions of neurons and trillions of synaptic connections that are the human brain constitute a truly impressive organ. In terms of what it can do, the human brain is in some ways unable to match the brain functioning of "lower" animals; in other ways, its capabilities are quite unrivaled. Salmon, caribou, and migrating birds, for example, have navigational abilities unparalleled in our own species, and even dogs and cats have senses of hearing and smell known, in human form, only to comic book superheroes. Yet, no other animal on the planet can communicate, solve problems, or think abstractly about itself and the future as we do. While these relative strengths and weaknesses can be attributed to the unique and complex structure of the human brain, neuroscientists also have traced these characteristics to the human brain's remarkable flexibility, what researchers call plasticity.

   Encased in a hard, protective skull that by the age of two is already 80 percent of its eventual adult size, the human brain has little room for size expansion even though the rest of the body, especially during adolescence, undergoes significant changes in physical form. Nevertheless, the human brain's plasticity allows for marked capacity changes because of usage, practice, and experience throughout a person's entire life.

   The idea that the human brain continues to develop and, some might say, improve over the course of one's life is a relatively new concept. Neuroscientists once believed that the basic structure and abilities of the adult brain were developed early in life and not subject to later change. Recent research, however, has debunked this myth; scientists have found that one's life experiences and environment not only mold the brain's particular architecture but also can continue to spark the expansion of its capacity to function.

5. The author's comparisons between the human brain and those of other animals are meant to:

   (A) Suggest that despite areas of weakness the human brain is the most sophisticated.

   (B) Emphasize the diversity of brain types found in the animal kingdom.

   (C) Reiterate that the human brain is not the only brain that displays remarkable plasticity.

   (D) Illustrate the unique characteristics and capabilities of the human brain.

6. The reference to "comic book superheroes" at the end of the first paragraph serves to:

   (A) Show that the sensory capabilities of cats and dogs are irrelevant when evaluating brain development.

   (B) Suggest that as humans we have always exaggerated our sensory capabilities.

   (C) Demonstrate that the human brain is not superior to but different from the brains of other animals.

   (D) Illustrate that, regardless of the remarkable sensory capabilities of cats and dogs, their brains have great weaknesses.

7. In context, the word *traced* (at the end of the first paragraph) means:

   (A) Connected.

   (B) Drawn.

   (C) Searched.

   (D) Copied.

GO ON TO THE NEXT PAGE

Questions 8–9 are based on the following passage.

The discovery of helium required the combined efforts of several scientists. Pierre-Jules Cesar Janssen first obtained evidence for the existence of helium during a solar eclipse in 1868, when he detected a new yellow line on his spectroscope while observing the sun. This experiment was repeated by Norman Lockyer who concluded that no known element produced such a line. However, other scientists were dubious, finding it unlikely that an element existed only on the sun. Then, in 1895, William Ramsay discovered helium on Earth after treating clevite, a uranium mineral, with mineral acids. After isolating the resulting gas, Ramsay sent samples to William Crookes and Norman Lockyer who identified it conclusively as the missing element helium.

8. The passage indicates that Ramsay's chief contribution to the discovery of helium was to:

    (A) Prove the validity of Janssen's experiment.

    (B) Find helium in uranium minerals.

    (C) Identify the element discovered by Crookes as helium.

    (D) Discover that helium naturally occurs on Earth.

9. The author of the passage suggests that the results of the work of Janssen and Lockyer were:

    (A) Repeated incorrectly by other scientists.

    (B) Thought by others to be the result of flawed methodologies.

    (C) Met with skepticism by other scientists.

    (D) Only valid during solar eclipses.

Questions 10–11 are based on the following passage.

Diamond is the hardest known material and has long been used in various industrial-shaping processes, such as cutting, grinding, and polishing. Diamond, sapphire, ruby (which is a sapphire with chromium "impurities"), and garnet are increasingly important in various applications. For example, diamond is used in sensors, diaphragms for audio speakers, and coatings for optical materials. Sapphire is used in gallium nitride-based LEDs; ruby is used in check valves; and synthetic garnet is used in lasers intended for applications in medical products.

10. The main idea of this passage can best be summarized with which of these titles?

    (A) The Timeless Allure of Precious Stones.

    (B) Nontraditional Uses of Diamonds.

    (C) Industrial Uses for Precious Stones.

    (D) Gem Hardness and Utility.

11. It can be inferred from this passage that:

    (A) Diamonds are more precious than sapphires.

    (B) Rubies come from the same type of stone as do sapphires.

    (C) Garnets are used in various industrial-shaping processes.

    (D) Precious stones are more costly than ever.

GO ON TO THE NEXT PAGE

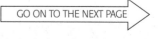

KAPLAN

Section 2: Vocabulary and Spelling

1. *Resignation* most nearly means:

    (A) Losing.

    (B) Waste.

    (C) Acceptance.

    (D) Pride.

2. *Tangible* most nearly means:

    (A) Real.

    (B) Open.

    (C) Graphic.

    (D) Costly.

3. *Feasible* most nearly means:

    (A) Workable.

    (B) Breakable.

    (C) Imperfect.

    (D) Evident.

4. *Impure* means the opposite of:

    (A) Harmonious.

    (B) Integral.

    (C) Unalloyed.

    (D) Assiduous.

5. *Scale* means the opposite of:

    (A) Enlarge.

    (B) Collapse.

    (C) Weigh.

    (D) Descend.

6. *Levity* means the opposite of:

    (A) Inequality.

    (B) Gravity.

    (C) Laxity.

    (D) Credulity.

7. Optimistic : Hope ::

    (A) Playwrights : Creativity.

    (B) Flying : Fear.

    (C) Sculpted : Talent.

    (D) Sage : Wisdom.

8. Agenda : Meeting ::

    (A) Show : Television.

    (B) Map : Plan.

    (C) Program : Play.

    (D) Organize : Detail.

9. Forge : Signature ::

    (A) Originate : Store.

    (B) Fake : Meal.

    (C) Counterfeit : Money.

    (D) Cut : Paper.

GO ON TO THE NEXT PAGE

Choose the word that is misspelled.

10. (A) Nuetral.
    (B) Perceived.
    (C) Efficient.
    (D) Analysis.

11. (A) Acessible.
    (B) Endure.
    (C) Magnified.
    (D) Comprehension.

12. (A) Surreal.
    (B) Obsolete.
    (C) Negligance.
    (D) Infused.

In the next four questions, find the sentences that contain a misspelled word. If there are no mistakes, choose (D).

13. (A) The hole is not noticeable.
    (B) We will conduct a formal inquiry.
    (C) Dana is an excelent athlete.
    (D) No mistake.

14. (A) What time will the room be availible?
    (B) Smoking is not allowed in public places.
    (C) We used various fruits in the salad.
    (D) No mistake.

15. (A) His proposal for a new park was very interesting.
    (B) Our school cafateria always opens at 8:00 in the morning.
    (C) The secretary typed very quickly.
    (D) No mistake.

16. (A) Please try not to interupt me when I'm speaking.
    (B) Are you sure this information is accurate?
    (C) This knitting pattern is very complicated.
    (D) No mistake.

GO ON TO THE NEXT PAGE

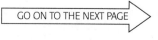

Section 3: Mathematics

1. If $100 + x = 100$, then $x = ?$

    (A) -100

    (B) -10

    (C) 0

    (D) 10

2. The percent decrease from 12 to 9 is equal to the percent decrease from 40 to what number?

    (A)   3

    (B)   10

    (C)   25

    (D)   30

3. On a certain planet, if each year has 9 months and each month has 15 days, how many full years have passed after 700 days on this planet?

    (A)   1

    (B)   2

    (C)   3

    (D)   5

4. $\left(\frac{1}{5} + \frac{1}{3}\right) \div \frac{1}{2} = ?$

    (A) $\frac{1}{8}$

    (B) $\frac{1}{4}$

    (C) $\frac{4}{15}$

    (D) $\frac{16}{15}$

5. Marty has exactly 5 blue pens, 6 black pens, and 4 red pens in his knapsack. If he pulls out one pen at random from his knapsack, what is the probability that the pen is either black or red?

    (A)   1 out of 5

    (B)   1 out of 3

    (C)   1 out of 2

    (D)   2 out of 3

6. Bill has to type a paper that is p pages long, with each page containing w words. If Bill types an average of x words per minute, how many hours will it take him to finish the paper?

    (A) $60wpx$

    (B) $\frac{wx}{60p}$

    (C) $\frac{wpx}{60}$

    (D) $\frac{wp}{60x}$

7. At a certain school, if the ratio of teachers to students is 1 to 10, which of the following could be the total number of teachers and students?

    (A)   100

    (B)   121

    (C)   144

    (D)   222

8. If $r = 3$ and $s = 1$, then $r^2 - 2s = ?$

    (A)   2

    (B)   4

    (C)   6

    (D)   7

9. A machine caps 5 bottles every 2 seconds. At this rate, how many bottles will be capped in 1 minute?

    (A)   75

    (B)   150

    (C)   225

    (D)   300

10. If $\frac{2}{x} + \frac{5}{3} = 2$, what is the value of x?

    (A)   6

    (B)   2

    (C) $\frac{4}{5}$

    (D) $\frac{-4}{5}$

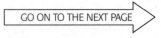

GO ON TO THE NEXT PAGE

11. If a sweater sells for $48 after a 25% markdown, what was its original price?

    (A) $56

    (B) $60

    (C) $64

    (D) $68

12. Which of the following must be equal to 30% of x?

    (A) $\dfrac{3x}{1,000}$

    (B) $\dfrac{3x}{100}$

    (C) $\dfrac{3x}{10}$

    (D) $3x$

13. A certain phone call costs 75¢ for the first 3 minutes plus 15¢ for each additional minute. If the call lasted x minutes and x is an integer greater than 3, which of the following expresses the cost of the call, in dollars?

    (A) $0.75(3) + 0.15x$

    (B) $0.75(3) + 0.15(x + 3)$

    (C) $0.75 + 0.15(3 - x)$

    (D) $0.75 + 0.15(x - 3)$

14. $(2 \times 10^4) + (5 \times 10^3) + (6 \times 10^2) + (4 \times 10^1) = ?$

    (A) 20,564

    (B) 25,064

    (C) 25,604

    (D) 25,640

15. If $2n + 3 = 5$, then $4n = ?$

    (A) 1

    (B) 2

    (C) 4

    (D) 8

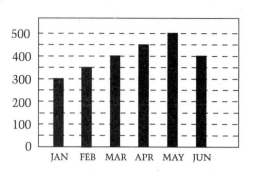

NUMBER OF BOOKS BORROWED

FROM MIDVILLE LIBRARY

16. According to the graph above, the number of books borrowed during the month of January was what fraction of the total number of books borrowed during the first six months of the year?

    (A) $\dfrac{1}{8}$

    (B) $\dfrac{1}{7}$

    (C) $\dfrac{1}{6}$

    (D) $\dfrac{3}{16}$

17. A business is owned by 4 women and 1 man, each of whom owns an equal share. If one of the women sells $\frac{1}{2}$ of her share to the man, and another woman keeps $\frac{1}{4}$ of her share and sells the rest to the man, what fraction of the business will the man own?

    (A) $\dfrac{1}{3}$

    (B) $\dfrac{9}{20}$

    (C) $\dfrac{11}{20}$

    (D) $\dfrac{2}{3}$

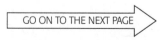

GO ON TO THE NEXT PAGE

KAPLAN

Section 4: Science

1. Animals that consume plants are called:

   (A) Saprophytes.
   (B) Herbivores.
   (C) Carnivores.
   (D) Omnivores.

2. Which of the following kingdoms is considered the most primitive?

   (A) Fungi.
   (B) Protista.
   (C) Archaebacteria.
   (D) Plantae.

3. A bottle of perfume is opened in the back of a classroom. A short time later, the teacher detects the odor. Once the liquid was exposed to the air in the room, how did the vapors get from the perfume bottle to the teacher's nose?

   (A) Osmosis.
   (B) Diffusion.
   (C) Dilution.
   (D) Dialysis.

4. During mitosis, distribution of one copy of each chromosome to each of the resulting cells virtually guarantees

   (A) Reduction of the chromosome number to half of the original chromosome number.
   (B) Formation of daughter cells with identical DNA sequences.
   (C) Cell growth.
   (D) Maximum cell size.

5. Which of the following is the name for the muscular tissue that contracts to permit air to enter the lungs?

   (A) Trachea.
   (B) Alveoli.
   (C) Esophagus.
   (D) Diaphragm.

6. Air entering the lungs of a tracheotomy patient through a tracheotomy (a tube inserted directly into the trachea) is colder and drier than normal, which often causes lung crusting and infection. This occurs primarily because the air:

   (A) Enters the respiratory system too rapidly to be filtered.
   (B) Is not properly humidified by the larynx.
   (C) Does not flow through the nasal passageways.
   (D) Does not flow past the mouth and tongue.

7. Which of the following is the location for the exchange of oxygen and carbon dioxide through thin membrane walls?

   (A) Alveoli.
   (B) Trachea.
   (C) Nasal cavity.
   (D) Diaphragm.

8. What is the function of a lysosome's membrane?

   (A) It isolates an acidic environment for the lysosome's hydrolytic enzymes from the neutral pH of the cytoplasm.
   (B) It is continuous with the nuclear membrane, thereby linking the lysosome with the endoplasmic reticulum.
   (C) It is used as an alternative site of protein synthesis.
   (D) The cytochrome carriers of the electron transport chain are embedded within it.

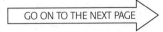
GO ON TO THE NEXT PAGE

9. Oogenesis is the process by which:

   (A) Primary oocytes produce sperm.
   (B) Primary oocytes produce eggs.
   (C) The egg implants in the uterus.
   (D) The egg is released from the ovary.

10. In a neutral atom:

    (A) The number of electrons is greater than the number of protons.
    (B) The number of electrons is less than the number of protons.
    (C) The number of electrons is equal to the number of protons.
    (D) There are no electrons.

11. Which of the following indicates the relative randomness of molecules in the three states of matter?

    (A) Solid > liquid < gas
    (B) Liquid < solid < gas
    (C) Liquid > gas > solid
    (D) Gas > liquid > solid

12. Which of the following states of matter has the highest average translational kinetic energy?

    (A) Solid.
    (B) Liquid.
    (C) Gas.
    (D) None of the above.

13. An element that contains a full outer shell is called a:

    (A) Metal.
    (B) Nonmetal.
    (C) Metalloid.
    (D) Noble gas.

14. Which of the following waves on the electromagnetic spectrum has the highest frequency?

    (A) Microwaves.
    (B) X-rays.
    (C) Visible light.
    (D) Radio waves.

15. Which of the following best explains the recoil action of a shooting gun?

    (A) Newton's First Law of Motion.
    (B) Newton's Second Law of Motion.
    (C) Newton's Third Law of Motion.
    (D) Newton's Law of Gravitation.

16. Which of the following states the law of charges?

    (A) Like charges repel each other and unlike charges attract each other.
    (B) Unlike charges repel each other and like charges attract each other.
    (C) All charges repel each other.
    (D) All charges attract each other.

END OF TEST. STOP

KAPLAN

Diagnostic Quiz Answer Key

Reading Comprehension	Vocabulary and Spelling	Mathematics	Science
1. A	1. C	1. C	1. B
2. C	2. A	2. D	2. C
3. C	3. A	3. D	3. B
4. C	4. C	4. D	4. B
5. D	5. D	5. D	5. D
6. C	6. B	6. D	6. C
7. A	7. D	7. B	7. A
8. D	8. C	8. D	8. A
9. C	9. C	9. B	9. B
10. C	10. A	10. A	10. C
11. B	11. A	11. C	11. D
	12. C	12. C	12. C
	13. C	13. D	13. D
	14. A	14. D	14. B
	15. B	15. C	15. C
	16. A	16. A	16. A
		17. B	

Answers and Explanations

Reading Comprehension

1. A

Remember that inference questions keep you close to the text as you draw a conclusion. When evaluating the implications of an author's description, consider what particular aspects of the description are relevant in the context. The author states that sloths move "from branch to branch almost imperceptibly," implying that their movements are so slow or gradual that they're difficult to detect. (A) is a good fit for your prediction. (B) is out of scope; the passage does not indicate whether or not such slowness is intentional, only that sloths tend to move slowly. (C) is extreme; although the passage states that sloths are rarely sighted, it does not go so far as to suggest that they are impossible to observe. (D) is a distortion; the author never states that sloths are unable to move faster.

2. C

Rather than answering reference questions such as this one from memory, always use the clues provided in the question to guide you through the text. The question notes two characteristics of the three-toed sloth: lack of speed and a tendency to hang upside down. In introducing these traits, the passage says that some of the sloth's characteristics "seem to run counter to the instincts displayed by almost all wild animals," so the correct choice will note that these are differences between sloths and almost all other wild animals. (A) is extreme; although the passage indicates that these characteristics distinguish sloths from other wild animals, "entirely unique" is too strong a statement. (B) is a distortion; the passage never states why sloths were long mistaken for a species of monkey. (C) is a good match for your prediction. (D) is an irrelevant detail; the passage does not suggest that eating, sleeping, or mating upside down is detrimental to sloths.

3. C

The author notes that biomes are distinguished primarily by the kind of plants that are *most prevalent* and offers the temperate grassland as an example of a biome. As a result, you can infer that the "grasses and scrub brush" mentioned are the plants that occur most frequently in the temperate grassland. "Control" (A) matches the primary definition for *dominate* but does not make sense in the paragraph. "Rule over" (B) is a common meaning of the word *dominate* that

does not fit here. (C) matches neatly, but even if you were unaware of this meaning for *overwhelm*, you could still have reached it by process of elimination. Although grasses and scrub brush are the most prevalent features, this doesn't mean that they take all attention away from other features of the biome, so "overshadow" (D) is incorrect.

4. C

Remember, valid inferences do not stray far from the text. The passage says that grasses and scrub brush dominate the landscape of temperate grassland biomes, and that these areas "remain relatively dry throughout the year." Look for a statement that follows directly from these facts. (A) is extreme; passage states that grasses and scrub brush are prevalent in the biome but never indicates that this biome is the only area where these plants are found. (B) is also extreme; the passage doesn't indicate that these plants can thrive only in dry climates, just that they do thrive in this biome. (C) makes sense; if the plants thrive in an area that is always dry, they must not require too much water. (D) is extreme as well; the passage describes these particular plants as structurally simple, but this does not mean that all grasses and scrub brush are structurally simple.

5. D

It is important to keep in mind the general tone of a reading passage, because you can usually eliminate incorrect answer choices based on their mismatch with the author's tone or meaning. Here, although the author mentions some of the unrivaled strengths of the human brain, nowhere in the text is one animal's brain described as superior to another's. The last sentence in the first paragraph, beginning "While these relative strengths and weaknesses…" clearly illustrates this nonjudgmental tone and indicates that the author is comparing the brain capabilities of various animals to describe how the human brain differs and can be distinguished. (A) is a distortion; this choice does not match the tone of the text, which does not describe one animal's brain as more sophisticated than another's. (B) is a misused detail; while the author's comparisons may have this effect, the diversity of brain types is neither mentioned nor emphasized in the passage. (C) is out of scope; the author mentions only the human brain as having plasticity. (D) is a great fit for your prediction.

6. C

Before making your answer selection, make sure to consider the surrounding context. The reference is being used as an example that supports the preceding sentence: "In terms of what it can do, the human brain is in some ways unable to match the brain functioning of 'lower' animals; in other ways, its capabilities are quite unrivaled." In other words, it supports the idea that the brain capabilities of different animals vary so dramatically that it is hard to compare one to another, which matches (C). Choice (A) is a distortion; while the paragraph does not focus on cats and dogs, nowhere is it suggested that this information is irrelevant. Choice (B) is out of scope; the paragraph does not discuss how humans have historically represented our sensory capabilities. Choice (D) is out of scope; the paragraph does not mention any "great weaknesses" of the brains of cats and dogs.

7. A

In a context question, don't worry too much about what you know of any given word; instead, focus only on how this word fits within the sentence where it is used. In this case, notice that earlier in the sentence, the word *attributed* is used in essentially the same way as the cited word—that is, connecting the characteristics and capabilities of the human brain with the concept of plasticity. "Connected" (A) is a great match for your prediction. "Drawn" (B) fits with the primary definition of the word *traced* but not its context in the passage. "Searched" (C) matches another meaning of the cited word, but the author is implying more than just the idea of a search. "Copied" (D) is another meaning of *traced* but does not fit its specific meaning here.

8. D

Ramsay appears toward the middle of the passage after the author mentions that scientists doubted helium exists only on the sun. Since Ramsay's experiment with naturally occurring Earth minerals occurs in the next sentence, the correct answer would be something that cites discovering helium on Earth, and (D) fits this well.

9. C

The passage states that Janssen and Lockyer observed the sun using their spectroscopes and discovered a new yellow line that belonged to an unknown element. Reading the next sentence reveals that Janssen and Lockyer's work was doubted by many other scientists (C).

10. C

The passage discusses industrial uses for precious stones, so the correct answer, choice (C), should pretty much jump out at you.

11. B

The passage notes parenthetically that a ruby is a sapphire with chromium "impurities," so one can logically infer that both gems come from the same kind of stone, choice (B).

Vocabulary and Spelling

1. C

Sometimes, if you are having trouble with a word, such as *resignation* here, try coming up with a different form of the same word—another part of speech—and then working on a synonym for the related word. For instance, if you come up with *resigned*, you might be able to make an easier sentence, such as: He was *resigned* to defeat. And from this you figure out that resignation most nearly means *acceptance*.

2. A

Even if you only have a vague notion of the meaning of *tangible*, you might have a sense that something *tangible* can be felt or seen, as oppose to intangible objects, which cannot. From that, you should be able to pick *real* (A) as the closest match.

3. A

When the question doesn't provide a context, try to come up with your own. Maybe you've heard something like: "The plan is feasible." Which answer choice best describes a plan? *Feasible* does mean *workable* or viable.

4. C

Since the *im-* prefix means *not*, then something *impure* is not pure. The correct answer choice will be a synonym for *pure*. *Unalloyed* means *not alloyed,* or *unmixed.* If you did not know what *unalloyed* meant, you could have tried to eliminate other answer choices to help you make an educated guess.

5. D

The answer choices tell you that *scale* is being used as a verb. To scale is to climb up, as in *scale a mountain*. The correct answer choice will mean *climb down. Descend* means to *climb down*. This is the correct answer. If you needed to guess, you could eliminate *collapse* and *weigh*, since they have no clear opposites.

6. B

Levity means *lightness* or *humor*. The correct answer choice will be a word that means *seriousness* or *lack of humor*. *Gravity* is not only the force that holds us to Earth, but it also means *seriousness*. This is the correct answer.

7. D

Optimistic means full of hope; *sage* means full of wisdom.

8. C

An *agenda* is a plan for a meeting, and a *program* is a plan for a play.

9. C

One *forges* a *signature* and one *counterfeits money*.

10. A

The correct spelling is *neutral*.

11. A

The correct spelling is *accessible*.

12. C

The correct spelling is *negligence*.

13. C

The correct spelling is *excellent*.

14. A

The correct spelling is *available*.

15. B

The correct spelling is *cafeteria*.

16. A

The correct spelling is *interrupt*.

Mathematics

1. C

Subtract 100 from both sides of the equation $100 + x = 100$ to find that $x = 0$.

2. D

Let x represent the number that 40 must be reduced to so that the percent decrease from 40 to x will equal the percent decrease from 12 to 9. Percent decrease means the same thing as fractional decrease, except that a percent decrease describes the fractional decrease with a fraction that has a denominator of 100.

Let's work with fractional decreases. When a positive number decreases to a smaller positive number, the fractional decrease is $\frac{\text{Original value} - \text{New value}}{\text{Original value}}$. The decrease from 12 to 9 is $12 - 9 = 3$, so the fractional decrease from 12 to 9 is $\frac{12 - 9}{12} = \frac{3}{12}$. Reduce $\frac{3}{12}$ to $\frac{1}{4}$. Now you want to define x so the fractional decrease from 40 to x is also $\frac{1}{4}$. If 40 decreases from 40 to x, the decrease is $40 - x$. Therefore, the fractional decrease from 40 to x is $\frac{40 - x}{40}$. Since you want the fractional decrease from 40 to x to be $\frac{1}{4}$, set up the equation $\frac{40 - x}{40} = \frac{1}{4}$.

Let's solve this equation for x:

$$\frac{40 - x}{40} = \frac{1}{4}$$

Cross-multiply: $(40 - x)4 = 40(1)$

Simplify both sides: $160 - 4x = 40$

Subtract 40 from both sides: $120 - 4x = 0$

Add $4x$ to both sides: $120 = 4x$

Divide both sides by 4: $30 = x$

Thus, $x = 30$, which is the number that 40 must decrease to in order to have a fractional decrease that equals the fractional decrease from 12 to 9.

Note that it was not necessary to work with any percent decrease to solve this question. Just for the sake of the discussion, let's convert $\frac{1}{4}$ to a percent. To convert a fraction or decimal to a percent, multiply that fraction or decimal by 100%: $\frac{1}{4} = \frac{1}{4} \times 100\% = 25\%$. Remember, when a positive number decreases to a smaller positive number that the fractional decrease is $\frac{\text{Original value} - \text{New value}}{\text{Original value}}$. To convert this fractional decrease to a percent decrease, multiply the fractional decrease by 100%: $\frac{\text{Original value} - \text{New value}}{\text{Original value}} \times 100\%$.

3. D

Each month on this planet has 15 days, so 700 days = (700 days) ÷ (15 days per month) = $\frac{700}{15}$ months = $\frac{140}{3}$ months on this planet. Let's keep the format of $\frac{140}{3}$ months the way it is right now, so the division later on will be easier. Each year on this planet has 9 months, so 700 days expressed as years $= \left(\frac{140}{3} \text{ months}\right) \div$ (9 months per year) $= \frac{140}{3 \times 9}$ years $= \frac{140}{27}$ years $= 5\frac{5}{27}$ years. So on this planet, 700 days is $5\frac{5}{27}$ years. Therefore, 5 full years have passed.

4. D

Calculate what's in parentheses first. To add the fractions $\frac{1}{5}$ and $\frac{1}{3}$ you need a common denominator. Find this by starting with the smallest positive multiple of 5, which is 1×5, or 5, and then looking at the next positive multiples of 5, which are $2 \times 5, 3 \times 5, 4 \times 5, \ldots$, until you find a multiple of 3:

- $1 \times 5 = 5$ is not a multiple of 3.
- $2 \times 5 = 10$ is not a multiple of 3.
- $3 \times 5 = 15$ is obviously a multiple of both 5 and 3 since it contains factors of 5 and 3.

Thus, $15 = 3 \times 5$ is a multiple of 3—it is actually the smallest positive multiple of 5 and 3.

Therefore, $\frac{1}{5} + \frac{1}{3} = \frac{3}{15} + \frac{5}{15} = \frac{3+5}{15} = \frac{8}{15}$, and $\left(\frac{1}{5} + \frac{1}{3}\right) \div \frac{1}{2} = \frac{8}{15} \div \frac{1}{2}$.

Now, to divide fractions, invert the one after the division sign and multiply: $\frac{8}{15} \div \frac{1}{2} = \frac{8}{15} \times \frac{2}{1} = \frac{8 \times 2}{15 \times 1} = \frac{16}{15}$.

5. D

An event is a set of possible outcomes. When we are concerned with the probability of an event, E, each outcome that is an element of the set E is called a desired outcome. When all the possible outcomes are equally likely, the probability of event E is defined as the number of desired outcomes divided by the number of possible outcomes.

In this question, there are 5 blue pens, 6 black pens, and 4 red pens in the knapsack. Thus, there are $5 + 6 + 4 = 15$ pens in the knapsack. If Marty pulls out 1 pen, there are 15 different pens he might pick, or 15 outcomes. The question asks the probability of one pen picked being either black or red. There are 6 black pens and 4 red pens. The number of desired outcomes is $6 + 4 = 10$. So the probability that the pen picked will be black or red is $\frac{10}{15}$, which can be reduced to $\frac{2}{3}$, or 2 out of 3.

6. D

Pick numbers for p, w, and x that work well in the problem, then solve the question with the numbers you selected. Any answer choice that does not equal the value of your solution for the values of the variables you selected can be eliminated.

Let $p = 3$ and let $w = 100$. So there are 3 pages with 100 words per page, therefore there are (100 words per page)(3 pages) = 300 words total. Say Bill types 5 words a minute, so $x = 5$. Since he types 300 words at rate of 5 words per minute, he types 300 words in (300 words) ÷ (5 words per minute) = 60 minutes, which equals 1 hour. It takes him 1 hour to type the paper. The only answer choice that equals 1 when $p = 3$, $w = 100$, and $x = 5$ is choice (D).

Here is an algebraic solution. Bill has to type a paper that is p pages long with each page containing w words. So the entire paper contains (w words per page)(p pages) = wp words. Bill types an average of x words per minute. Now the question wants you to determine how many hours it will take Bill to type the wp words. Let's determine Bill's rate of typing in words per hour: x words per minute = (x word per minute) × (60 minutes per hour) = $60x$ words per hour. Bills types at a rate of $60x$ words per hour. So the number of hours it takes Bill to type wp words is (wp words) ÷ ($60x$ words per hour) = $\frac{wp}{60x}$ hours. Again, choice (D) is correct.

7. B

The ratio of teachers to students is 1 to 10, so there might be only 1 teacher and 10 students, 50 teachers and 500 students, or any reasonable positive integer number of teachers and any reasonable positive integer number of students that are in the ratio of 1 to 10. That means the teachers and students can be divided into groups of 11, with 1 teacher and 10 students in each group. Think of it as a school with a large number of classrooms, all with 1 teacher and 10 students, for a total of 11 people in each room. So the total number of teachers and students in the school must be a multiple of 11. If you look at the answer choices, you'll notice that only 121, choice (B), is a multiple of 11: $121 = 11 \times 11$. Therefore, choice (B) must be correct.

8. D

This is a straightforward substitution problem. Plug in the given values and remember your order of operations (PEMDAS). Since $r = 3$ and $s = 1$, $r^2 - 2s = (3)^2 - 2(1) = 9 - 2 = 7$.

9. B

Since the machine caps 5 bottles every 2 seconds, the machine caps bottles at the rate of (5 bottles) ÷ (2 seconds), or 2.5 bottles per second. The question requires finding how many bottles will be capped in 1 minute, so let's convert 1 minute to seconds: 1 minute = 60 seconds. So in 60 seconds, the machine caps (2.5 bottles per second) × (60 seconds) = 150 bottles.

10. A

Solve the equation $\frac{2}{x} + \frac{5}{3} = 2$ for x.

$$\frac{2}{x} + \frac{5}{3} = 2$$

Subtract $\frac{5}{3}$ from both sides: $\quad \frac{2}{x} = 2 - \frac{5}{3}$

Begin to simplify the right side: $\quad \frac{2}{x} = \frac{6}{3} - \frac{5}{3}$

Continue to simplify the right side: $\quad \frac{2}{x} = \frac{6-5}{3}$

Continue to simplify the right side: $\quad \frac{2}{x} = \frac{1}{3}$

Cross-multiply: $\quad (2)(3) = (x)(1)$

Simplify both sides: $\quad 6 = x$

Thus, $x = 6$.

11. C

Let x dollars represent the original price. After a 25% markdown, the cost of the sweater is 100% − 25% = 75% of the original price. Next, convert 75% to a fraction. To convert a percent to a fraction or decimal, divide the percent by 100%: $75\% = \frac{75\%}{100\%} = \frac{75}{100} = \frac{3}{4}$. Thus, $\frac{3}{4}x$ dollars is the reduced price. The reduced price is also given as $48. So $\frac{3}{4}x = 48$. Divide both sides by $\frac{3}{4}$: $x = 48 \div \frac{3}{4} = 48 \times \frac{4}{3} = 16 \times 4 = 64$. The original price was $64.

12. C

Let's convert 30% to a fraction. To convert a percent to a fraction or decimal, divide the percent by 100%: $30\% = \frac{30\%}{100\%} = \frac{30}{100} = \frac{3}{10}$. The word "of" means "times," or "multiply by." So 30% of x means 30% times x, or $\left(\frac{3}{10}\right)(x) = \frac{3x}{10}$.

13. D

The first 3 minutes of the phone call cost 75¢, or $0.75. If the entire call lasted x minutes, the rest of the call lasted $x - 3$ minutes. Each minute after the first 3 cost 15¢, or $0.15, so the rest of the call cost $0.15(x - 3)$. Thus, the cost of the entire call is $0.75 + 0.15(x - 3)$ dollars.

14. D

$2 \times 10^4 = 20{,}000$. $5 \times 10^3 = 5{,}000$. $6 \times 10^2 = 600$. $4 \times 10^1 = 40$.

So the sum is $20{,}000 + 5{,}000 + 600 + 40 = 25{,}640$.

15. C

All you have to do here is solve the equation, but instead of solving it for n, you have to solve it for $4n$. If $2n + 3 = 5$, then you can subtract 3 from both sides of the equation to get $2n = 2$. Multiplying both sides of this equation by 2 gives you $4n = 4$, choice (C).

16. A

Looking at the graph, you can see that the number of books borrowed in January was 300. To find the total number of books borrowed during the first six months of the year, add the values of each bar: 300 + 350 + 400 + 450 + 500 + 400 = 2,400 books.

So the fraction of books borrowed in January out of the total number of books borrowed during the first 6 months of the year is $\frac{300}{2{,}400}$, which can be reduced to $\frac{1}{8}$.

17. B

Rather than dealing with fractions of the business, let's say that each person owns one share, and each share is worth 20 dollars. At the beginning, each of the 4 women owns 20 dollars' worth, and the man owns 20 dollars' worth. One woman sells $\frac{1}{2}$ of her part of the business, which is $\frac{1}{2}$ (20 dollars) = 10 dollars' worth. Another woman sells $1 - \frac{1}{4} = \frac{4}{4} - \frac{1}{4} = \frac{3}{4}$ of her part of the business, which is $\frac{3}{4}$ (20 dollars) = 15 dollars' worth. Now the man owns (20 + 10 + 15) dollars' worth, or 45 dollars' worth. The total business is worth (20 dollars per share) × (5 shares) = 100 dollars. The fraction of the business that he owns is (45 dollars) ÷ (100 dollars), which is $\frac{45}{100}$, and can be reduced to $\frac{9}{20}$.

Science

1. B

Animals that consume plants are called herbivores.

2. C

The kingdom archaebacteria is considered the most primitive kingdom.

3. B

Diffusion is the tendency of molecules or ions to move from areas of higher concentration to areas of lower concentration until the concentration is uniform throughout the system. Diffusion explains how gases in the air spread out when released from a location where the concentration of their molecules is higher than in the space surrounding their source.

4. B

Mitosis is the process of nuclear cell division and chromosomal replication that results in two daughter nuclei with identical DNA sequences.

5. D

The diaphragm is a muscular band of tissue that contracts to permit air to enter the lungs.

6. C

When a patient breathes through a tracheotomy, the air entering the respiratory system bypasses a very important area—the nasal cavities. In an individual breathing normally, the extensive surfaces of the nasal passageways warm and almost completely humidify the air, and particles are filtered out by nasal air turbulence. Since the air reaching the lungs of a tracheotomy patient has not been warmed or humidified, lung crusting and infection often result.

7. A

The alveoli are the location for the exchange of oxygen and carbon dioxide within the lungs.

8. A

Lysosomes have an acidic interior to enhance the activity of lysosomal enzymes that degrade biomolecules. The lysosomal membrane separates the acidic interior of the lysosome from the rest of the cell, which has a neutral pH.

9. B

Oogenesis is the process whereby primary oocytes undergo meiosis to produce one egg (or ovum) and two or three polar bodies.

10. C

In a neutral atom, the number of negatively charged electrons is equal to the number of positively charged protons.

11. D

Because gas molecules have the greatest freedom to move around, gases have the greatest disorder. Liquids are more dense than gases and therefore the molecules experience stronger intermolecular attractions and are less free to move around. The arrangement of molecules in solids is the least random.

12. C

The random motion of a gas holds the most translational kinetic energy.

13. D

An element whose outer shell is full is called a noble gas.

14. B

Of the wave states listed, X-rays have the highest frequency in the electromagnetic spectrum (gamma rays have an even higher frequency).

15. C

The recoil action of a shooting gun is explained by Newton's Third Law of Motion; that is, for every action there is an equal and opposite reaction.

16. A

The law of charges states that like charges repel each other and unlike charges attract each other.

Interpreting the Results of the Diagnostic Quiz

Because this is a diagnostic quiz, it's important to do more than just calculate your overall score and move on. How you did on this quiz is not a clear reflection on how you will perform on Test Day. Remember, its purpose is to help you diagnose your strengths and weaknesses.

Strengths and Weaknesses

Take a minute or so to list the areas of the Nursing School Entrance Exams Diagnostic Quiz you were good at. They can be general (math) or specific (addition of negative numbers). Put down as many as you can think of.

Strong Test Subjects

_____

_____

_____

_____

_____

_____

_____

_____

_____

_____

Now, take more time to list areas of the test you need to improve on, are just plain bad at, or have failed at.

Weak Test Subjects

Taking stock of your strengths and weaknesses lets you know the areas you don't have to worry about and the ones that will demand extra attention and effort. It helps to know where to put the extra effort. You will feel better (and do better) when you face up to what you need to work on instead of neglecting it.

As you work through this book, refer back to your weaknesses list. Check off your weaknesses as you tackle each one of them. (Math? Nerves? Reading Comprehension?) Now we're going to focus on what you're good at. Sharpen your pencil. Go to your strengths list. Copy the general items on that list below. You're going to make them more specific. For example, if you listed math as a broad topic you feel strong in, you would get specific by including areas of this subject about which you are particularly knowledgeable.

If any new strengths come to mind, jot them down. Focus all of your attention and effort on your strengths. Don't underestimate yourself or your abilities. Give yourself full credit. At the same time, don't list strengths you don't really have. You'll only be fooling yourself.

Strengths: From General to Specific

General Test-Taking Strengths

_____

_____

_____

_____

_____

_____

Specific Subject Strengths

_____

_____

_____

_____

_____

_____

After you've stopped, look over your list. Did you write down more things than you thought you knew? Is it possible you know more than you've given yourself credit for? Could that mean you've found a number of areas in which you feel strong?

You just took an active step toward helping yourself. Increased feelings of confidence work wonders on Test Day. If you are ready to begin your review, turn to Part Three now.

Chapter Three: **Reading Comprehension Review**

You may be thinking you don't need to review the lessons in this chapter. You already know how to read, right? After all, you have already read the first two chapters of this book! However, there is a big difference between knowing how to read, and being able to interpret, understand, and remember everything you read. The lessons in this chapter teach you how to be a more efficient reader. In turn, the strategies section of this book shows you how to handle the kinds of reading comprehension questions you are likely to face on your nursing school entrance exam. Don't forget to complete the review questions at the end of this chapter to make sure you have understood everything you have read so far!

(K) (H) READING COMPREHENSION LESSON

As you probably know, the way you read during a test is not exactly how you read in everyday life. In general, you usually read to learn or for pleasure. It's a pretty safe bet that you are not reading test passages for fun. If you do enjoy them, great! However, it should be clear that you are not reading these passages for enjoyment. You are reading them to answer questions and earn points. Here are some tips on how to get the most out of the passages you are reading.

Mark It Up
Use your test booklet (or scrap paper, if your test is computer based) to your advantage. Do not take a lot of notes, but indicate the main idea of the whole passage or specific paragraphs. Your notes will help you find the information you need to answer the questions later.

Focus on the First Third of the Passage
Although you may not find the passages on the test interesting, they are well organized. This means the author is very likely to present important information at the beginning of the passage. Chances are you will be able to answer the main idea questions based on the first third of the passage.

Use the Paragraph Topics

The first two sentences of each paragraph should tell you what it's about. The rest of the paragraph is likely to be more detail-heavy. Just as you should pay more attention to the beginning of the passage, you should also pay more attention to the beginning of each paragraph.

Don't Worry If You Get Stuck

If there's something in the passage you don't understand, don't waste time reading it over and over again. As long as you have a general idea of where the details are, you don't have to know what they are. Remember, later you can go back and look at paragraphs or notes you have made. This is another example of why marking up passages is so useful. You can circle or underline details that seem important. Furthermore, as long as you have made a note of the paragraph topic, you should be able to go back and find details within it. Details about a particular topic will always be located in the paragraph that deals with that topic.

Summarizing, Researching, and Making Inferences

The following skills will also help you with Reading Comprehension sections on Test Day.

Summarizing: For the purpose of the test, summarizing means being able to analyze a single phrase to capture what the entire passage is about.

Researching: Research is important in helping you answer detail questions. Researching means knowing where to look for the details. Generally, if you jot down paragraph topics, you should have a good idea where to locate the details.

Inferring: Making an inference means coming to a conclusion based on information that is hinted at, but not directly stated.

How to Read a Passage

You may not know it, but how we read depends upon why we're reading. When you're reading a Reading Comprehension passage on an exam, your goal is to correctly answer each question about that passage. Contrary to what you might expect, to reach that goal, you don't need to read the passage word by word. Instead, your best bet is to carefully skim the passage.

How do you skim as a reader? Rather than read the passage word for word, you scan it for important information such as names (proper names of people, places, and things are easy to identify because they are capitalized), dates, numerical figures, and words that suggest action.

Serious Skimming

Each Reading Comprehension passage is written with a distinct purpose. The author wants to make a point, describe a situation, or convince you of his or her ideas. Test-makers commonly ask you questions about the main idea of a passage or its tone. Common prompts for these question types include:

- The main idea of the passage is:
- The passage is primarily about:
- An appropriate title for this passage would be:
- The tone of the passage can best be described as:

The best way to anticipate these questions is to use active reading. Active reading does not mean reading a passage word-for-word. It means reading lightly but with a focus—in other words, serious skimming. This strategy will allow you to grasp quickly the main ideas of a passage and identify its tone. As you skim through each passage, keep the following questions in mind:

- What is this passage about?
- What is the point of the passage?
- What is the author trying to say?
- Why did he or she write this?
- What are the two or three most important things mentioned in this passage?

Remember not to worry about remembering every detail from a passage. You want to get a sense of the general outline; you can go back into the passage for the details.

Components of the Serious Skimming Technique

- Skim the passage to get the author's drift. Don't read the passage thoroughly. It's a waste of time.
- As you skim, search for important points. Don't wait for important information to jump out at you.
- Don't get caught up in details. The questions will often supply them for you or tell you exactly where to find them.

Kinds of Reading Comprehension Questions

When you read passages on a test, you're reading for a specific purpose: to be able to correctly answer as many questions as possible. Fortunately, most tests tend to use the same kinds of Reading Comprehension questions over and over again, so whatever the passage is about and however long it may be, you can expect the same four basic question types:

- Main Idea
- Detail
- Inference
- Vocabulary-in-Context

Main Idea Questions

Main Idea questions test how well you understand the passage as a whole. They ask about:

- The main point or purpose of a passage or individual paragraphs
- The author's overall attitude or tone
- The logic underlying the author's argument
- How ideas relate to each other in the passage

If you're stumped on a Main Idea question, even after reading the passage, do the Detail questions first. They can help you fill in the Main Idea.

Detail Questions

Detail questions ask about localized bits of information—usually specific facts or details from the passage. These questions may give you a line reference—a clue to where in the passage you'll find your answer. Beware of answer choices that seem to reasonably answer the question but don't make sense in the context of the passage or that are true but refer to a different section of the text.

Detail questions test:

- Whether or not you understand significant information that's stated in the passage
- Your ability to locate information within a text
- Your ability to differentiate between main ideas and specific details

Inference Questions

Some Reading Comprehension questions begin with, "it can be inferred that the author…" To infer is to draw a conclusion based on reasoning or evidence. For example, if you wake up in the morning and there's three feet of fresh snow on the ground, you can safely infer that it snowed during the night.

Often, writers will use suggestion or inference rather than stating ideas directly. But they will also leave you plenty of clues so you can figure out just what they are trying to convey. Inference clues include word choice (diction), tone, and specific details. For example, say a passage states that a particular idea was perceived as revolutionary. You might infer from the use of the word *perceived* that the author believes the idea was not truly revolutionary but seen that way.

Thus, Inference questions test your ability to use information in the passage to come to a logical conclusion. The key to Inference questions is to stick to the evidence in the text. Most Inference questions have pretty strong clues, so avoid any answer choices that seem far-fetched. If you can't find any evidence in the passage, then it probably isn't the right answer.

Make sure you read Inference questions carefully. Multiple answer choices may seem true; however, if particular answers can't be inferred from the passage and don't correspond to the passage as a whole or the specific part of the passage cited in the question, then they can't be the correct answer.

Vocabulary-in-Context Questions

Vocabulary-in-Context questions test your ability to infer the meaning of a word from the context in which it appears. The words tested are usually fairly common words with more than one meaning. That's the trick.

Many of the answer choices will be definitions of the tested word, but only one will work in context. Sometimes one of the answer choices will jump out at you. It will be the most common meaning of the word in question—but it's rarely right. You can think of this as the obvious choice. Say *curious* is the word being tested. The obvious choice is *inquisitive*. But *curious* also means "odd"; if that is the context the word appears in, that's the correct answer.

Using context to find the answer will help keep you from falling for this kind of trap. But you can also use these obvious choices to your advantage. If you get stuck on a Vocabulary-in-Context question, you can eliminate the obvious choice and guess from the remaining answers.

(K) (H) SAMPLE QUESTIONS

Questions 1–4 are based on the following passage.

A real-life invisibility cloak? Scientists think it's possible. In fact, a theory for how one might work already exists. Researchers believe that they can make light "bend" around an object in the same way that water flows around a rock in a river by using a special material—or metamaterial. A metamaterial is any man-made substance that doesn't act like anything else in nature. In this case, researchers are trying to create a metamaterial that will bend light waves instead of reflect them. To do this, researchers say, the material must be made of objects that are smaller than light waves.

The possibility of creating metamaterials was first envisaged in 1967 by the Russian scientist Victor Veselago. However, it wasn't until 2006 that a team of U.S. and British scientists could use this idea to create a metamaterial capable of bending microwaves. The following year, Vladimir Shalaev of Purdue University published a design for a cloak that could bend red light waves. Most recently, Duke University scientists made two exciting announcements. The first was that they were able to create a cloak that worked with a wider range of waves. The second was that the metamaterial used was cheap and easy to make.

Main Idea:

1. This passage is primarily about:

   (A) The science behind invisibility cloaks.

   (B) The importance of Victor Veselago's idea to the creation of an invisibility cloak.

   (C) Why scientists have yet to create a true invisibility cloak.

   (D) Scientists' efforts to create a real invisibility cloak.

Detail:

2. According to the passage, a metamaterial that could bend microwaves was created by:

(A) Victor Veselago.

(B) Scientists at Duke University.

(C) U.S. and British scientists.

(D) Vladimir Shalaev.

Inference:

3. It can be inferred from paragraph 2 of the passage that:

(A) U.S. and British scientists competed with each other to see who could create a metamaterial that could bend microwaves first.

(B) There is currently a great deal of interest surrounding the creation of an invisibility cloak.

(C) A metamaterial that can bend only red light waves is essentially useless.

(D) Scientists and researchers aren't getting any closer to creating a metamaterial that can bend light waves.

Vocabulary-in-Context:

4. The word "envisaged" in paragraph 2 most likely means:

(A) Produced.

(B) Seen.

(C) Imagined.

(D) Criticized.

Sample Question Answers and Explanations

1. D

The first paragraph describes scientists' theory about how an invisibility cloak might be created. The second paragraph describes a sequence of events that shows how scientists are getting closer to creating an actual invisibility cloak. Both paragraphs focus on the efforts that scientists have made toward creating such a cloak. (D) is the correct choice.

2. C

The easiest way to find an answer for a detail question is to go back into the passage to look for the information. Paragraph 2 states that a team of U.S. and British scientists created a metamaterial that could bend microwaves. (C) is the right answer.

3. B

The second paragraph names a number of different scientists and universities that are involved in trying to design invisibility cloaks. This suggests that many people are interested in achieving such a goal. (B) is the correct choice.

4. C

The fact that the metamaterials that Veselago created were only "possibilities" rules out choices (A) and (B). If you plug in the two remaining choices, you will find that (C), imagined, better fits the context of the paragraph, which shows a series of events bringing scientists closer to the invention of an invisibility cloak.

(K) (H) READING COMPREHENSION STRATEGIES

Here are some of the strategies that will help you on Test Day.

Kaplan's 5-Step Method for Reading Comprehension Questions

From the lesson, you learned that skimming is a vital component of Kaplan's 5-Step Method for Reading Comprehension Questions. Once you have skimmed the passage, apply our system of attacking the questions.

- Read the question stem.
- Locate the material you need.
- Predict the answer.
- Scan the answer choices.
- Select your answer.

Step 1. Read the Question Stem

You can't answer the question correctly if you haven't read it. It's as simple as that. So make sure to really read it carefully. Make sure you understand exactly what the question is asking. Is it a Main Idea question? Detail? Inference? Vocabulary? Are you looking for an overall main idea or a specific piece of information? Are you trying to determine the author's attitude or the meaning of a particular word?

Step 2. Locate the Material You Need

If you are given a line reference, read the material surrounding the line mentioned. It will clarify exactly what the question is asking and provide you with the context you need to answer the question correctly.

If you're not given a line reference, scan the text to find the section of the text the question applies to, then quickly reread those few sentences. Keep the main point of the passage in mind.

Step 3. Predict the Answer

Don't spend time making up a precise answer. You need only a general sense of what you're after so you can recognize the correct answer quickly when you read the choices.

Step 4. Scan the Answer Choices

Scan the choices, looking for one that fits your idea of the right answer. If you don't find an ideal answer, quickly eliminate wrong choices by checking over the passage again. Rule out choices that are too extreme or go against common sense. Get rid of answers that sound reasonable but don't make sense in the context of the passage or the question. Don't pick far-fetched inferences, and make sure there is evidence for your inference in the passage. Remember, to infer the correct answer, look at what is strongly implied in the passage.

Step 5. Select Your Answer

You've eliminated the obvious wrong answers. One of the remaining choices should fit your ideal. If you're left with more than one contender, consider the passage's main idea, and make an educated guess.

Long Passage Strategies

Some of the passages on your nursing school entrance exam are going to be longer. There are a few things to keep in mind when you read the long passages. Consider these as strategies that will help you master the section.

Question Order

For longer passages, Reading Comprehension questions are usually organized in a specific order. In general, order of questions corresponds with the passage; so it is safe to assume the first few questions ask about the beginning of the passage, the center questions about the middle, and the last few questions about the end.

Map It

Longer passages cover many aspects of a topic. For example, the first paragraph might introduce the subject, the second paragraph might present one viewpoint, and the third paragraph might argue for a different viewpoint. Within each of these paragraphs, there are several details that help the author convey a message.

Because there is a lot to keep track of, it is always smart to mark up long passages if you can.

- Write simple notes in the margin as you read.
- Underline key points.
- Write down the purpose of each paragraph.
- Concentrate on places where the author expresses an opinion. Most Reading Comprehension questions hinge on opinions and viewpoints, not facts.

These notes are your passage map, which can help you find the part of the passage that contains the information you need. The process of creating your passage map also forces you to read actively. Because you are constantly trying to identify the author's viewpoint, as well as the purpose of each sentence and paragraph, you will be working hard to understand what's happening in the passage. This translates into points on the test.

Now that you have read the lesson and strategies for Reading Comprehension questions, it's time to answer some review questions to make sure you have understood what you've read.

REVIEW QUESTIONS

The following questions are not meant to mimic actual test questions. Instead, these questions will help you review the concepts and terms covered in this chapter.

1. True or False? The reason you are reading should affect how you read.

2. Fill in the blank. The main idea of a passage is usually found _____.

3. Match the words with their definitions.

   ____ Summarizing

   ____ Researching

   ____ Inferring

   A. Knowing where to look for details.
   B. Coming to a conclusion based on information that is hinted at.
   C. Analyzing a single phrase to capture the meaning.

4. Write at least four questions you should be asking yourself when reading.

   _____

   _____

   _____

   _____

   _____

5. All of the following are types of Reading Comprehension questions EXCEPT:

   (A) Detail.
   (B) Inference.
   (C) Underlining.
   (D) Main Idea.

6. True or False? Detail questions test your ability to differentiate between main ideas and specific details.

7. Fill in the blank. _____ questions test your ability to draw a conclusion based on reasoning.

8. When you are mapping a passage, you should do all of the following EXCEPT:

   (A) Write simple notes in the margin as you read.
   (B) Write down the purpose of each paragraph.
   (C) Underline key points.
   (D) Concentrate on places where the author goes into specific detail about an element of the passage.

9. True or False? The order of questions generally follows the order of the passage.

10. Write Kaplan's 5-Step Method for Reading Comprehension Questions in order.

    1. _____
    2. _____
    3. _____
    4. _____
    5. _____

REVIEW ANSWERS

1. True. You wouldn't read your favorite novel in the same manner you would read a Reading Comprehension passage. Remember, you are reading to earn points, not for enjoyment or to learn anything.

2. The main idea is usually found in the first third of a passage.

3. The correct definitions are:
   - Summarizing means analyzing a single phrase to capture what the entire passage is about.
   - Researching means knowing where to look for details.
   - Inferring means coming to a conclusion based on information that is hinted at.

4. Your answers may vary, but here are some possible answers:
   - What is this passage about?
   - What is the point of this?
   - What is the author trying to say?
   - Why did the author write this?
   - What are the two or three most important things in this passage?

5. Underlining is not a question type.

6. True. Detail questions test your ability to differentiate between main ideas and specific details.

7. Inference questions test your ability draw a conclusion based on reasoning.

8. The correct answer is (D), because you should not concentrate on places where the author goes into specific detail. Instead, you should concentrate on places where the author expresses an opinion.

9. True. The order of the questions generally follows the order of the passage.

10. The correct order is:
    1. Read the question stem.
    2. Locate the material you need.
    3. Predict the answer.
    4. Scan the answer choices.
    5. Select your answer.

Chapter Four: **Vocabulary, Spelling, and Grammar Review**

As a nursing student—and eventually when you are a nurse—correct spelling and an understanding of complicated vocabulary will be essential aspects of your work. Having a strong grasp on spelling, vocabulary, prefixes, and root words will be key. Examine the word *hypothyroidism* (an underactive thyroid condition) for a moment. Just by changing two letters, the underactive thyroid condition becomes *hyperthyroidism* (an overactive thyroid condition). The treatment for these conditions is very different, and mixing them up could be a serious mistake. Similarly, mixing up pronouns or similar-sounding words can lead to confusion in medical situations where clarity and accuracy are critical. This is why nursing schools need to know you have a good foundation of spelling and vocabulary skills. The best way to learn spelling, vocabulary, and grammar is by practicing and memorizing.

Make sure to check out the additional study aids for this chapter in the Learning Resources section of the book.

K H VOCABULARY LESSON

Your Vocabulary

To get a sense of your vocabulary strength, take a few minutes to go through the following list of 15 words and see how many you know. Write your definition to the right of each word. Then, check the definitions on the next page.

Resolute _____

Terse _____

Vanquish _____

Cautious _____

Lethargic _____

Sullen _____

Distraught _____

Legible _____

Fawn (v.) _____

Jeer (n.) _____

Adrift _____

Query _____

Impure _____

Disinterested _____

Pathetic _____

Here are the definitions:

Resolute:	Determined
Terse:	Short, abrupt
Vanquish:	To defeat or conquer in battle
Cautious:	Careful in actions and behaviors
Lethargic:	Sluggish, inactive, apathetic
Sullen:	Depressed, gloomy
Distraught:	Extremely troubled; agitated with anxiety
Legible:	Possible to read or decipher
Fawn (v.):	To act in a servile manner
Jeer (n.):	Taunt, ridicule
Adrift:	Wandering aimlessly; afloat without direction
Query:	A question; to call into question
Impure:	Lacking in purity; containing something unclean
Disinterested:	Impartial; unbiased
Pathetic:	Sad, pitiful, tending to arouse sympathy

If you got 11 or more definitions correct, your vocabulary is above average. Congratulations! If you got 10 or fewer correct, the techniques and tools in this chapter will teach you ways to improve your vocabulary and help you make the most out of words you already know.

A Vocabulary-Building Plan

A great vocabulary can't be built overnight, but you can begin building a good vocabulary with a little bit of time and effort. Here are some strategies for how to do that.

Look It Up

Challenge yourself to find at least five words a day that are unfamiliar to you. You could find these words while listening to a news broadcast or reading a magazine or novel. In fact, books that you choose to read for enjoyment normally contain three to five words per page that are unfamiliar to you. Write down these words, look them up in the dictionary, and record their definitions in a notebook.

But don't only write the word's definition. Below your definition, use the word in a sentence. This will help you to remember the word and anticipate possible context questions.

Study Word Roots and Prefixes

Many difficult vocabulary words are made up of roots, prefixes, and suffixes. (See Part Seven: Learning Resources for some common roots and prefixes.) Understanding the meaning of any of these parts of a word can help guide you to a correct definition. For example, if you know that the prefix *bio-* means "life," then you might be able to decode the definition of *biodegradable*, which means "able to be broken down by living things." If you've studied a foreign language in school, your knowledge in that area can also help you decipher the meaning of a prefix or word root.

Think Like a Thesaurus

On any test it's better to know a little bit about a lot of words than to know a lot about a few words. So, try to think like a thesaurus rather than a dictionary. For instance, instead of just studying the definition of *lackluster*, study the words associated with *lackluster* (such as *drab, dull, flat, lifeless, lethargic, listless, sluggard, somnolent*) in a thesaurus. By grouping words of similar definition, you can get 12 words for the price of one definition.

Personalize the Way You Study Vocabulary

Most students do not learn best by reading passively from texts. Taking an active role in your learning helps you focus and retain more new information. That said, it's important to find a study method that works best for you and to stick to it.

Use Flashcards

Write down new words or word groups and run through them whenever you have some spare time. Write the word or word group on one side of an index card and a short definition on the other side.

Make a Vocabulary Notebook

List words in the left-hand column and their meanings in the right-hand column. Cover up or fold over the page to test yourself. See how many words you can define from memory.

Create Memory Devices

That is, try to come up with hooks to lodge new words into your head. Create visual images, silly sentences, rhymes, whatever, to build associations between words and their definitions.

Trust Your Hunches

Vocabulary knowledge is not an all-or-nothing proposition. Don't write off a word you see just because you can't recite its definition. There are many levels of vocabulary knowledge.

- Some words you know so well you can rattle off their dictionary definitions.
- Some words you "sort of" know. You can't define them precisely and you probably wouldn't use them yourself, but you understand them when you see them in context.
- Some words you barely recognize. You know you've heard them before, but you're not sure where.
- Some words you've never, ever seen before.

If the word before you falls in the second or third category, go with your hunch. The following techniques may help you to get a better fix on the word.

Try To Recall Where You've Heard the Word Before

If you can recall a phrase in which the word appears, that may help you choose the correct answer. Take a look at the following example. Remember that you don't need to know the dictionary definition to solve a question like this one. A sense of where you've heard a word before may be sufficient.

> *Clandestine* most nearly means:
>
> (A) Amicable
> (B) Spirited
> (C) Auspicious
> (D) Secret

You may not have known the definition of *clandestine*, but you may have heard the word used in phrases like "*clandestine activity*" on the news or in spy films. In that case, you may have gotten a sense of the meaning, which is "covert" or "secret." Choice (D) is the correct answer.

Think Positive and Negative

Sometimes just knowing the "charge" of a word—that is, whether a word has a positive or negative sense—will be enough to earn you points on a test. Take the word *auspicious*. Let's assume you don't know its dictionary definition. Ask yourself: Does *auspicious* sound positive or negative? How about *callow*? Negative words often just sound negative. Positive words, on the other hand, tend to sound more friendly. If you said that *auspicious* is positive, you're right. It means "favorable or hopeful." And if you thought that *callow* is negative, you're also right. It means "immature or unsophisticated."

You can also use prefixes to help determine a word's charge. *Mal-, de-, dis-, dys-, un-, in-, im-,* and *mis-* often indicate a negative, while *pro-, ben-, magn-,* and *eu-* are often positives. Some words are neutral and don't have a charge. But if you can get a sense of the word's charge, you can probably answer some questions on that basis alone.

In the example below, begin by getting a sense of the "charge" of the word in italics.

> *Rankle* most nearly means:
>
> (A) Exhort
> (B) Impress
> (C) Relieve
> (D) Irk

Word sense is a very subjective thing, but in this case, most people—even if they can't come up with an exact definition of *rankle*—can just tell by the sound of the word that it has some sort of negative connotation. In this case, just having that sense should be enough for you to pick the correct answer.

Choices (B) and (C) are clearly too positive for either to be the right answer. And choice (A) is neither positive nor negative, which also can't be right if you're sure the word is negative. *Rankle*, like *irk*, means "to annoy or irritate." So you shouldn't become *rankled* if you don't know the exact definition of a word. Try to come up with the word's charge instead. It may be enough to find the correct answer.

🅚 🅗 VOCABULARY STRATEGIES

Here are some strategies that will help you on Test Day.

Kaplan's 3-Step Method for Synonyms
- Define the stem word.
- Find the answer choice that best fits your definition.
- If no choice fits, think of other definitions for the stem word and go through the choices again.

Let's use the Kaplan 3-Step Method for the sample synonym question found earlier in the chapter.

> *Genuine* most nearly means:
>
> (A) Authentic
> (B) Valuable
> (C) Ancient
> (D) Damaged

Step 1. Define the Stem Word

What does *genuine* mean? Something genuine is something real, such as a real Picasso painting, rather than a forgery. Your definition might be something like this: *Something genuine can be proven to be what it claims to be.*

Step 2. Find the Answer Choice That Best Fits Your Definition

Go through the answer choices one by one to see which one fits best. Your options are: *authentic, valuable, ancient,* and *damaged.* Something genuine could be worth a lot or not much at all, old or new, or in good shape or bad. The only word that really means the same thing as *genuine is* (A) *authentic.*

Step 3. If No Choice Fits, Think of Other Definitions for the Stem Word and Go Through the Choices Again

In the example above, one choice fits. Now, take a look at the following example:

> *Grave* most nearly means:
>
> (A)   Regrettable
> (B)   Unpleasant
> (C)   Serious
> (D)   Careful

When you applied Step 1 to this example, maybe you defined *grave* as a burial location. You looked at the choices and didn't see any words like *tomb* or *coffin.* What to do? Use the idea presented in Step 3; go back to the stem word, and think about other definitions. Have you ever heard the word *grave* used any other way? If someone were in a "grave situation," what would that mean? *Grave* can also mean *serious* or *solemn,* so (C) *serious* fits perfectly. If none of the answer choices seems to work with your definition, there may be a second definition you haven't considered yet.

Avoiding a Pitfall

Kaplan's 3-Step Method for Synonyms should be the basis for tackling every question, but there are a few other things you need to know to perform your best on synonym questions. Fortunately, there is only one pitfall to watch out for.

Choosing Tempting Wrong Answers

Test makers choose wrong answer choices very carefully. Sometimes that means throwing in answer traps that will tempt you but aren't right. Be a savvy test taker; don't fall for these distracters!

What kinds of wrong answers are we talking about here? In synonym questions, there are two types of answer traps to watch out for: answers that are almost right, and answers that sound like the stem word. Let's illustrate both types to make the concept concrete.

> *Delegate* most nearly means:
>
> (A)   Delight
> (B)   Assign
> (C)   Decide
> (D)   Manage

Favor most nearly means:

(A) Award

(B) Prefer

(C) Respect

(D) Improve

In the first example, choices (A) and (C) might be tempting, because they all start with the prefix *de-*, just like the stem word, *delegate*. It's important that you examine all the answer choices, because otherwise you might choose (A) and never get to the correct answer, which is (B). In the second example, you might look at the word *favor* and think, oh, that's something positive. It's something you do for someone else. It sounds a lot like choice (A), *award*. Maybe you pick (A) and move on. If you did that, you would be falling for a trap! The correct answer is (B) *prefer*, since *favor* is being used as a verb, and *to favor* someone or something is to like it better than something else—in other words, to prefer it. If you don't read through all of the choices, you might be tricked into choosing a wrong answer.

At this point, you have a great set of tools for answering most synonym questions. You know how to approach them and you know some traps to avoid. But what happens if you don't know the word in the question? Here are some techniques to help you figure out the meaning of a tough vocabulary word and answer a difficult synonym question.

What to Do if You Don't Know the Word

- Look for familiar roots and prefixes.
- Use your knowledge of foreign languages.
- Remember the word used in a particular context.
- Figure out the word's charge.

Let's examine each technique more closely:

Look for Familiar Roots and Prefixes

Having a good grasp of how words are put together will help you tremendously on synonym questions, particularly when you don't know a vocabulary word. If you can break a word into pieces you do understand, you'll be able to answer questions you might have thought too difficult to tackle. Look at the words below. Circle any prefixes or roots you know.

Benevolence   Conspire

Insomnia   Verify

Inscribe

Bene- means "good"; *somn-* has to do with sleep; *scribe* has to do with writing; *con-* means "doing something together"; and *ver-* has to do with truth. So, for example, if you were looking for a synonym for *benevolence*, you'd definitely want to choose a positive, or "good" word.

KAPLAN

Use Your Knowledge of Foreign Languages

Remember, any knowledge of a foreign language, particularly if it's one of the Romance languages (French, Spanish, Italian), can help you decode lots of vocabulary words. Look at the example words below. Do you recognize any foreign language words in them?

Facilitate

Dormant

Explicate

In Italian, *facile* means "easy"; in Spanish, *dormir* means "to sleep"; and in French, *expliquer* means "to explain." A synonym for each of these words would have something to do with what they mean in their respective languages.

Remember the Word Used in a Particular Context

Sometimes a word might look strange to you when it is sitting on the page by itself, but if you think about it, you realize you've heard it before in a phrase. If you can put the word into context, even if that context is cliché, you're on your way to deciphering its meaning.

Illegible most nearly means:

(A) Illegal

(B) Twisted

(C) Unreadable

(D) Eligible

Have you heard this word in context? Maybe someone you know has had his or her handwriting described as illegible. What is illegible handwriting? The correct answer is (C). Remember to try to think of a definition first, before you look at the answer choices. Some of the answer choices in this example are tricks. Which wrong answers are tempting, meant to remind you of the question word?

Here's another example:

Laurels most nearly means:

(A) Vine

(B) Honor

(C) Lavender

(D) Cushion

Is "don't rest on your laurels" a phrase you've ever heard or used? What do you think it might mean? The phrase "don't rest on your laurels" originated in ancient Greece, where heroes were given wreaths of laurel branches to signify their accomplishments. Telling people not to rest on their laurels is the same thing as telling them not to get too smug; rather than living off the success of one accomplishment, they should strive for improvement. The answer is (B).

Figure Out the Word's Charge

Even if you know nothing about the word, have never seen it before, don't recognize any prefixes or roots, and can't think of any word in any language that it sounds like, you can still take an educated guess by trying to define the word's charge. Remember the discussion found earlier in the chapter about deciding if a word has a positive or negative charge? Well, on all synonym questions, the correct answer will have the same charge as the stem word, so use your instincts about word charge to help you when you're stuck on a tough word.

Not all words are positive or negative; some are neutral. But, if you can define the charge, you can probably eliminate some answer choices on that basis alone. Word charge is a great technique to use when answering antonym questions, too.

Ⓚ Ⓗ SPELLING LESSON

Spelling is a difficult skill to teach. We'll start by reviewing two types of questions you may face on Test Day. Then, you'll see a list of the most commonly misspelled words, as well as a list of words that are often confused for one another or used interchangeably. Use these lists as well as the spelling rules found in this lesson to improve your spelling skills. (*See* Part Seven: Learning Resources for frequently misspelled words and words commonly confused for one another.)

Two Types of Spelling Questions

There are essentially two types of spelling questions on your nursing school entrance exam. The first type is a multiple-choice question that gives you a list of four words. Only one of the words is spelled incorrectly; to answer the question correctly, you will have to choose the word that is misspelled.

Here's an example:

- (A) Regret
- (B) Unpleasent
- (C) Solemn
- (D) Cautious

In this case, the correct answer is (B). The correct spelling is *unpleasant*.

The other type is also a multiple-choice question. However, instead of giving you a list of just four words, you are provided four sentences, and one of the sentences contains a misspelled or misused word. This question type can be tricky. Take a look at the following example to find out why.

- (A) I was genuinely surprised to hear the good news.
- (B) The girl was upset when she was asked to meet with the principle of the school.
- (C) My favorite cuisine is Mexican food.
- (D) Growing up, my brother was extremely timid and shy.

The correct answer is (B). You may say to yourself that every word is spelled correctly, which is partially true. In this case, the word *principle* is spelled correctly. However, it is the wrong word for the sentence. The head of a school is a *principal*, so (B) contains the misspelled word.

(K) (H) SPELLING STRATEGIES

Although there aren't any steps for answering spelling questions, there are six rules you can memorize, along with the lists found in Part Seven. Sounding things out may help, or it may not, especially if you are not certain of the word's pronunciation.

Rule 1: *i* before *e*, except after *c*, and except when it sounds like *a* as in *neighbor* and *weigh*.

> Example: *Receive, transient, feign*

Rule 2: When a word of more than one syllable ends in a single vowel and a single consonant, the word's emphasis is usually on the final syllable; to add a suffix that begins with a vowel, the consonant preceding should be doubled.

> Example: *Occur, occurring*
> *Prefer, preferred*

Rule 3: If the final syllable has no accent, do not double the consonant.

> Example: *Benefit + -ing = Benefiting*

Rule 4: If a word ends with a silent *e*, drop the *e* before adding a suffix that begins with a vowel.

> Example: *Hope, hoping*
> *Like, liking*

Rule 5: Do not drop the *e* when the suffix begins with a consonant.

> Example: *Manage, management*
> *Like, likeness*
> *Use, useless*

Rule 6: When *y* is the last letter in a word and the *y* is preceded by a consonant, change the *y* to *i* before adding any suffix other than those beginning with *i*.

> Example: *Pretty, prettier*
> *Hurry, hurried*
> *Deny, denied*

Spelling is one area where knowing your own strengths and weaknesses is important. If you tend to have trouble spelling, you may decide to go against your instinct when selecting an answer choice. In other words, if a word looks right to you, but you know you are a terrible speller, you may guess that the word is actually spelled incorrectly. Vice versa, if a word sounds wrong to you, but you admit you're not sure of its pronunciation, you may decide that word is actually correct. Finally, if you are not certain whether or not a word is spelled correctly, take your best guess and move on.

Ⓚ Ⓗ GRAMMAR LESSON AND STRATEGIES

Just thinking about the rules of grammar can be enough to send some test takers into panic mode. But here's some good news: You're probably better at grammar than you think. After spending many years reading, we've all developed a keen sense of what looks correct on the page. However, even if you can tell when something is wrong, you might not be able to explain *why*, and you might not know the technical terms grammarians use to describe certain parts of speech. Fortunately, the grammar questions you encounter on your nursing exam will deal mainly with relatively common errors and terms that we will review in this section.

Note for Kaplan exam test takers: Grammar-related questions are covered under the Writing section of your test.

Parts of the Sentence

A noun, as you know, is a person, place, thing, or idea. A noun that is the focus of a sentence is known as the subject of the sentence. In the sentence "John walked his dog," "John" is clearly the focus, because he is the one doing something. "John" is the subject. The rest of the sentence, "walked his dog," is known as the **predicate** of the sentence, and it includes all the action performed by the subject. But "dog" is a noun too, right? Yes. But "dog" is not the subject of the sentence; "dog" is a **direct object**, or the thing directly affected by the **verb** of the sentence: "walked."

Let's look at a slightly different sentence: "John gave his dog a bone." Almost everything is the same as in the previous sentence: "John" is the subject; he performs an action in the predicate ("gave"); and his "dog" is there again, too. However, notice that "dog" does not relate directly to the verb "gave." Did John give his dog to someone? No . . . he gave something ("bone") *to* his dog. So in this case, "bone" is the direct object, and "dog" is the **indirect object**. One easy way to spot indirect objects is to look for the words *to* or *for* before the object. Sometimes, as in the sentence above, you won't see the word *to*; however, you could rewrite the sentence with the word *to* so that the meaning is the same, and the indirect object becomes clearer: "John gave a bone to his dog."

Personal pronouns are easy to spot, because there are only a handful to remember:

Subject Pronoun	Object Pronoun
I	Me
He	Him
She	Her
They	Them
We	Us
You	You
It	It
Who	Whom

Pronouns take the place of nouns or of groups of words acting together as a noun. Here's the most important thing about pronouns: You have to know *what noun is being replaced* by the pronoun. Look at this pair of sentences:

Jack woke up at 7 a.m. He walked his dog.

Because the first sentence is about Jack, you know that "he" in the second sentence is standing in as a replacement for "Jack." The noun that a pronoun replaces is called the **antecedent**. In this case, "Jack" is the antecedent of "he." Here's why it's important to know the antecedent for a pronoun: You have to make sure you've chosen the right pronoun for the job. If Jack is male, the pronoun *she* would not be the correct replacement. Assuming Jack is just one person, the pronoun *they* would also be incorrect.

In the preceding table, you can also see that the pronouns in the left column are related to those in the right column. The pronouns on the left are known as *subject pronouns*, because they take the place of nouns being used in the subject position of a sentence. The pronouns on the right are *object pronouns*, because they replace nouns being used as objects in the sentence. The bottom two pronouns, *you* and *it*, can be used as either subject or object pronouns.

Possessive pronouns and possessive determiners show the "owner" of an object—in other words, what or whom something belongs to. While pronouns take the place of a noun, determiners appear before a noun to show possession. In the sentence "Jack walked his dog," the possessive determiner "his" tells us that the dog belongs to Jack. Here are the most important possessive determiners and pronouns you need to know:

Possessive Determiner	Possessive Pronoun
My	Mine
His	His
Her	Hers
Their	Theirs
Our	Ours
Your	Yours
Its	Its

Even though these words show possession, notice that they do not require apostrophes. *This is important,* because it's one of the most common types of errors to appear in grammar testing. Remember: The word *its* always means "belonging to it," while *it's* always means "it is."

Adjectives are simply words that modify nouns or pronouns. They provide a better description of the thing in question, and they generally appear right before the thing they modify. Here's where it can get confusing: Some words are only adjectives, like *big* or *soft*, but there are lots of other kinds of words—including verbs and nouns—that can also act as adjectives. One of the trickiest, and therefore important to remember for grammar tests, is the **participle**. A participle is a verb form, usually ending in *-ing* or *-ed*, that is used to modify a noun. Here are some examples: "*working* lunch," "*wrecked* car," "*traveling* companion."

You probably already know that **adverbs** are words or phrases that modify verbs. You might also remember that words ending in -*ly* are generally adverbs, such as *quickly* or *skillfully*. But keep in mind that adverbs can also modify adjectives ("*very* ugly sweater") or even other adverbs ("performed *quite* poorly on the test").

Prepositions indicate relationships—usually relationships of location or time. Words like *under, between, by,* and *throughout* are prepositions. Prepositions often appear in prepositional phrases, which include an object of the preposition as well: *under the water; behind the fence; at home.* These phrases function like adjectives or adverbs. The object of the preposition cannot also be the subject of the sentence.

Conjunctions are used to connect words, phrases, and clauses. The most common conjunctions are *and, or, but,* and *so.* These are called **coordinating conjunctions**. It's also important to remember the two sets of **correlative conjunctions**: *either/or* and *neither/nor.* When used as conjunctions, these always occur in pairs: *Either* is always followed later in the sentence by *or,* and *neither* is always followed by *nor.*

Two final terms that might sound confusing, but are actually quite simple, are **predicate adjective** and **predicate nominative**. The word *predicate* tells you right away where these are found in the sentence. A predicate adjective is simply an adjective that describes the subject, but is found after a linking verb. Here is an example: *Harriet was **sleepy**.* Similarly, a predicate nominative provides a new "name" for the subject, often by providing a position, title, or relationship. For example: *Harriet was a **professor**. That man by the cashier is my **father**.*

Sentence Types

Remember that there are four different types of sentences. You might encounter a question that uses the names for these sentence types. They are:

Declarative. This is the most common sentence type. Declarative sentences present information in a straightforward manner.

> Example: *Jack cleaned up the kitchen.*

Interrogative. This type of sentence asks a question and therefore ends with a question mark. Interrogative sentences often begin with words associated with questions, such as *who, what,* or *where,* but they can also begin with verbs, such as *did* or *have.*

> Examples: *Who cleaned up the kitchen?*
> *Have they cleaned up the kitchen yet?*

Exclamatory. These are sentences that express sudden emotion. They end with an exclamation mark. Sometimes exclamatory sentences begin with *what, how,* or other words often used in questions—just like interrogative sentences. In these cases, you will need to determine whether the sentence is expressing sudden emotion (exclamatory) or asking a question (interrogative).

> Example: *What a clean kitchen this is!*

Imperative. These sentences are perhaps the trickiest, because they often do not appear to be complete sentences. Imperative sentences are commands or requests, and the subject generally is an implied word: *you.*

Example:　*Please clean the kitchen.*

Common Errors

Incorrect Verb Forms

One of the most common grammatical errors you are likely to encounter is the use of incorrect verb forms. Because some nonstandard verb forms have been accepted in various dialects and informal speech, these incorrect verb forms might even sound correct to you. Here are some examples of commonly used—but incorrect—verb forms, along with correct usage.

Incorrect:　I *been* watching that show since I was little.
Correct:　I *have been* watching that show since I was little.

Incorrect:　She *seen* her friends down at the pool.
Correct:　She *saw* her friends down at the pool.

Incorrect:　They *was* on the opposite side of the street from the accident.
Correct:　They *were* on the opposite side of the street from the accident.

Incorrect:　He *done* a great job cleaning out the garage.
Correct:　He *did* a great job cleaning out the garage.

Subject-Verb Agreement

One type of error you are very likely to encounter on a nursing exam is an error of agreement between the subject and verb of a sentence. Put simply, singular subjects require singular verb forms, and plural subjects require plural verb forms. It sounds simple—and most of the time, it *is* simple. Here are two examples:

Reyna has a degree in accounting.
　　(Reyna is a single person, so the singular verb *has* is used.)

The three interns have degrees in art.
　　(The three interns form a plural subject, so the plural verb *have* is used.)

Sometimes, however, another noun might get in the way and make things confusing. Look at this example:

The guy with three parrots was hanging out in the quad.

Three parrots appears immediately before the verb, but the three parrots are not the subject of the sentence—*the guy* is the subject. Therefore, the verb must be singular.

How about a situation where a single noun refers to a group of people? Words like these, such as *team, committee,* or *family,* are known as collective nouns. Even though a committee could have 30 members, it is still only one committee, and it therefore requires a singular verb.

Example:　*The 15-member crew has a competition next week.*

Some sentences have compound subjects. If the subjects are connected by the word *and*, then they require a plural verb, even if both subjects are singular.

> Example: *Paul and Laura are going to the party.*

If two or more singular subjects are connected by words like *nor* or *or*, the verb should be singular.

> Example: *Neither Patsy nor Sam is working tonight.*

In cases where one subject is singular and one subject is plural, and the subjects are connected by *nor* or *or*, match the verb to the nearer of the subjects.

> Example: *Either the honor students or the swim team is going to receive the extra fundraising cash.*

Pronoun Usage

Just as a verb must agree with the subject of a sentence, a pronoun must agree with the noun that it replaces. Also, pronouns can replace nouns other than the subject. A singular noun must be replaced with a singular pronoun, while a plural noun requires a plural pronoun. Review the pronoun tables shown earlier in this chapter under "Parts of the Sentence," and remember: Subject pronouns are used to replace the subject in a sentence or clause, and object pronouns are used in the predicate of a sentence or clause. Using this knowledge about pronouns, identify which of the two sentences below is correct:

> *Her and Jaime went to the cafeteria together.*
> *She and Jaime went to the cafeteria together.*

The pronoun in question is either *her* or *she*. Because the pronoun in this example serves as part of the subject of the sentence, a subject pronoun must be used. Therefore, the correct sentence is the second sentence.

Who/Whom

This distinction is a tricky one for many people. In spoken speech, *whom* rarely makes an appearance, and when it does, it's sometimes used incorrectly by people attempting to sound "correct." *Who* and *whom* are actually pronouns, and they are used mainly (though not always) to form questions; like other pairs of pronouns, one is considered a subject pronoun (*who*) and one is considered an object pronoun (*whom*). One simple rule can help you remember when to use *whom*: If you can replace the word in question with *him*, *her*, *we*, *them*, or *us* in the sentence or clause, use *whom*. Try applying this rule to the sentence below:

> *(Who/Whom) do you believe regarding the car accident?*

Think about how you would answer this question. Would you respond by saying "I believe her" or "I believe she"? "I believe her" is the correct response, which means *whom* is the correct pronoun to use in the sentence.

That/Which

This is another tricky distinction, since spoken speech is often structured differently from written speech and this problem arises less often. Both *that* and *which* are used to introduce clauses. Here's the key difference: *That* is used to introduce restrictive clauses, while *which* is used to introduce nonrestrictive clauses. What does this mean? *That* is used when the clause is an essential part of the sentence, and *which* is used when the clause is not essential to the meaning of the sentence. Here are some examples:

> The sedan *that* was parked in the driveway belonged to Nancy. (The clause "that was parked in the driveway" is essential, because it specifies which sedan is being discussed.)

> The sedan, *which* was metallic green, was parked in the driveway. (The clause "which was metallic green" is not essential; it merely provides additional information about the sedan. If you removed the clause from the sentence, the meaning of the sentence would not be altered.)

If you're having trouble recognizing restrictive versus nonrestrictive clauses, here's another method that works quite well: If the clause is set off from the rest of the sentence with commas, use *which*. If the clause is not set off from the rest of the sentence with commas, use *that*.

i.e. or e.g.?

The abbreviations i.e. and e.g. are common in written text, particularly in technical material, so it's important to understand the difference between the two. Here's an easy way to distinguish between them: *i.e.* can be replaced by the phrase "in other words," while *e.g.* can be replaced by "for example." If you are unsure which abbreviation to use, try inserting one of these two phrases instead, and the answer should become clear. Here are some examples:

> *There are many good reasons for the current lunch policy (e.g., safety, convenience, etc.).*
> *The voter registration form was mailed without a completed signature—i.e., it was invalid.*

Note that when either *i.e.* or *e.g.* is used, it must be followed by a comma, as shown in the preceding examples.

Between/Among

Both *between* and *among* are prepositions that cover similar ground. Both can be used to express location, choice, or distribution. *Between* is used with two things, while *among* is used with three or more things. The key here is that *between* is used when referring to separate and distinct things, while *among* refers to things without clear distinction or separation because they make up a group. Here are some examples:

> *The choice between a station wagon and a sport utility vehicle can be a difficult one.*
> *She had to choose from among the available options.*
> *The cat was hiding among the shrubs and trees.*

Note that in the third example, *shrubs* and *trees* are not separate and distinct things—they are groups of things.

Comma Usage

When it comes to punctuation, the comma is perhaps the most misused mark of all. This is not surprising, since commas are useful in so many different situations and are governed by so many specific rules. Here are a few of the most important rules to remember regarding comma usage.

Use a comma:

- Before a coordinating conjunction when connecting two independent clauses.

    Example: *I like to fish, and I like to spend time on the water.*

- Between items in a series when there are more than two items.

    Example: *She bought balloons, candles, streamers, and a cake.*

- Before and after a nonrestrictive clause.
  (Sometimes, parentheses or dashes can be used instead.)

    Example: *The mayor, who was a big fan of Winston Churchill, decided that the statue should remain.*

- Between two or more adjectives used with the same noun.

    Example: *The fearsome, hairy beast lunged toward them.*

Do not use a comma:

- Between two complete sentences without a coordinating conjunction. If there is no coordinating conjunction, the sentences should be separated by a period.

    Incorrect: *I went to the grocery store across town, my favorite yogurt was not in stock.*
    Correct: *I went to the grocery store across town. My favorite yogurt was not in stock.*

- Between the final adjective and noun when two or more adjectives modify the same noun.

    Incorrect: *The steaming, wheezing, machine sputtered along the track.*
    Correct: *The steaming, wheezing machine sputtered along the track.*

Style Issues

The HESI exam also covers a handful of style issues that should be avoided by writers. If you're taking the HESI exam, you might encounter questions that ask about examples of these style issues. These are the particular writing style issues that should be avoided:

Clichés. Clichés are informal, overused expressions that most native speakers understand but that lack precision and may prove confusing to nonnative speakers. Some examples include "his bark was worse than his bite" and "I slept like a log." Although clichés are colorful, in standard speech and writing they should be eliminated in favor of clearer and more precise terms.

Euphemisms. Euphemisms are words or expressions meant to stand in for other terms that might be considered vulgar, upsetting, or offensive. For example, the phrase *passed away* is used in place of the word *died*. In most cases, euphemisms should be avoided because they can be ambiguous and lack the precision of the terms they replace.

Profanity. Profanity and insults should always be avoided in professional communication, except in rare instances where you might be required to transcribe the exact words that a person used (such as in an incident report).

Sexist language. Sexist language generally shows gender bias through word choice. For example, if the head of a committee is called the *chairman*, it is assumed that the position can only be held by an adult male. Similarly, if a term such as *garbage man* is used to refer to a hypothetical garbage collector, rather than an actual, specific person who is male, then the language is sexist. Avoid using gender-specific terms whenever possible, and mention gender only when the information is necessary.

Textspeak. *Textspeak*, or conversational use of terms that arise in the context of text messaging, has become far more common in everyday language with the rise of smartphones. For the exam, remember that many terms that might be acceptable in text messages, including acronyms such as *OMG* or *BRB*, remain unacceptable in professional communication.

Now that you have read the lessons and strategies for Vocabulary, Spelling, and Grammar, test how much you learned by answering the following review questions.

REVIEW QUESTIONS

The following questions are not meant to mimic actual test questions. Instead, these questions will help you review the concepts and terms covered in this chapter.

1. True or False? Determining a word's charge is an effective strategy for spelling questions.

2. Synonym questions test your knowledge of words with:

   (A) Similar meanings.
   (B) Opposite meanings.
   (C) Similar spellings.
   (D) Alternative spellings.

3. *Tacit* most nearly means:

   (A) Official.
   (B) Tactile.
   (C) Unstated.
   (D) Charming.

4. True or False? In spelling, if the final syllable has no accent, you do not double the consonant when adding the suffix *-ing*.

5. Fill in the blank. The rule is: *i* before *e*, except after *c*, _____.

6. True or False? To figure out a word's charge to answer antonym questions, you should always look for an answer choice that has the same charge as the question.

7. *Ghastly* most nearly means:

   (A) Fun.
   (B) Lazy.
   (C) Torrid.
   (D) Awful.

8. *Acute* means the opposite of:

   (A) Conspicuous.
   (B) Relevant.
   (C) Aloof.
   (D) Dull.

9. *Malicious* means the opposite of:

   (A) Hurtful.
   (B) Mild.
   (C) Refined.
   (D) Benevolent.

10. Choose the word that is misspelled:

    (A) Regulation.
    (B) Catergory.
    (C) Conflagration.
    (D) Incident.

REVIEW ANSWERS

1. False. You should determine a word's charge (deciding whether a word is positive, negative, or neutral) in order to find a synonym or antonym of a word.

2. **A** Synonyms test your knowledge of words with similar meanings.

3. **C** *Tacit* most nearly means "unstated."

4. True. For example, *benefit* becomes *benefiting*.

5. The rule is: *i* before *e*, except after *c*, except when it sounds like *a* as in *neighbor* and *weigh*.

6. False. Because you are looking for the opposite of the word in the question, you should look for a word with an opposite word charge among the answer choices.

7. **D** *Ghastly* most nearly means "awful."

8. **D** *Dull* is the opposite of *acute*.

9. **D** *Malicious* is the opposite of *benevolent*.

10. **B** The correct spelling is *category*.

Chapter Five: **Writing Review**

The Kaplan Nursing Admission Test contains a section labeled Writing. Although you are not required to do any writing for it, this section assesses your ability to understand and apply the basic mechanics of writing. Skill areas include how to organize and develop a written passage, the best way to structure a paragraph, and how to correct basic mistakes involving writing mechanics. Some of the questions in the Writing section may address spelling and grammar issues; these topics are reviewed in Chapter Four: Vocabulary, Spelling, and Grammar Review, and are not covered here.

(K) ASSESSING PASSAGE DEVELOPMENT

The key to understanding passage development is understanding *what kind* of passage you are looking at. Being able to identify the type of writing used for a specific passage can tell you a great deal about how a passage is structured. There are four basic types of writing you are likely to see in reading passages:

1. Expository
2. Descriptive
3. Persuasive
4. Narrative

Expository writing is intended to inform the reader. A great variety of information can be imparted in expository writing—anything from explaining how photosynthesis works to detailing a dress code policy. Most of the passages that you will encounter on your nursing entrance exam are likely to be expository writing.

Descriptive writing is intended to give a detailed look at a specific topic. Such a passage typically includes many sensory details, since those help the author to paint a mental picture for the reader. Indeed, the purpose of descriptive writing is to create a detailed image or idea in the mind of the reader.

Persuasive writing is intended to express a viewpoint on a topic. In persuasive writing, the author's purpose is to persuade the reader to adopt a certain position regarding a topic.

Persuasive writing uses arguments to support a particular point of view or to refute an opposing point of view, often accompanied by statistics, reasoning, and appeals to emotion. When you read a piece of persuasive writing, it should be clear from the passage exactly how the writer feels about the topic in question.

Narrative writing is intended to tell a story. While it can include elements of other types of writing, its main purpose is to carry the reader on a journey. Narrative writing is normally organized along chronological lines, with each new paragraph telling the reader what happens next. Narrative writing includes fiction and also nonfiction biographies.

(K) ASSESSING PARAGRAPH STRUCTURE AND LOGIC

Every reading passage has multiple levels of structure. The passage as a whole is organized in a certain way to support its purpose (to inform, to create a mental image, to persuade, or to tell a story). In addition, each paragraph is structured to support its main idea. If you have read Chapter Three: Reading Comprehension Review, you already know to look for main ideas in paragraphs and in passages as a whole. Further clues to the purpose of each paragraph in a passage are the five basic text structures:

1. Cause and effect
2. Compare/contrast
3. Description
4. Order/sequencing
5. Problem-solution

As you will see, there is some overlap between the four writing types and the five basic text structures, and some text structures are more common in certain kinds of writing. Let's review each of the structures and their applications.

The cause-and-effect structure draws connections between a situation or event and one or more things that helped bring about that situation or event. Sometimes, the paragraph might be structured like a mystery, introducing the effect first and only later revealing the cause. The cause-and-effect structure is most commonly found in expository writing.

The compare/contrast structure presents the similarities and/or differences between two or more things, people, ideas, etc. The compare/contrast structure is common in expository writing, but you might find it in the other forms of writing as well.

The description text structure, as you might expect, is used to present a detailed description of a topic in order to paint a mental picture for the reader. This structure is most common in descriptive writing, but it can be found often in narrative writing.

The order/sequencing structure is used to present information in chronological or step-by-step order. It can be used to describe a process, as in expository writing, or to simply relate events, as in narrative writing.

The problem-solution structure presents a challenge, problem, or question, and then offers a solution. Sometimes, the author might evaluate several possible solutions. The problem-solution structure is a key element in a great deal of persuasive writing, though it also appears in expository writing.

Now it's time to apply these tools to identify the structure of a sample passage. Read the paragraph below and answer the question that follows.

> Both alligators and crocodiles can be found in southern Florida, particularly in the Everglades National Park. Alligators and crocodiles do look similar but there are several physical characteristics that differentiate the two giant reptiles. The most easily observed difference between alligators and crocodiles is the shape of the head. A crocodile's skull and jaws are longer and narrower than an alligator's. When an alligator closes its mouth, its long teeth slip into sockets in the upper jaw and disappear. When a crocodile closes its mouth, its long teeth remain visible, protruding outside the upper jaw. In general, if you can still see a lot of teeth even when the animal's mouth is closed, you are looking at a crocodile.
>
> What type of text structure is used in this paragraph?
>
> (A) Cause and effect
> (B) Compare/contrast
> (C) Order/sequencing
> (D) Problem-solution

The paragraph focuses on how to tell the difference between a crocodile and an alligator. In other words, the paragraph *compares and contrasts* the physical appearance of the two animals. Choice (B) is correct.

Ⓚ "FIXING" READING PASSAGES

In this section of the test, many of the questions will focus on the best way to "fix" or improve a passage in some way. All sentences and sentence parts in the passages will be marked by a number, and the questions will refer to those numbers. Some of these questions will relate to grammar, spelling, and punctuation, as covered in Chapter Four: Vocabulary, Spelling, and Grammar Review. Others will ask you to rearrange or edit existing passages to improve their structure, for instance, by selecting the best location to add a sentence or by choosing a sentence to remove because it is unnecessary. The correct answer choice will maintain the passage's structure and purpose.

Take a look at the paragraph below and answer the question that follows.

> [1]Ecology—the study of the relationships among organisms, and between organisms and their environment—is a relatively new branch of science. [2]The name itself was coined by a German biologist, Ernst Haeckel, in 1866. [3]Haeckel postulated the living world is a community where each species has a distinctive role to play. [4]Haeckel had another major theory that was widely

accepted at the time, but has since lost support from the scientific community. [5]One of the major focuses of ecological study today is fieldwork analyzing relationships within an ecosystem, or a collection of communities, such as a tropical rainforest or a coral reef. [6]The results of such studies have provided conservationists and wildlife managers with important new insights, though many questions remain unanswered.

Which sentence provides unnecessary or irrelevant information and should be removed?

(A)   Sentence 2

(B)   Sentence 3

(C)   Sentence 4

(D)   Sentence 6

Looking at the paragraph, you can see that it gives information about the meaning, history, and modern-day focus of a certain topic (ecology). As discussed earlier, writing that primarily imparts information is expository writing—and indeed, this passage is a piece of expository writing about ecology and its origins. Therefore, any sentence that is not about ecology and its origins is irrelevant. The only sentence that is not about ecology or its origins is sentence 4, which mentions another theory put forth by the biologist Ernst Haeckel. This sentence is irrelevant and should be removed; therefore, choice (C) is the correct answer.

Now that you have read the lessons and strategies for the Writing section, see how much you have learned by answering the following review questions.

REVIEW QUESTIONS

Questions 1–2 are based on the following passage.

[1]Most people think the Hula-Hoop was a fad born in the 1950s, but in fact people were doing much the same thing with circular hoops made from grapevines and stiff grasses all over the ancient world. [2]More than 3,000 years ago, children in Egypt played with large hoops of dried grapevines. [3]The toy was propelled along the ground with a stick or swung around at the waist. [4]The word *hula* became associated with the toy in the early 1800s when British sailors visited the Hawaiian Islands and noted the similarity between hooping and hula dancing. [5]In 1957, an Australian company began making wood rings for sale in retail stores. [6]The item attracted the attention of Wham-O, a fledgling California toy manufacturer. [7]The plastic Hula-Hoop was introduced in 1958 and was an instant hit.

1. Where should the following sentence be added?

    During the fourteenth century, a "hooping" craze swept England and was as popular among adults as kids.

    (A) After sentence 2.
    (B) After sentence 3.
    (C) After sentence 4.
    (D) After sentence 5.

2. Which of the following best describes how the information in the paragraph is presented?

    (A) In order of importance.
    (B) By geographic region.
    (C) In chronological order.
    (D) By comparing and contrasting.

Questions 3–4 are based on the following passage.

[1]Migration of animal populations from one region to another is called faunal interchange. [2]Concentrations of species across regional boundaries vary, however, prompting zoologists to classify routes along which penetrations of new regions occur. [3]A corridor, like the vast stretch of land from Alaska to the southeastern United States, is equivalent to a path of least resistance. [4]Relative ease of migration often results in the presence of related species along the entire length of a corridor; bear populations, unknown in South America, occur throughout the North American corridor. [5]However, fossils show that bears were present in South America hundreds of thousands of years ago. [6]A desert or other barrier creates a filter route, allowing only a segment of a faunal group to pass. [7]A sweepstakes route presents so formidable a barrier that penetration is unlikely. [8]It differs from other routes, which may be crossed by species with sufficient adaptive capability. [9]As the name suggests, negotiation of a sweepstakes route depends almost exclusively on chance, rather than on physical attributes and adaptability.

3. Which sentence contains unnecessary or irrelevant information and should be removed?

    (A) Sentence 2.
    (B) Sentence 4.
    (C) Sentence 5.
    (D) Sentence 8.

4. What is the main purpose of this passage?

    (A) To inform.
    (B) To persuade.
    (C) To entertain.
    (D) To describe.

Questions 5–6 are based on the following passage.

[1]A pioneering figure in modern sociology, French social theorist Emile Durkheim examined the role of societal cohesion on emotional well-being. [2]Believing scientific methods should be applied to the study of society, Durkheim studied the level of integration of various social formations and the impact that such cohesion had on individuals within a group. [3]He postulated that social groups with high levels of integration serve to buffer their members from frustrations and tragedies that could otherwise lead to desperation and self-destruction. [4]Integration, in Durkheim's view, generally arises through shared activities and values.

[5]Durkheim distinguished between *mechanical solidarity* and *organic solidarity* in classifying integrated groups. [6]Mechanical solidarity dominates in groups in which individual differences are minimized and group devotion to a common aim is high. [7]Durkheim identified mechanical solidarity among groups with little division of labor and high rates of cultural similarity, such as among traditional and geographically isolated groups. [8]Organic solidarity, in contrast, prevails in groups with high levels of individual differences, such as those with a highly specialized division of labor. [9]In such groups, individual differences are a powerful source of connection, rather than of division. [10]Because people engage in highly differentiated ways of life, they are by necessity interdependent. [11]In these societies, there is greater freedom from some external controls, but such freedom occurs in concert with the interdependence of individuals, not in conflict with it.

[12]Durkheim realized societies may take many forms and consequently that group allegiance can manifest itself in a variety of ways. [13]I myself have witnessed this in my own life experiences. [14]In both types of societies outlined above, however, Durkheim stressed that adherence to a common set of assumptions about the world was a necessary prerequisite for maintaining group integrity and avoiding social decay.

5. Which sentence contains unnecessary or irrelevant information and should be removed?

    (A) Sentence 2.

    (B) Sentence 6.

    (C) Sentence 9.

    (D) Sentence 13.

6. What is the main function of the second paragraph?

    (A) To explain Durkheim's theories of societal integration.

    (B) To compare and contrast mechanical solidarity and organic solidarity.

    (C) To argue that Durkheim's theories are scientifically significant.

    (D) To present the problem of societal integration and offer a solution.

Questions 7–10 are based on the following passage.

[1]It is possible to date a book by examining the paper it is printed on. [2]After the mid-nineteenth century, machine-made paper, constructed from wood pulp instead of rags, became the standard material for publishers.

[3]Machine-made paper is more acidic and more brittle than hand-made paper. Particularly brittle paper may provide clues to the date of publication. [4]Paper made during specific eras may be more brittle and fragile than paper made during the years immediately before and after. [5]For example, paper made in the United States during World War II—when conservation efforts impacted paper production—has discolored to a shade of dark yellow-brown and is so brittle it must be handled very gingerly to prevent cracking. [6]Books were first stored horizontally with their front covers facing up, then vertically with the fore-edge facing out, before the now-familiar spine-out arrangement became common.

[7]The amount and type of chemicals applied to the paper help establish its manufacture date. [8]Handmade and early machine-made paper was treated before it was printed so its fibers would not absorb the ink. [9]This treatment, called sizing, was made from gelatin and was used to render the surface ready to be printed. [10]Freshly made paper was dipped in a vat of sizing for centuries, until German papermakers found that adding alum and rosin to the raw mixture of fibers yielded paper that was sufficiently resistant to ink. [11]Other chemical treatments that may be applied to paper include bleaching and coating for illustration.

7. Where should the following sentence be added?

   Beginning in the fourteenth century, paper was made by hand from undyed linen or hemp rags.

   (A) Before sentence 2.
   (B) Before sentence 6.
   (C) Before sentence 9.
   (D) Before sentence 11.

8. What is the main function of the third paragraph?

   (A) To compare and contrast different types of sizing.
   (B) To describe how the presence of chemicals can help date paper.
   (C) To show a cause-and-effect relationship between paper's content and brittleness.
   (D) To present a problem associated with paper and present a solution to that problem.

9. Which sentence contains unnecessary or irrelevant information and should be removed?

   (A) Sentence 2.
   (B) Sentence 6.
   (C) Sentence 9.
   (D) Sentence 11.

10. What is the main purpose of this passage?

    (A) To entertain.
    (B) To describe.
    (C) To inform.
    (D) To persuade.

REVIEW ANSWERS

1. **B**   Looking at the paragraph, you can see that the details are arranged chronologically, beginning with the oldest and ending with the most recent. This makes it easy to figure out where the new sentence should be placed: Between the information on ancient Egypt and the information about British sailors in the 1800s. However, sentence 3 must directly follow sentence 2 to maintain a logical structure. This means that the new sentence must be placed after sentence 3.

2. **C**   The details included in the paragraph are presented in chronological order, beginning with the oldest events and ending with the most recent. The use of dates in many of the sentences is a good indicator that you are looking at something arranged by time.

3. **C**   The paragraph describes several routes along which animals migrate; most of the sentences address this topic. The sentence about bears living in South America in prehistoric times does not relate to the repeated idea of migration routes, so it is unnecessary and should be removed.

4. **A**   This paragraph contains a variety of detailed information about migration routes, which suggests that its purpose is to inform. Expository writing is meant to inform, and you already know that expository writing passages are the most common type. To confirm the hypothesis that this is an expository passage, consider the other possible purposes of the passage one by one. The paragraph does not seem to be aimed at persuading (B) or entertaining (C) the reader. While the information in the paragraph might be considered descriptive in a general sense, it does not include sensory details that would paint a mental picture for the reader (D).

5. **D**   This question is a little tricky. Although personal observation and opinion might be appropriate and relevant in some reading passages, sentence 13 does not fit with the rest of the passage and its neutral, informational tone; therefore, it is unnecessary and should be removed. Statements of personal opinion are commonly found in persuasive writing and even narrative writing, but are usually avoided in expository passages such as this one.

6. **B**   To determine the function of the second paragraph, take a look at the details that it presents. The paragraph describes both mechanical solidarity and organic solidarity, and it identifies their differences. The paragraph even uses the phrase "in contrast," which is a great clue that you are reading a compare/contrast text structure. Although the paragraph does explain some of Durkheim's theories of societal integration (A), this answer option applies more broadly to the passage as a whole, not specifically to the second paragraph. This passage is neutral and informational, not argumentative or persuasive (C). The passage does not present social integration as a problem (D).

7. **A**   The passage begins by introducing the possibility that paper can be used to determine the age of a book. The second sentence describes paper-making since the mid-nineteenth century. Because the new sentence refers to a time period prior to this (the fourteenth century), it should be inserted before sentence 2.

8. **B** The third paragraph discusses chemical processes used in paper production over time, and the first sentence describes the paragraph's thesis: Chemicals found in the paper can be used to estimate its manufacture date. Although the paragraph mentions different types of sizing, it does not compare or contrast them (A), nor does it show a cause-and-effect relationship between content and brittleness (C); brittleness is discussed in paragraph 2. The passage likewise does not present a problem and solution associated with paper (D).

9. **B** This passage is concerned with paper and its manufacture. Although sentence 6 also addresses customs associated with books over time, it is concerned with changes in the way books are shelved rather than the makeup of their paper, so it is not relevant to the rest of the passage.

10. **C** Although this passage describes some of its topics (such as yellow-brown pages that crack upon handling), it does not principally provide a sensory experience for the reader. It principally focuses on details of paper history and manufacture. This passage is intended to inform.

PART FOUR

Mathematics Review

Chapter Six: **Mathematics Review**

Mathematics is likely to be the longest section on your nursing school entrance exam. It also happens to be the subject most test takers feel is their weakest. This chapter offers a review of mathematics, from the most fundamental operations of addition and subtraction through the types of basic algebra and geometry you are likely to encounter on Test Day. You will also find strategies for answering math questions, as well as questions to reinforce principles you have reviewed. Don't forget to check out the "Math in a Nutshell" study aid in Part Seven: Learning Resources.

K H ARITHMETIC

The math skills tested on your nursing school entrance exam include basic computation, using integers, fractions, decimals, and percentages. You need to have a firm grasp of arithmetic concepts such as number properties, factors, divisibility, units of measure, ratio and proportion, percentages, and averages. These skills may be tested in basic operations or in word problems. Even if you feel that you know them, spend time on this section. The more you practice, the more comfortable you will feel working with numbers on your test.

First, take a look at a few definitions.

Number Type	Definition	Examples
Real Numbers	*Any number that can name a position on a number line, regardless of whether that position is negative, positive, or zero.*	-75% $.5$ $\frac{3}{4}$ $-5\ -4\ -3\ -2\ -1\ \ 0\ \ 1\ \ 2\ \ 3\ \ 4\ \ 5$
Rational Numbers	*Any number that can be written as a ratio of two integers, including integers, terminating decimals, and repeating decimals.*	$5 = \frac{5}{1}, 2 = \frac{2}{1}, 0 = \frac{0}{1}, -6 = -\frac{6}{1}$ $2\frac{50}{100}$, or $\frac{250}{100}$ $\frac{1}{3}$ (.33333)

Number Type	Definition	Examples
Integers	*Any of the positive counting numbers (which are also known as natural numbers), the negative numbers, and zero.*	Positive integers: 1, 2, 3… Negative integers: −1, −2, −3… Neither negative nor positive: zero
Fractions	*A **fraction** is a number that is written in the $\frac{A}{B}$ form where A is the numerator and B is the denominator. An **improper fraction** is a number that is greater than 1 (or less than −1) that is written in the form of a fraction. An improper fraction can be converted to a **mixed number**, which consists of an integer (positive or negative) and a fraction.*	$-\frac{5}{6}, \frac{3}{17}, \frac{1}{2}, \frac{899}{901}$ $-\frac{65}{64}, \frac{9}{8}, \frac{57}{10}$ $-1\frac{1}{64}, 1\frac{1}{8}, 5\frac{7}{10}$
Positive/Negative	*Numbers greater than zero are positive numbers; numbers less than zero are negative; zero is neither positive nor negative.*	Positive: 1, 5, 900 Negative: −64, −40, −11, $-\frac{6}{13}$
Even/Odd	*An even number is an integer that is a multiple of 2. NOTE: Zero is an even number. An odd number is an integer that is not a multiple of 2.*	Even numbers: −6, −2, zero, 4, 12, 190 Odd numbers: −15, −1, 3, 9, 453
Prime Numbers	*An integer greater than 1 that has no factors other than 1 and itself; 2 is the only even prime number.*	2, 3, 5, 7, 11, 13, 59, 83
Consecutive Numbers	*Numbers that follow one after another, in order, without any skipping.*	Consecutive integers: 3, 4, 5, 6 Consecutive even integers: 2, 4, 6, 8, 10 Consecutive multiples of 9: 9, 18, 27, 36
Factors	*A positive integer that divides evenly into a given number with no remainder.*	The complete list of factors of 12: 1, 2, 3, 4, 6, 12
Multiples	*A number that a given number will divide into with no remainder.*	Some multiples of 12: zero, 12, 24, 60

Odds and Evens

Even ± Even = Even $2 + 2 = 4$

Even ± Odd = Odd $2 + 3 = 5$

Odd ± Odd = Even $3 + 3 = 6$

Even × Even = Even $2 \times 2 = 4$

Even × Odd = Even $2 \times 3 = 6$

Odd × Odd = Odd $3 \times 3 = 9$

Positives and Negatives

There are a few things to remember about positives and negatives.

Adding a negative number is basically subtraction.

$6 + (-4)$ is really $6 - 4$, or 2.
$4 + (-6)$ is really $4 - 6$, or -2.

Subtracting a negative number is basically addition.

$6 - (-4)$ is really $6 + 4$, or 10.
$-6 - (-4)$ is really $-6 + 4$, or -2.

Multiplying and dividing positives and negatives is like all other multiplication and division, with one catch. To figure out whether your product is positive or negative, simply count the number of negatives you had to start. If you had an odd number of negatives, the product is negative. If you had an even number of negatives, the product is positive.

$6 \times (-4) = -24$ (1 negative → negative product)
$(-6) \times (-4) = 24$ (2 negatives → positive product)
$(-1) \times (-6) \times (-4) = -24$ (3 negatives → negative product)

Similarly,

$-24 \div 3 = -8$ (1 negative → negative quotient)
$-24 \div (-3) = 8$ (2 negatives → positive quotient)

Factors and Multiples

To find the prime factorization of a number, keep breaking it down until you are left with only prime numbers.

To find the prime factorization of 168:

$168 = 4 \times 42$
$= 4 \times 6 \times 7$
$= 2 \times 2 \times 2 \times 3 \times 7$

To find the greatest common factor (GCF) of two integers, break down both integers into their prime factorizations and multiply all prime factors they have in common. The greatest common factor is the largest factor that divides into each integer.

For example, if you're looking for the greatest common factor of 40 and 140, first identify the prime factors of each integer.

$40 = 4 \times 10$
$= 2 \times 2 \times 2 \times 5$

$$140 = 10 \times 14$$
$$= 2 \times 5 \times 2 \times 7$$
$$= 2 \times 2 \times 5 \times 7$$

Next, see what prime factors the two numbers have in common and then multiply these common factors.

Both integers share two 2s and one 5, so the GCF is $2 \times 2 \times 5$, or 20.

If you need to find a common multiple of two integers, you can always multiply them. However, you can use prime factors to find the least common multiple (LCM). To do this, multiply all of the prime factors of each integer as many times as they appear. Don't worry if this sounds confusing; it becomes pretty clear once it's demonstrated. Take a look at the example to see how it works.

To find a common multiple of 20 and 16:

$$20 \times 16 = 320$$

320 is a common multiple of 20 and 16, but it is not the *least* common multiple.

To find the least common multiple of 20 and 16, first find the prime factors of each integer:

$$20 = 2 \times 2 \times 5$$
$$16 = 2 \times 2 \times 2 \times 2$$

Now, multiply each prime integer the greatest number of times it appears in each integer:

$$2 \times 2 \times 2 \times 2 \times 5 = 80$$

The Order of Operations

You need to remember the order in which arithmetic operations must be performed. PEMDAS (or Please Excuse My Dear Aunt Sally) may help you remember the order.

Please = Parentheses

Excuse = Exponents

My Dear = Multiplication and Division (from left to right)

Aunt Sally = Addition and Subtraction (from left to right)

$$3^3 - 8(3 - 1) + 12 \div 4$$
$$= 3^3 - 8(2) + 12 \div 4$$
$$= 27 - 8(2) + 12 \div 4$$
$$= 27 - 16 + 3$$
$$= 11 + 3$$
$$= 14$$

Divisibility Rules

If you've forgotten—or never learned—divisibility rules, spend a little time with this chart. Even if you remember the rules, take a moment to refresh your memory. There are no easy divisibility rules for 7 and 8.

Divisible by	The Rule	Example: 558
2	The last digit is even.	A multiple of 2 because 8 is even.
3	The sum of the digits is a multiple of 3.	A multiple of 3 because 5 + 5 + 8 = 18, which is a multiple of 3.
4	The last 2 digits comprise a 2-digit multiple of 4.	NOT a multiple of 4 because 58 is not a multiple of 4.
5	The last digit is 5 or zero.	NOT a multiple of 5 because it doesn't end in 5 or zero.
6	The last digit is even AND the sum of the digits is a multiple of 3.	A multiple of 6 because it's a multiple of both 2 and 3.
9	The sum of the digits is a multiple of 9.	A multiple of 9 because 5 + 5 + 8 = 18, which is a multiple of 9.
10	The last digit is zero.	NOT a multiple of 10 because it doesn't end in zero.

Properties of Numbers

Here are some essential laws or properties of numbers.

Commutative Property for Addition

When adding two or more terms, the sum is the same regardless of which number is added to which.

$$3 + 2 = 2 + 3$$
$$a + b = b + a$$

Associative Property for Addition

When adding three terms, the sum is the same, regardless of which two terms are added first.

$$2 + (5 + 3) = (2 + 5) + 3$$
$$a + (b + c) = (a + b) + c$$

Commutative Property for Multiplication

When multiplying two or more terms, the result is the same regardless of which number is multiplied by which.

$$2 \times 4 = 4 \times 2$$
$$ab = ba$$

KAPLAN

Associative Property for Multiplication

When multiplying three terms, the product is the same regardless of which two terms are multiplied first.

$$2 \times (4 \times 3) = (2 \times 4) \times 3$$
$$a \times (b \times c) = (a \times b) \times c$$

Distributive Property of Multiplication Over Addition

When multiplying groups, the product of the first number, and the sum of the second and third number, is equal to the sum of the product of the first and second number, as well as the product of the first and third number.

$$a(b + c) = ab + ac$$
$$3 \times (7 + 18) = 3 \times 7 + 3 \times 18$$

Fractions and Decimals

Generally, it's a good idea to reduce fractions when solving math questions. To do this, simply cancel all factors that the numerator and denominator have in common.

$$\frac{28}{36} = \frac{4 \times 7}{4 \times 9} = \frac{7}{9}$$

To add fractions, get a common denominator and then add the numerators.

$$\frac{1}{4} + \frac{1}{3} = \frac{3}{12} + \frac{4}{12} = \frac{3 + 4}{12} = \frac{7}{12}$$

To subtract fractions, get a common denominator and then subtract the numerators.

$$\frac{1}{4} - \frac{1}{3} = \frac{3}{12} - \frac{4}{12} = \frac{3 - 4}{12} = \frac{-1}{12}$$

To multiply fractions, multiply the numerators and multiply the denominators.

$$\frac{1}{4} \times \frac{1}{3} = \frac{1 \times 1}{4 \times 3} = \frac{1}{12}$$

To divide fractions, invert the second fraction and multiply. In other words, multiply the first fraction by the reciprocal of the second fraction.

$$\frac{1}{4} \div \frac{1}{3} = \frac{1}{4} \times \frac{3}{1} = \frac{1 \times 3}{4 \times 1} = \frac{3}{4}$$

Comparing Fractions

To compare fractions, multiply the numerator of the first fraction by the denominator of the second fraction to get a product. Then, multiply the numerator of the second fraction by the denominator of the first fraction to get a second product. If the first product is greater, the first fraction is greater. If the second product is greater, the second fraction is greater.

Here's an example:

Compare $\frac{2}{5}$ and $\frac{5}{8}$

1. Multiply the numerator of the first fraction by the denominator of the second.

    $2 \times 8 = 16$

2. Multiply the numerator of the second fraction by the denominator of the first.

    $5 \times 5 = 25$

3. The second product is greater, therefore, $\frac{5}{8}$ (the second fraction), is greater than $\frac{2}{5}$.

To convert a fraction to a decimal, divide the numerator by the denominator. For example, to convert $\frac{8}{25}$ to a decimal, divide 8 by 25.

$$\frac{8}{25} = 0.32$$

To convert a decimal to a fraction, first set the decimal over 1. Then, move the decimal point over as many places as it takes until it is immediately to the right of the digit farthest to the right. Count the number of places that you moved the decimal. Then, add that many zeros to the 1 in the denominator.

$$0.3 = \frac{0.3}{1} = \frac{3.0}{10} \text{ or } \frac{3}{10}$$

$$0.32 = \frac{0.32}{1} = \frac{32.0}{100} \text{ or } \frac{8}{25}$$

Common Percent Equivalencies

Being familiar with the relationships among percents, decimals, and fractions can save you time on Test Day. Don't worry about memorizing the following chart. Simply use it to review relationships you already know (e.g., $50\% = 0.50 = \frac{1}{2}$) and to familiarize yourself with some that you might not already know. To convert a fraction or decimal to a percent, multiply by 100%. To convert a percent to a fraction or decimal, divide by 100%.

Fraction	Decimal	Percent
$\frac{1}{20}$	0.05	5%
$\frac{1}{10}$	0.10	10%
$\frac{1}{8}$	0.125	12.5%
$\frac{1}{6}$	$0.16\overline{6}$	$16\frac{2}{3}\%$

KAPLAN

Fraction	Decimal	Percent
$\frac{1}{5}$	0.20	20%
$\frac{1}{4}$	0.25	25%
$\frac{1}{3}$	$0.33\overline{3}$	$33\frac{1}{3}\%$
$\frac{3}{8}$	0.375	37.5%
$\frac{2}{5}$	0.40	40%
$\frac{1}{2}$	0.50	50%
$\frac{3}{5}$	0.60	60%
$\frac{2}{3}$	$0.66\overline{6}$	$66\frac{2}{3}\%$
$\frac{3}{4}$	0.75	75%
$\frac{4}{5}$	0.80	80%
$\frac{5}{6}$	$0.83\overline{3}$	$83\frac{1}{3}\%$
$\frac{7}{8}$	0.875	87.5%

Rounding

You might be asked to estimate or round a number on the test. Rounding might also help you determine an answer choice. There are a few simple rules to rounding. Look at the digit to the right of the number in question. If it is a 4 or less, leave the number in question as it is and replace all the digits to the right with zeros.

For example, round off 765,432 to the nearest 100. The 4 is the hundreds digit, but you have to look at the digit to the right of the hundreds digit, which is the tens digit, or 3. Since the tens digit is 3, the hundreds digit remains the same and the tens and ones digits both become zero. Therefore, 765,432 rounded to the nearest 100 is 765,400.

If the digit to the right of the number in question is 5 or greater, increase the number by 1 and replace all the digits to the right with zeros.

For example, 837 rounded to the nearest 10 is 840. If 2,754 is rounded to the nearest 100, it is 2,800.

Place Units

Rounding requires that you know the place unit value of the digits in a number.

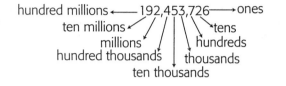

Symbols of Inequality

An inequality is a mathematical sentence in which two expressions are joined by symbols such as ≠ (not equal to), > (greater than), < (less than), ≥ (greater than or equal to), ≤ (less than or equal to). Examples of inequalities are:

$5 + 3 \neq 7$	5 plus 3 is not equal to 7
$6 > 2$	6 is greater than 2
$8 < 8.5$	8 is less than 8 and a half
$x \leq 9 + 6$	x is less than or equal to 9 plus 6
$c \geq 10$	c is greater than or equal to 10. (c is an algebraic variable. That means it varies and could be any number greater than or equal to 10.)

Exponents and Roots

An exponent indicates the number of times that a number (or variable) is to be used as a factor. On your nursing school entrance exam you'll usually deal with numbers or variables that are squares (a variable multiplied by itself) and cubes (a variable multiplied by itself 3 times).

You should remember the squares of 1 through 10.

Square = A number raised to the exponent 2 (also known as the second power)		Cube = A number raised to the exponent 3 (also known as the third power)	
2^2	$2 \times 2 = 4$	2^3	$2 \times 2 \times 2 = 8$
3^2	$3 \times 3 = 9$	3^3	$3 \times 3 \times 3 = 27$
4^2	$4 \times 4 = 16$	4^3	$4 \times 4 \times 4 = 64$
5^2	$5 \times 5 = 25$	5^3	$5 \times 5 \times 5 = 125$
6^2	$6 \times 6 = 36$	6^3	$6 \times 6 \times 6 = 216$
7^2	$7 \times 7 = 49$	7^3	$7 \times 7 \times 7 = 343$
8^2	$8 \times 8 = 64$	8^3	$8 \times 8 \times 8 = 512$
9^2	$9 \times 9 = 81$	9^3	$9 \times 9 \times 9 = 729$
10^2	$10 \times 10 = 100$	10^3	$10 \times 10 \times 10 = 1,000$

To add or subtract terms consisting of a coefficient (the number in front of the variable) multiplied by a power (a power is a base raised to an exponent), both the base and the exponent must be the same. As long as the bases and the exponents are the same, you can add the coefficients. For example:

$x^2 + x^2 = 2x^2$ can be added. The base (x) and the exponent (2) are the same.

$3x^4 - 2x^4 = x^4$ can be subtracted. The base (x) and the exponent (4) are the same.

$x^2 + x^3$ cannot be combined. The exponents are different.

$x^2 + y^2$ cannot be combined. The bases are different.

To multiply terms consisting of coefficients multiplied by powers having the same base, multiply the coefficients and add the exponents.

$$2x^5 \times (8x^7) = (2 \times 8)(x^{5+7}) = 16x^{12}$$

To divide terms consisting of coefficients multiplied by powers having the same base, divide the coefficients and subtract the exponents.

$$6x^7 \div 2x^5 = (6 \div 2)(x^{7-5}) = 3x^2$$

To raise a power to an exponent, multiply the exponents.

$$(x^2)^4 = x^{2 \times 4} = x^8$$

A square root of a non-negative number is a number that, when multiplied by itself, produces the given quantity. The radical sign $\sqrt{}$ is used to represent the positive square root of a number, so $\sqrt{25} = 5$, since $5 \times 5 = 25$.

To add or subtract radicals, make sure the numbers under the radical sign are the same. If they are, you can add or subtract the coefficients outside the radical signs.

$$2\sqrt{2} + 3\sqrt{2} = 5\sqrt{2}$$

$\sqrt{2} + \sqrt{3}$ cannot be combined.

To simplify radicals, factor out the perfect squares under the radical, take the square root of the perfect square, and put the result in front of the radical sign.

$$\sqrt{32} = \sqrt{16 \times 2} = 4\sqrt{2}$$

To multiply or divide radicals, multiply (or divide) the coefficients outside the radical. Multiply (or divide) the numbers inside the radicals.

$$\sqrt{x} \times \sqrt{y} = \sqrt{xy}$$
$$3\sqrt{2} \times 4\sqrt{5} = 12\sqrt{10}$$
$$\frac{\sqrt{x}}{\sqrt{y}} = \sqrt{\frac{x}{y}}$$
$$12\sqrt{10} \div 3\sqrt{2} = 4\sqrt{5}$$
$$12 \div 3 = 4 \text{ and } \sqrt{10} \div \sqrt{2} = \sqrt{5}$$
$$\text{So, } 12\sqrt{10} \div 3\sqrt{2} = 4\sqrt{5}$$

To take the square root of a fraction, break the fraction into two separate roots and take the square root of the numerator and the denominator.

$$\sqrt{\frac{16}{25}} = \frac{\sqrt{16}}{\sqrt{25}} = \frac{4}{5}$$

The Power of 10

When a power of 10 (that is, the base is 10) has an exponent that is a positive integer, the exponent tells you how many zeros to add after the 1. For example, 10 to the 12th power (10^{12}) has 12 zeros.

When multiplying a number by a power of 10, move the decimal point to the right the same number of places as the number of zeros in that power of 10.

$$0.0123 \times 10^4 = 123$$

When dividing by a power of 10 with a positive exponent, move the decimal point to the left.

$$43.21 \div 10^3 = 0.04321$$

Multiplying by a power with a negative exponent is the same as dividing by a power with a positive exponent. Therefore, when you multiply by a number with a positive exponent, move the decimal to the right. When you multiply by a number with a negative exponent, move the decimal to the left.

For example:

$$10^3 = 1.000 = 1,000$$
$$2 \times 10^{-3} = 0.002$$

Percents

Remember these formulas: Part = Percent $\times$ Whole *or* Percent = $\frac{\text{Part}}{\text{Whole}}$

From Fraction to Percent

To find part, percent, or whole, plug the values you have into the equation and solve.

$$44\% \text{ of } 25 = 0.44 \times 25 = 11$$

42 is what percent of 70?

$$42 \div 70 = 0.6$$
$$0.6 \times 100\% = 60\%$$

To increase or decrease a number by a given percent, take that percent of the original number and add it to or subtract it from the original number.

To increase 25 by 60%, first find 60% of 25.

$$25 \times 0.6 = 15$$

KAPLAN

Then, add the result to the original number.

$$25 + 15 = 40$$

To decrease 25 by the same percent, subtract the 15.

$$25 - 15 = 10$$

Average

$$\text{Average} = \frac{\text{Sum of the Terms}}{\text{Number of the Terms}}$$

The formula to calculate the average of 15, 18, 15, 32, and 20 is:

$$\frac{15 + 18 + 15 + 32 + 20}{5} = \frac{100}{5} = 20.$$

Conversions

One of the most important math skills required for both the HESI and Kaplan exams is the ability to convert between fractions, decimals, and percentages. All of these numeric forms can be used to represent a part of a total. For example, half of a total quantity could be written $\frac{1}{2}$ as a fraction, 0.5 as a decimal, or 50% as a percentage. All of these numeric forms are equal, but converting between them can be tricky.

Converting Between Decimals and Percentages

Perhaps the easiest conversion is between decimals and percentages. Just remember that whole number percentages are equivalent to *the first two number places behind a decimal point*. In other words, 10% is equivalent to 0.10, while 5% is equivalent to 0.05. To convert a percentage to a decimal, just move the decimal point two places to the left. Likewise, to convert a decimal to a percentage, move the decimal point two places to the right. For example, 0.375 = 37.5%. When you need to perform calculations, always use the decimal form of the number and you will make the task easier.

Converting Between Fractions and Decimals/Percentages

When converting between fractions and percentages or decimals, remember the formula you learned in the Percents section:

$$\text{Percent} = \frac{\text{Part}}{\text{Whole}}$$

If you are asked to find the percentage equivalent of a fraction, simply perform the division already shown in the fraction. For example, $\frac{4}{5}$ is equivalent to $4 \div 5$. Dividing 4 by 5 yields 0.8, which is the correct answer in decimal form. If you're asked to find the percentage equivalent, the only additional step you need to do is move the decimal point two places to the right: 80%.

If you are asked to find the fraction equivalent of a percentage, just remember that all percentages are basically fractions of 100%. For example, 60% is equivalent to $\frac{60}{100}$, which can be reduced:

$$\frac{60}{100} = \frac{6}{10} = \frac{3}{5}.$$

Ratios, Proportions, and Rates

Ratios can be expressed in different forms.

One form is $\frac{a}{b}$.

If you have 15 dogs and 5 cats, the ratio of dogs to cats is $\frac{15}{5}$. (The ratio of cats to dogs is $\frac{5}{15}$.) Like any other fraction, this ratio can be reduced; $\frac{15}{5}$ can be reduced to $\frac{3}{1}$. In other words, for every three dogs, there's one cat.

Another form of expressing ratios is *a:b*.

The ratio of dogs to cats is 15:5 or 3:1. The ratio of cats to dogs is 5:15 or 1:3.

Pay attention to what ratio is specified in the problem. Remember that the ratio of dogs to cats is different from the ratio of cats to dogs.

A proportion is two ratios set equal to each other. To solve a proportion, cross-multiply and solve for the variable.

$$\frac{x}{6} = \frac{2}{3}$$
$$3x = 12$$
$$x = 4$$

A rate is a ratio that compares quantities measured in different units. The most common example is miles per hour. Use the following formula for such problems:

Distance = Rate × Time or $D = R \times T$

Remember, although not all rates are speeds, this formula can be adapted to any rate.

Units of Measurement

You will most likely see at least a few questions that include units of measurement on the test. You are expected to remember these basic units of measurement. Spend some time reviewing the list below.

Distance

1 foot = 12 inches
1 yard = 3 feet = 36 inches

Metric: 1 kilometer = 1,000 meters. 1 meter = 10 decimeters = 100 centimeters = 1,000 millimeters (Remember, the root *deci* is 10; the root *centi* is 100; the root *milli* is 1,000.)

Weight

1 pound = 16 ounces

Metric: A gram is a unit of mass. A kilogram is 1,000 grams.

Volume

1 cup = 8 ounces

2 cups = 1 pint
1 quart = 2 pints
4 cups = 1 quart
1 gallon = 4 quarts

Metric: A liter is a unit of volume. A kiloliter is 1,000 liters.

Temperature

–20°C = –4°F
–10°C = 14°F
0°C = 32°F
10°C = 50°F
20°C = 72°F
30°C = 86°F
40°C = 104°F

To convert between temperatures in degrees Celsius and degrees Fahrenheit, use the formula $F = \frac{9}{5}C + 32$, where C is the temperature in degrees Celsius and F is the temperature in degrees Fahrenheit. Be careful to place your number into the correct position in the formula, and remember your order of operations (PEMDAS). For example, to convert 37°C to degrees Fahrenheit, plug 37 into the C position in the formula:

$$F = \frac{9}{5}C + 32$$
$$F = (\frac{9}{5} \times 37) + 32$$
$$F = (66.6) + 32$$
$$F = 98.6$$

Use the same formula to convert a temperature in degrees Fahrenheit to degrees Celsius. For example, to convert –40°F to Celsius, plug –40 into the F position in the formula:

$$F = \frac{9}{5}C + 32$$
$$-40 = \frac{9}{5}C + 32 - 32$$
$$-40 - 32 = \frac{9}{5}C + 32 - 32$$
$$-72 = \frac{9}{5}C$$
$$\frac{5}{9} \times (-72) = C$$
$$-40 = C$$

You must be careful when approaching a problem that includes units of measurement. Be sure that the units are given in the same format. You may have to convert pounds to ounces or feet to yards (or vice versa) to arrive at the correct answer choice.

Converting to Military Time

In addition to recognizing common units of measure, you might be asked to convert standard "12-hour" time (which ends with "a.m." or "p.m.") to what is known as military time. Military time simply uses a 24-hour clock, which avoids any confusion that could be caused by a 12-hour clock. For example, does 8:30 mean 8:30 in the morning, or 8:30 at night? In military time, every time of day is a unique number.

Military time begins at 0000 hours, which is equivalent to midnight (the start of the day). Another distinction is that military time, unlike a 12-hour clock, does not use a colon between the hours and minutes; for example, 0100 hours is equivalent to 1:00 a.m. However, when seconds are included in military time, a colon is used to separate seconds from the rest of the time; for instance, 0420:30 hours is equivalent to 4:20 a.m. and 30 seconds. And whereas a conventional clock resets at noon, the military clock keeps counting: Noon is written as 1200 hours, 1:00 p.m. is written as 1300 hours, and so on. If you wanted to set an appointment for 9:30 p.m., the military time equivalent would be 2130 hours. Note that while military time covers a 24-hour period, "2400 hours" does not exist; because the clock resets to 0000 hours at midnight, the highest number in military time is 2359 hours.

A Word About Word Problems

You can expect to see a lot of word problems on the test. Some of them, however, will just be asking you to perform arithmetic equations. Your job is to find the math within the story.

Here's an example:

> A grocery store charges $1.59 for a liter of milk, $2.29 for a half pound of tomatoes, $1.25 for a jar of tomato paste, and $2.25 for a box of pasta. If Reggie buys 2 liters of milk, 1 pound of tomatoes, a jar of tomato sauce, and 2 boxes of pasta, what is his bill?
>
> (A) $10.88
> (B) $13.51
> (C) $11.22
> (D) $14.76

If you sort through the story, you realize that the question is asking you to add the amounts of each item that Reggie bought. Read the question carefully to make sure you have the correct number of each item he bought, then add the amounts.

$1.59 × 2 = $3.18 (The price of two liters of milk.)

$2.29 × 2 = $4.58 (The price given was per half pound; Reggie bought 1 full pound.)

$1.25 (The price of one jar of tomato paste.)

$2.25 × 2 = $4.50 (The price of two boxes of pasta.)

Now, add these numbers together to get the total.

3.18
4.58
1.25
4.50
───────
$13.51 (B)

Often, word problems can seem tricky because it may be hard to figure out precisely what you are being asked to do. It can be difficult to translate English into math. The following table lists some common words and phrases that turn up in word problems, along with their mathematical translation.

When you see:	Think:
Sum, plus, more than, added to, combined total	+
Minus, less than, difference between, decreased by	−
Is, was, equals, is equivalent to, is the same as, adds up to	=
Times, product, multiplied by, of, twice, double, triple	×
Divided by, over, quotient, per, out of, into	÷

🅚 🅗 ALGEBRA

Algebra has been called math with letters. Just like arithmetic, the basic operations of algebra are addition, subtraction, multiplication, division, and roots. Instead of numbers though, algebra uses letters to represent unknown or variable numbers. Why would you work with a variable? Let's look at an example.

> You buy 2 bananas from the supermarket for 50 cents total. How much does one banana cost?

That's a simple equation, but how would you write it down on paper if you were trying to explain it to a friend? Perhaps you would write: $2 \times ? = 50$ cents.

Algebra gives you a systematic way to record the question mark.

$2 \times b = 50$ cents or $2b = 50$ cents, where $b =$ the cost of 1 banana in cents.

Algebra is a type of mathematical shorthand. The most commonly used letters in algebra are a, b, c and x, y, z.

The number 2 in the term $2b$ is called a coefficient. It is a constant that does not change.

To find out how much you paid for each banana, you could use your equation to solve for the unknown cost.

$$2b = 50$$
$$\frac{2b}{2} = \frac{50}{2}$$
$$b = 25$$

Algebraic Expressions

An expression is a collection of quantities made up of constants and variables linked by operations such as $+$ and $-$.

Let's go back to our fruit example. Let's say you have 2 bananas and you give one to your friend. You could express this in algebraic terms as:

$$2b - b$$

$2b - b$ is an example of an algebraic expression, where $b = 1$ banana.

In fact, this example is a binomial expression. A *binomial* is an expression that is the sum of two terms. A term is the product of a constant and one or more variables. A *monomial* expression has only one term; a *trinomial* expression is the sum of three terms; a *polynomial* expression is the sum of two or more terms.

$2b$ = monomial
$2b - b$ = binomial
$2(b + x)$ = binomial, because $2(b + x) = 2b + 2x$
$2 + b^2 + y$ = trinomial or polynomial

On the test, an algebraic expression is likely to look something like this:

$$(11 + 3x) - (5 - 2x) = ?$$

In addition to algebra, this problem tests your knowledge of positives and negatives and the order of operations (PEMDAS).

The main thing you need to remember about expressions is that you can only combine like terms.

Let's talk about fruit once more. Let's say in addition to the 2 bananas you purchased you also bought 3 apples and 1 pear. You spent $4.00 total. If b is the cost of a banana, a is the cost of an apple, and p is the cost of a pear, the purchase can be expressed as $2b + 3a + p = 4.00$.

However, let's say that once again you forgot how much each banana cost. You could NOT divide $4.00 by 6 to get the cost of each item. They're different items.

While you cannot solve expressions with unlike terms, you *can* simplify them. For example, to combine monomials or polynomials, simply add or subtract the coefficients of terms that have the exact same variable. When completing the addition or subtraction, do not change the variables.

$$6a + 5a = 11a$$
$$8b - 2b = 6b$$
$$3a + 2b - 8a = 3a - 8a + 2b = -5a + 2b \text{ or } 2b - 5a$$

Coefficient: The number that comes before the variable. In $6x$, 6 is the coefficient.

Variable: The variable is the letter that stands for an unknown. In $6x$, x is the variable.

Term: The product of a constant and one or more variables.

Monomial: One term: $6x$ is a monomial.

Polynomial: Two or more terms: $6x - y$ is a polynomial.

Binomial: Two terms: $6x - y$ is a binomial.

Trinomial: Three terms: $6x - y + z$ is a trinomial.

To review:

$6a + 5a^2$ cannot be combined. Why not? The variables are not exactly alike; that is, they are not raised to the same exponent. (One is a, the other is a^2.)

$3a + 2b$ cannot be combined. Why not? The variables are not the same. (One is a, the other is b.)

Multiplying and dividing monomials is a little different. Unlike addition and subtraction, you can multiply and divide terms that are different. When you multiply monomials, multiply the coefficients of each term. (In other words, multiply the numbers that come before the variables.) Add the exponents of like variables. Multiply different variables together.

$$(6a)(4b) = (6 \times 4)(a \times b)$$
$$= 24ab$$

$$(6a)(4ab) = (6 \times 4)(a \times a \times b)$$
$$= (6 \times 4)(a^{1+1} \times b)$$
$$= 24a^2b$$

Use the FOIL method to multiply and divide binomials. FOIL stands for First Outer Inner Last.

$$(y + 1)(y + 2) = (y \times y) + (y \times 2) + (1 \times y) + (1 \times 2)$$
$$= y^2 + 2y + y + 2$$
$$= y^2 + 3y + 2$$

Equations

The key to solving equations is to do the same thing to both sides of the equation until you have your variable isolated on one side of the equation and all of the numbers on the other side.

$$8a + 4 = 24 - 2a$$

First, subtract 4 from each side so that the left side of the equation has only variables.

$$8a + 4 - 4 = 24 - 2a - 4$$
$$8a = 20 - 2a$$

Then, add $2a$ to each side so that the right side of the equation has only numbers.

Finally, divide both sides by 10 to isolate the variable.

$$\frac{10a}{10} = \frac{20}{10}$$
$$a = 2$$

Treat Both Sides Equally

Always perform the same operation to both sides to solve for a variable in an equation.

Sometimes you're given an equation with two variables and asked to solve for one variable in terms of the other. This means that you must isolate the variable for which you are solving on one side of the equation and put everything else on the other side. In other words, when you're done, you'll have x (or whatever the variable you're looking for is) on one side of the equation and an expression on the other side.

Solve $7x + 2y = 3x + 10y - 16$ for x in terms of y.

Since you want to isolate x on one side of the equation, begin by subtracting $2y$ from both sides.

$$7x + 2y - 2y = 3x + 10y - 16 - 2y$$
$$7x = 3x + 8y - 16$$

Then, subtract $3x$ from both sides to get all the x's on one side of the equation.

$$7x - 3x = 3x + 8y - 16 - 3x$$
$$4x = 8y - 16$$

Finally, divide both sides by 4 to isolate x.

$$\frac{4x}{4} = \frac{8y}{4} - \frac{16}{4}$$
$$x = 2y - 4$$

Substitution

If a problem gives you the value for a variable, just plug the value into the equation and solve. Make sure that you follow the rules of PEMDAS and are careful with your calculations.

If $x = 15$ and $y = 10$, what is the value of $4x(x - y)$?

Plug 15 in for x and 10 in for y.

$$4(15)(15 - 10) = ?$$

Then, find the value.

$$(60)(5) = 300$$

Inequalities

Solve inequalities like you would any other equation. Isolate the variable for which you are solving on one side of the equation and everything else on the other side of the equation.

$$4a + 6 > 2a + 10$$
$$4a - 2a > 10 - 6$$
$$2a > 4$$
$$a > 2$$

The only difference here is that instead of finding a specific value for a, you get a range of values for a. That is, a can be any number greater than 2. The rest of the math is the same.

There is, however, one *crucial* difference between solving equations and inequalities. **When you multiply or divide an inequality by a negative number, you must change the direction of the sign.**

$$-5a > 10$$
$$\frac{-5a}{-5} > \frac{10}{-5}$$
$$a < -2$$

If this seems confusing, think about the logic. You're told that -5 times something is greater than 10. This is where your knowledge of positives and negatives comes into play. You know that negative $\times$ positive $=$ negative and negative $\times$ negative $=$ positive. Since -5 is negative and 10 is positive, -5 has to be multiplied by something negative to get a positive product. Therefore, a has to be *less* than -2, not *greater* than it. If $a > -2$, then any value for a that is greater than -2 should make $-5a$ greater than 10. Say a is 20; $-5a$ would be -100, which is certainly NOT greater than 10.

Algebra Word Problems

Understanding algebra word problems is probably one of the most useful math skills you can have. The great thing about word problems is that they're not only important on Test Day, they're also useful in everyday life. Whether you're figuring out how much a piece of clothing will cost you with sales tax, or calculating your earnings, algebraic word problems help you figure out unknown amounts.

Word Problems with Formulas

Some of the more challenging word problems may involve translations with mathematical formulas. For example, you might see questions dealing with averages, rates, or areas of geometric figures. (More about geometry later.) For example:

> If a truck driver travels at an average speed of 50 miles per hour for 6.5 hours, how far will the driver travel?

To answer this question, you need the distance formula:

> Distance = Rate × Time or $D = R \times T$

Once you know the formula, you can plug in the numbers:

> $D = 50 \times 6.5$
> $D = 325$ miles

Here's another example:

> Thomas took an exam with 60 questions on it. If he finished all the questions in two hours, how many minutes on average did he spend answering each question?

To answer this question, you need the average formula:

> $\text{Average} = \dfrac{\text{Sum of Terms}}{\text{Number of Terms}}$

Then plug in the numbers:

> $x = \dfrac{(2 \text{ hours} \times 60 \text{ minutes})}{60 \text{ questions}} = \dfrac{120}{60} = 2$ minutes per question

You may have noticed there's a trick in this question as well. Do you see it? The time it took for Thomas to finish the exam is given in *hours*, but the question is asking how many *minutes* each question took. Be sure to read each the question carefully so you don't fall for tricks like this.

Working with a Question

Sometimes you do not need to use a formula to solve a word problem. You need to know how to work with the question. Remember to translate the words into math.

When you see:	Think:
Sum, plus, more than, added to, combined total	+
Minus, less than, difference between, decreased by	−
Is, was, equals, is equivalent to, is the same as, adds up to	=
Times, product, multiplied by, of, twice, double, triple	×
Divided by, over, quotient, per, out of, into	÷
What, how much, how many, a number	$x, n, a, b,$ etc.

KAPLAN

🄺 🄷 MATHEMATICS STRATEGIES

Multiple-choice questions are the kind of questions you are most likely to see on your nursing school entrance exam. They are simply questions followed by answer choices. All the questions in this book are followed by four answer choices, although the number of choices on the test may vary depending on the exam your school requires. Fortunately, on this question type the correct answer is right in front of you—you just have to pick it out. Just like on any other exam, the key to working quickly and efficiently through the math section is to think about the question before you start looking for the answer. Kaplan has developed a special process for tackling math questions.

Kaplan's 4-Step Method for Math Questions

1. Read the question.
2. Decide to skip or do the problem.
3. Look for the fastest approach.
4. Make an educated guess.

Step 1: Read the Question

This is obvious. If you try to solve the question without knowing all the facts, you'll most likely come up with the wrong answer.

Step 2: Decide to Skip or Do the Problem

If a question leaves you seriously scratching your head, circle it and move on. Spend your time on the questions you can do, and then at the end of the section, if you have more time, go back to the difficult problems. Remember, easy questions are usually worth as much as difficult ones.

Step 3: Look for the Fastest Approach

All the information you will need to answer the question is right there in front of you. You never need outside knowledge to answer a question. Your job is to figure out the best way to use that information. There's more than one way to use given information. Look for shortcuts. Sometimes the most obvious way of finding a solution is also the longest way. Take the following question for example:

> At a diner, Joe orders 3 doughnuts and a cup of coffee and is charged $4.30.
> Stella orders 2 doughnuts and a cup of coffee and is charged $3.45. What is
> the price of 2 doughnuts?
>
> (A) $0.85
> (B) $0.95
> (C) $1.70
> (D) $2.05

The information about the costs of doughnuts and coffee could be translated into two distinct equations using the variables d and c. You could start by finding c in terms of d, then you could plug the values into the other equation.

But if you stop for a minute and look for a shortcut, you'll see there's a faster way: The difference in price between 3 doughnuts and a cup of coffee and 2 doughnuts and a cup of coffee is the price of one doughnut. So the cost of one doughnut can be figured out by subtracting the two costs:

$$\$4.30 - \$3.45 = \$0.85.$$

Notice that's choice (A). Don't get caught in the trap! The price of one doughnut is $0.85, but if you read the question carefully you'll see that it's asking for the price of two doughnuts, which is $2 \times \$0.85$, or $1.70. Choice (C) is the correct answer.

Step 4: Make an Educated Guess

In the previous example, you were able to find the correct answer through several simple steps. However, if you've tried solving a problem and are stuck, cut your losses. Eliminate any wrong answer choices you can, make an educated guess, and move on.

Kaplan's Other Strategies

There are also other special Kaplan strategies you might use, such as picking numbers and backsolving.

Picking Numbers

This strategy is based on the idea that instead of always trying to wrap your head around abstract variables, you can pick numbers for them. This way you end up making calculations with real numbers and you can really see the answer. The strategy of picking numbers works especially well with even/odd questions. For example:

If a is an odd integer and b is an even integer, which of the following must be odd?

(A) $2a + b$

(B) $a + 2b$

(C) ab

(D) a^2b

By picking numbers to represent a and b, you may come to the solution more easily. When you are adding, subtracting, or multiplying even and odd numbers, you can generally assume that what happens with one pair of numbers happens with similar pairs of numbers. Let's say, for the time being, that $a = 3$ and $b = 2$. Plug those values into the answer choices, and there's a good chance that only one choice will be odd:

(A) $2a + b = 2(3) + 2 = 8$

(B) $a + 2b = 3 + 2(2) = 7$

(C) $ab = (3)(2) = 6$

(D) $a^2b = (3^2)(2) = 18$

KAPLAN

Choice (B) is the only odd answer when the numbers 2 and 3 are used to represent the variables; thus, it is fair to assume that it must be the only odd-answer choice, no matter what odd number you plug in for *a* and even number you plug in for *b*. The answer is (B).

Picking numbers is a helpful strategy in several other situations, such as when:

- The answer choices for problems involving percentages are all percents.
- The answer choices for word problems are algebraic expressions.

Here are a few rules to remember when picking numbers:

- Pick easy numbers rather than ones that might be used or suggested in the problem. Keep the numbers small and manageable. You should avoid zero and 1; these often give several answers that are possibly correct.
- Remember that you have to try all the answer choices. If more than one works, pick another set of numbers.
- Don't pick the same number for more than one variable.
- Always pick 100 for questions involving percents.

Backsolving

With some math questions, it's easier to work backward from the answer choices than to try and trudge through the question. Basically, with backsolving, you are plugging the answer choices back into the question until you find a solution. This method works best when the question is a complex word problem and the answer choices are numbers, or when your only other choice is to set up multiple algebraic equations.

Backsolving is not ideal:

- If the answer choices include variables.
- If the answer choices are radicals or fractions (plugging them in takes too much time).

Here's an example of how backsolving works:

> A music club draws 27 patrons. If there are 7 more males than females in the club, how many patrons are male?
>
> (A)   8
> (B)   10
> (C)   14
> (D)   17

Try each of the answers as a substitute for the number of males in the club. Plugging in choice (C) gives you 14 males in the club. Since there are 7 more males than females, there are 7 females in the club, but $14 + 7 < 27$, so 14 doesn't work. You know the solution has to be higher, so you can eliminate (A), (B), and (C). Already you've found the right answer. Now, if you plug in (D) you see that it gives you 17 males and 10 females. $17 + 10 = 27$. That's the right answer.

Now that you have reviewed the best math strategies, it's time to test how much you have learned by answering the following review questions.

REVIEW QUESTIONS

The following questions are not meant to mimic actual test questions. Instead, these questions will help you review the concepts and terms covered in this chapter.

1. Match the number type with its definition.

    _____ Real numbers

    _____ Rational numbers

    _____ Consecutive numbers

    (A) Any number that can be written as a ratio of two integers, including integers, terminating decimals, and repeating decimals.

    (B) Numbers that follow one after another, in order, without any skipping.

    (C) Any number that can name a position on a number line regardless of whether that position is positive, negative, or zero.

2. Fill in the blank. When you multiply an even number by an odd number the product is

    _____.

3. True or False? The product of three negative numbers is positive. _____

4. Define the term Greatest Common Factor.

    _____

5. Write the steps of the Order of Operations.

    _____

    _____

    _____

    _____

    _____

6. True or False? To convert a fraction to a decimal, you divide the numerator by the denominator.

7. Write the formula for calculating an average.

    _____

8. Fill in the blank. In algebra, the _____ is the letter that stands for an unknown.

9. Write the formula used to calculate distance when dealing with rate, distance, and time.

    _____

10. What is 20% of 10% of 500?

    (A) 5

    (B) 10

    (C) 15

    (D) 20

11. If $x = 3$, $y = 8$, and $z = 2$, then what is the value of $3x^2 + 5(3 - y) - 2z$?

    (A) −20

    (B) −2

    (C) 12

    (D) 48

12. $4\frac{3}{8} - 2\frac{5}{12} =$

    (A) $\frac{27}{24}$

    (B) $1\frac{1}{24}$

    (C) $1\frac{23}{24}$

    (D) 2

13. Which fraction is equivalent to 25%?

    (A) $\frac{5}{18}$

    (B) $\frac{2}{9}$

    (C) $\frac{2}{10}$

    (D) $\frac{3}{12}$

REVIEW ANSWERS

1. **C** Real numbers are any number that can name a position on a number line regardless of whether that position is positive, negative, or zero.

   A Rational numbers are any number that can be written as a ratio of two integers. The first integer in the ratio can be positive, negative, or zero. The second integer in the ratio can be positive or negative, however, it cannot be zero, since we cannot divide by zero. Rational numbers include integers, terminating decimals, and repeating decimals.

   B Consecutive numbers are numbers that follow one after another, in order, without any skipping.

2. When you multiply an even number by an odd number the product is even.

3. False. The product of three negative numbers is negative.

4. The Greatest Common Factor is the largest factor that goes into two or more integers.

5. Parentheses
   Exponents
   Multiplication and Division (from left to right)
   Addition and Subtraction (from left to right)

6. True. To convert a fraction to a decimal, you divide the numerator by the denominator.

7. Average $= \dfrac{\text{Sum of the terms}}{\text{Number of terms}}$

8. In algebra, the variable is the letter that stands for an unknown.

9. Distance $=$ Rate $\times$ Time

10. **B** This question is a little bit tricky because it requires you to find a percent of a percent. First, convert each percent to a fraction. To convert a percent to a fraction or decimal, divide the percent by 100%:

    $20\% = \dfrac{20\%}{100\%} = \dfrac{20}{100} = \dfrac{2}{10} = \dfrac{1}{5}$

    $10\% = \dfrac{10\%}{100\%} = \dfrac{10}{100} = \dfrac{1}{10}$

    Therefore, 20% of 10% of 500 $=$

    $\dfrac{1}{5} \times \dfrac{1}{10} \times 500 = \dfrac{1}{5} \times \left(\dfrac{1}{10} \times 500\right) = \dfrac{1}{5} \times 50 = 10.$

11. **B** Since $x = 3$, $y = 8$, and $z = 2$, you can simply substitute the given values for each variable into the expression $3x^2 + 5(3 - y) - 2z$:
    $3(3)^2 + 5(3 - 8) - 2(2)$
    $= 3(9) + 5(-5) - 2(2)$
    $= 27 - 25 - 4$
    $= 2 - 4 = -2.$

12. **C** First, convert $4\frac{3}{8}$ and $2\frac{5}{12}$ into improper fractions:

    $4\dfrac{3}{8} = \dfrac{4 \times 8 + 3}{8} = \dfrac{32 + 3}{8} = \dfrac{35}{8}$

    $2\dfrac{5}{12} = \dfrac{2 \times 12 + 5}{12} = \dfrac{24 + 5}{12} = \dfrac{29}{12}$

    So $4\frac{3}{8} - 2\frac{5}{12} = \frac{35}{8} - \frac{29}{12}$. To subtract, find a common denominator, which here is a multiple of 8 and 12. You can find a positive multiple of 8 and 12 by starting with the smallest positive multiple of 12, which is $1 \times 12 = 12$, and then looking at the next positive multiples of 12, which are $2 \times 12, 3 \times 12, 4 \times 12, 5 \times 12, \ldots$, until you find a multiple of 8:

    - $1 \times 12 = 12$ is not a multiple of 8.
    - $2 \times 12 = 24$ is a multiple of 8, since $24 = 3 \times 8.$

    The positive multiple of 8 and 12 you found, 24, is actually the smallest positive multiple of 8 and 12.

    Therefore,

    $\dfrac{35}{8} - \dfrac{29}{12} = \dfrac{105}{24} - \dfrac{58}{24} = \dfrac{105 - 58}{24} = \dfrac{47}{24} = 1\dfrac{23}{24}.$

13. **D** First, convert 25% to a fraction. To convert a percent to a fraction or decimal, divide the percent by 100%: $25\% = \dfrac{25\%}{100\%} = \dfrac{25}{100} = \dfrac{1}{4}.$

    Since $\frac{1}{4}$ is not one of the answer choices, see if any of the answer choices can be reduced to $\frac{1}{4}$. The fractions $\frac{5}{18}$, choice (A), and $\frac{2}{9}$, choice (B), cannot be further reduced, while $\frac{2}{10}$, choice (C), can be reduced to $\frac{1}{5}$. Only $\frac{3}{12}$, choice (D), can be reduced to $\frac{1}{4}$.

| PART FIVE |

Science Review

- Biology Review
- Anatomy and Physiology Review
- Physical Science Review

Chapter Seven: **Biology Review**

In preparing for your nursing school entrance exam, it is important to have a grasp of the fundamentals of Biology. This chapter covers everything from the structure of cells through genetics and beyond.

BUILDING BLOCKS FOR THE TEST

Use this chapter as a road map or your core set of building blocks. Just as it's easier in mathematics to start with addition and work your way up to algebra, it is easier to learn biology starting with cells and then move up to evolution and diversity. Since our review lessons are already organized this way, you should avoid skipping around in a chapter. Instead, you should review each lesson from beginning to end.

(K) (H) BIOLOGY LESSON

One way to solve a puzzle is to put together the pieces in larger and larger assemblies until the entire puzzle is complete. Biologists try to gain understanding about living systems in a similar way, by studying life at many levels and then putting all of the pieces together in one complete picture.

Looking at biology from this perspective, molecules are studied for further knowledge of the workings of cells, which explain how tissues, organs, and organisms function. From those facts, we can explain how and why populations and ecosystems operate as they do, as well as evolutionary changes that have created the great diversity of life on Earth today.

In the beginning of this lesson we will discuss molecules and the workings of cells. This will form the foundation for later parts of this lesson, which concern organisms, genetics, ecology, and evolution. By the final section of this lesson, it will be possible to view life not as a set of isolated facts, but as a rich, interconnected network.

The important topics of Anatomy and Physiology appear on both nursing exams. They will be covered in the next chapter.

Ⓚ Ⓗ CELLULAR BIOLOGY

Biological Chemistry

At the elemental level, all life is composed primarily of carbon, hydrogen, oxygen, nitrogen, phosphorous, and sulfur, with traces of other elements such as iron, iodine, magnesium, and calcium—these are all essential components for living organisms. Salts like sodium chloride are also essential components of life. Chemicals that do not contain carbon—such as sodium chloride, nitrogen, and phosphorus—are called **inorganic compounds**.

Chemicals that contain carbon are called **organic compounds**, and include the major types of biological molecules (that is, molecules that support life) found in all organisms, including proteins, lipids, carbohydrates, and nucleic acids. Before we explore these molecules, let's look at a vastly important and seldom-appreciated molecule fundamental for all life: water.

Water

Life is not possible without water. The presence of liquid water allowed life to evolve and to persist on Earth. The way water molecules are structured gives water unique properties that allow it to play its particular role. Each water molecule is composed of one atom of oxygen and two hydrogen atoms that are attached at an angle. Water's ability to absorb heat means that water remains in a liquid form over a range of temperatures common on our planet. Another important feature of water is that the solid form of water, ice, is less dense than its liquid form. This is due to a special type of bonding that takes place in water called hydrogen bonding.

Hydrogen bonding gives water other unique properties as well. Because of the uneven distribution of its electron density, water is considered a "polar" molecule: Near the end with the oxygen atom, it has a partial negative charge, while near the hydrogen atoms, it has a partial positive charge. The polarity of the water molecule is one reason that water is so good at dissolving so many different substances, earning water the title "the universal solvent." Also as a consequence of its polarity, water exhibits both cohesive and adhesive properties; cohesion allows water molecules to "stick together," while adhesion allows water to stick to other substances. You might never have thought of it this way before, but at the molecular level, water is most definitely sticky!

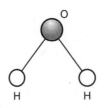

Other Biological Molecules

There are a few other biological molecules you should be familiar with. These are carbohydrates, lipids, proteins, enzymes, and nucleic acids. A description of each follows.

Carbohydrates

Carbohydrates are a main class of biological molecules. Another name for carbohydrates is **saccharides**. Carbohydrates are composed of carbon, hydrogen, and oxygen; they include sugars and starches. Carbohydrates provide short-term energy for metabolism and can be converted into lipids for long-term energy storage. The simplest forms of carbohydrates are monosaccharides; these are sugars, such as glucose and fructose, that cannot be broken down into simpler sugars. Monosaccharides are the building blocks of larger carbohydrates such as disaccharides (for instance, lactose) and polysaccharides (for instance, cellulose). Carbohydrates also provide structural support for cells and organisms. Cellulose, for example, forms the cell wall of plants, and is the single most abundant biological molecule on Earth.

Lipids (Fats and Oils)

Like carbohydrates, **lipids** are composed of carbon, hydrogen, and oxygen; but lipids are very distinct from carbohydrates in their structure and function. Lipids have much lower oxygen content than carbohydrates and are less oxidized, storing more energy than carbohydrates. Lipids tend to repel water. Lipids are a long-term energy source. The significance of this is important to understand. When you ingest carbohydrates and lipids, your body first uses carbohydrates for energy. If you take in more carbohydrates than necessary, the body will store them as fatty acids, which are eventually re-synthesized as lipids called triglycerides and can lead to increased cholesterol levels.

Phospholipids make up a special class of lipids that repel water at one end (the tail) but attract water at the other (the head). This special property gives phospholipids the ability to form a durable membrane that is difficult to pass through: the phospholipid bilayer. In this structure, each layer consists of a dense array of phospholipids with the heads outward. The lipid bilayer is what makes up much of the cellular membrane in living cells.

Steroids are also lipids, though their structure differs from that of other lipids. Cholesterol is the most common steroid, and it is a key component of cell membranes. Other steroids include testosterone and progesterone, which play critical roles in sexual reproduction.

Proteins

Carbohydrates and lipids provide both energy and structure for cells. There is much more to life, however, than these functions. Cells continually carry out a broad range of functions in order to grow, reproduce, and survive, which are important characteristics of life. **Proteins** provide cells with the ability to carry out these functions; below you will find a list of several of these functions.

Type of Protein	Functions	Examples
Hormonal	Chemical messengers	Insulin, glucagon
Transport	Transports other substances	Hemoglobin, carrier proteins
Structural	Physical support	Collagen
Contractile	Movement	Actin, myosin
Antibodies	Immune defense	Immunoglobulins, interferons
Enzymes	Biological catalysts	Amylase, lipase, ATPase

Enzymes

Enzymes act as catalysts for all biochemical reactions, making them essential for living organisms. Enzymes increase reaction rates by lowering activation energy. Activation energy is the minimum amount of energy needed to start a reaction. Every chemical reaction begins with reactants and proceeds to products. The reactants have a certain amount of energy contained in their bonds, and the products contain a unique amount of energy as well.

Nucleic Acids

Nucleic acids are another class of the essential biological molecules found in all living organisms. They act as informational molecules, and include deoxyribonucleic acid (DNA) and ribonucleic acid (RNA). All organisms (except for some viruses, which most people do not classify as truly living) use DNA as their **genome** (an organism's chromosomal set). The structure and function of nucleic acids will be addressed in a separate section about genome expression.

How Cells Get Energy to Make ATP

One of the essential features of life is the ability to capture and harness energy from the environment and use this energy to build, move, grow, and replicate. What energy is used and where does it come from?

Organisms eat carbohydrates and fats that contain chemical energy, digesting these molecules to trap their chemical energy in a molecule called adenosine triphosphate (ATP). Cells use ATP to do most activities that require energy input to occur. Processes requiring energy input will not occur on their own, catalyzed or not. In fact, without energy input, most of the molecules fundamental to life tend to move in the other direction, toward oxidation and a loss of structure. By capturing food energy and converting it into ATP, life uses energy to drive forward all of the reactions it needs to perform. This process is known as **cellular respiration**.

Where does ATP come from? Cells in humans and other organisms use a common set of biochemical reactions to make ATP, including pathways such as **glycolysis**, the **Krebs cycle**, and **electron transport**. The process of generating energy in the form of ATP begins with the glucose molecule. In humans, glucose is present in the blood as a fuel for all cells. Cells take in glucose, leading to the glycolytic pathway that is the first step in the path to ATP.

Glycolysis

A **metabolic pathway** is a linked series of biochemical reactions that have a common purpose. Glycolysis is a very ancient pathway in the evolution of life, present in all of the kingdoms of life, from bacteria to humans. Glycolysis is important because it is the first biochemical pathway in the capture of energy from glucose, which makes ATP. The **glycolytic pathway** consists of ten steps, each catalyzed by an enzyme uniquely evolved to catalyze that reaction. You will not need to know all of the individual reactions or the individual enzymes, but being familiar with the idea of metabolic pathways and the function of glycolysis is a good idea. Glycolysis takes glucose, a sugar molecule with six carbon atoms, and breaks it into two pyruvate molecules, each with three carbons, that capture energy in different ways. Energy is captured to make NADH, an energy carrier the cell uses to make ATP through electron transport.

Fermentation

In glycolysis, NAD^+ is required, and it is converted to NADH. Obviously, NAD^+ must be regenerated or glycolysis would run out of it and stop, halting ATP production as well (and probably the life of the cell or organism involved). NAD^+ is regenerated in one of two ways. In the first, in the presence of oxygen, NADH goes on to the electron transport chain and is used to produce more ATP, as described in the sections that follow; during this process it is converted back to NAD^+. The second way to regenerate NAD^+ occurs in the absence of oxygen or in anaerobic organisms that do not use oxidative metabolism. This alternate pathway is called **fermentation**.

Fermentation allows glycolysis to continue even in the absence of oxygen. In fermentation, NADH is regenerated back to NAD^+ in the absence of oxygen to allow glycolysis to continue to produce ATP, producing either ethanol or lactic acid as by-products.

Aerobic Respiration

Although glycolysis produces two ATP and two NADH for every molecule of glucose, this is not where the eukaryotic cell extracts most of its energy from glucose. Glycolysis is only the beginning; **aerobic respiration** is the rest of the story. During aerobic respiration, glucose is fully combusted by the cell as an energy source, going through the **Krebs cycle** and electron transport to trap energy ultimately used to make ATP.

To accomplish this more efficient form of energy production, pyruvate from glycolysis is oxidized all the way to carbon dioxide in a pathway called the Krebs cycle. The Krebs cycle and the other steps of oxidative metabolism occur in mitochondria. It is not important to know all the details about the Krebs cycle, but you should understand that the Krebs cycle is a series of reactions linked in a circle that extracts energy from the products of glycolysis to make the high-energy electron carriers. Finally, **electron transport** is the mechanism used to convert the energy held by these carriers into a more useful form that ultimately results in ATP production.

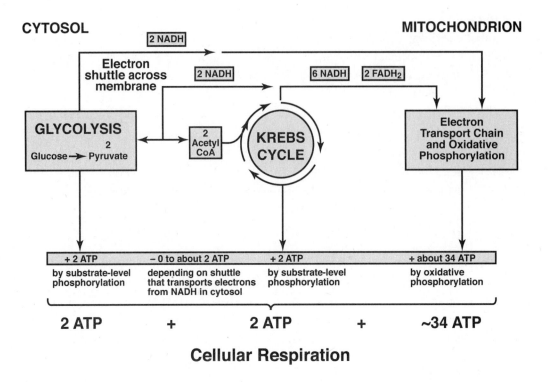

Cellular Respiration

Photosynthesis

Photosynthesis is the foundation of all ecosystems because it is the primary source of energy. Plants are **autotrophs**, or self-feeders, that use photosynthesis to generate their own chemical energy from the energy of the sun. There are also many prokaryotic and eukaryotic photosynthetic organisms, such as algae, that contribute significantly to biological production. The chemical energy that plants get from the sun is used to produce the glucose that can be burned in mitochondria to make ATP, which is then used to drive all of the energy-requiring processes in a plant, including the production of proteins, lipids, carbohydrates, and nucleic acids. Animals eat plants to extract this energy for their own metabolic needs. In this way, photosynthesis supports almost all living systems.

In plants, photosynthesis occurs in the **chloroplast**, an organelle that is specific to plants. In prokaryotes, there are no chloroplasts, and photosynthesis occurs throughout the cytoplasm. Chloroplasts are found mainly in the cells of the **mesophyll**, green tissue in the interior of leaves. A leaf contains pores in its surface called **stomata** that allow carbon dioxide in and oxygen out, facilitating photosynthesis in the leaf. Chloroplasts have an inner and outer membrane; within the inner membrane there is a fluid called the **stroma**. Photosynthesis involves the reduction of carbon dioxide (CO_2) to a carbohydrate. It can be characterized as the reverse of respiration, in that the reduction of CO_2 produces glucose instead of the oxidation of glucose making CO_2. Oxygen, one of the by-products of photosynthesis, is of keen interest to all of us air-breathers since we need it to survive.

H THE GENOME AND GENE EXPRESSION

Plants, animals, and bacteria may differ in their form, biochemistry, and lifestyle, but they all share a common molecular structure that underlies the inheritance and expression of traits. All living organisms inherit traits from their parent organisms, and these traits are encoded by the molecule called DNA. By comparing the features of parents with their children, humans throughout history have known intuitively that animals transfer traits from one generation to another. Many years ago, Gregor Mendel (discussed further in Classical Genetics) pioneered studies of the genetic behavior of traits passed between generations of pea plants. The discovery of the identity of the molecules that store and transfer genetic information is relatively recent, however. **Genes** encode these physical traits. Many scientists once believed that proteins were the main source of genetic material. That theory was based on the fact that nucleic acids such as DNA have such simple components. As such, it was difficult for many scientists to believe DNA could carry such complex information. Through many elegant experiments, however, it was proven that DNA is the foundation of genetic material. Furthermore, with the elucidation of DNA by Watson and Crick in 1953, it became clear how and why DNA has its role as the source of genetic material.

The basic outline of information flow in living organisms is sometimes called the **Central Dogma**. The Central Dogma includes several concepts, which are the foundation of modern molecular biology.

Principles of Central Dogma

1. DNA contains an organism's genetic material—the genes that are responsible for the physical traits (phenotype) observed in all living organisms.

2. DNA is replicated from existing DNA to produce new genomes.

3. RNA is produced when a gene segment of DNA is read by RNA. Through the process of **transcription**, RNA acquires a complementary gene sequence.

4. The gene sequence carried by RNA is read and appropriated into a sequence of amino acids, which form protein. This process of protein synthesis is called **translation**.

DNA Basics

Although DNA is a complex molecule, there are key concepts surrounding it you should understand. DNA is a double-stranded polymer built from simple building blocks called **nucleotides**, of which there are four types: **adenine** (A), **guanine** (G), **thymine** (T), and **cytosine** (C). It is important to note that adenine (A) always pairs with thymine (T), and cytosine (C) always pairs with guanine (G).

The Genetic Code

Part of the Central Dogma is that DNA contains genes that are transcribed to create messenger RNA (mRNA) which is in turn translated to make proteins. How do the four base pairs in DNA encode the 20 amino acids found in a protein polypeptide chain? The order of the four base pairs in DNA is the basis of this encoded information and is called the **genetic code**.

Mutation

In a **mutation**, nucleotides are added, deleted, or substituted to change the sequence of a gene. In some cases, inappropriate amino acids are created and a mutated protein is produced. Genetic diseases are caused by these gene mutations. There will be more information about mutation later in the lesson.

RNA

The Central Dogma states that RNA is produced while DNA is read during transcription. Like DNA, RNA is a polymer of nucleotides. Both DNA and RNA are nucleic acids; the structure of RNA is very similar to single-stranded DNA. However, there are some important differences between DNA and RNA. These differences include the use of ribose in the RNA backbone rather than deoxyribose; the presence of the base uracil in RNA rather than thymine; and the fact that RNA is usually single-stranded, while DNA is usually double-stranded.

There are three types of RNA with distinct functions: **messenger** RNA (mRNA), **ribosomal** RNA (rRNA), and **transfer** RNA (tRNA). In short, mRNA encodes gene messages that are to be decoded during protein synthesis to form proteins; rRNA is a part of the structure of ribosomes and is involved in translation (protein synthesis); and tRNA plays a role in protein synthesis.

Ⓚ Ⓗ CELL STRUCTURE AND ORGANIZATION

Cell Theory

Modern biology has shown that the cell is so inherent in the way we view life that it is easy to overlook its importance. Cells were unknown until the seventeenth century, after the development of the microscope allowed scientists to see cells for the first time. In 1838, Matthias Schleiden and Theodor Schwann proposed that all life was composed of cells, while Rudolph Virchow proposed in 1855 that cells arise only from other cells. The **cell theory** based on these ideas unifies all biology at the cellular level and may be summarized as follows:

- All living things are composed of cells.
- The cell is the basic unit of structure and organization in all living things.
- Cells arise only from pre-existing cells.

Prokaryotic Versus Eukaryotic Cells
Prokaryotic Cells

Prokaryotes include archaebacteria and eubacteria, which are unicellular organisms with a simple cell structure. These organisms have an outer lipid bilayer cell membrane, but do not contain any membrane-bound organelles, unlike their cousins the eukaryotes. Prokaryotes have no true nucleus and their genetic material consists of a single, circular molecule of DNA concentrated in an area of the cell called the nucleoid region. Bacteria also have a cell wall, cell membrane, cytoplasm, ribosomes, and, sometimes, flagella, that are used for locomotion.

Prokaryotes conduct respiration in the cell membrane. This is due to the fact that there are no other membranes present for ATP (energy) synthesis to take place.

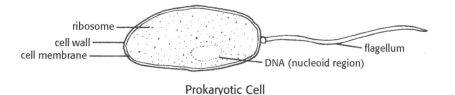

Prokaryotic Cell

Archaebacteria, which typically exist in extreme environments that lack oxygen, can differ significantly from this structure (e.g., types of lipids in cell membranes, composition of cell walls, etc.).

Eukaryotic Cells

All multicellular organisms (for example: you, a tree, a mushroom) and all protists (amoebas or paramecia) are composed of **eukaryotic cells**. A eukaryotic cell is enclosed within a lipid bilayer cell membrane, as are prokaryotic cells. Unlike prokaryotes, however, eukaryotic cells contain organelles, which are membrane-bound structures within a cell with specific functions isolated in separate compartments. The organelle membrane and interior are separated from the rest of the cell, allowing organelles to perform distinct functions isolated from other activities, which is not possible in prokaryotes.

The presence of membrane-enclosed organelles prevents incompatible processes from mixing together, allows stepwise processes to be more strictly regulated, and makes processes more efficient by making them happen in a single, constrained place. **Cytoplasm** is the liquid inside a cell that surrounds organelles.

Although both animal and plant cells are eukaryotic, they differ in a number of ways. For example, plant cells have a cell wall and chloroplasts, while animal cells do not. Centrioles, located in the centrosome, are found in animal cells but not in plant cells.

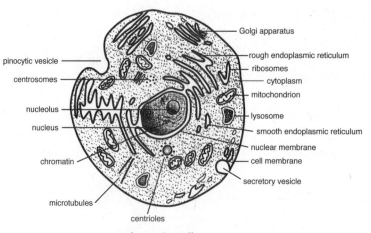

Eukaryotic Cell

Summary of Cell Properties				
Structure	**Nucleus?**	**Genetic Material?**	**Cell Wall?**	**Cell Membrane?**
Eukaryote	Yes	DNA	Yes/No	Yes
Prokaryote	No	DNA	Yes	Yes
Structure	**Membrane Organelles?**	**Ribosomes?**		
Eukaryote	Yes	Yes		
Prokaryote	No	Yes*		

*Ribosomes in prokaryotes are smaller and have a different subunit composition than those in eukaryotes.

Plasma Membrane

The **plasma membrane** is not an organelle but is an important component of cellular structure. The plasma membrane (also called the **cell membrane**) encloses the cell and exhibits **selective permeability**; it regulates the passage of materials into and out of the cell. To carry out the biochemical activities necessary to sustain life, some molecules must be retained inside the cell and other materials must be kept out of the cell. This is what the selective permeability of the membrane provides.

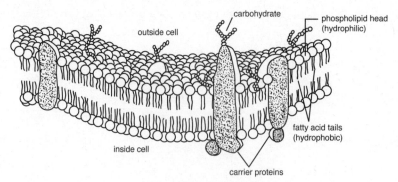

The Plasma Membrane

Organelles

Eukaryotic cells have specialized membrane-bound structures called **organelles** that carry out particular functions for the cell. Organelles include the nucleus, endoplasmic reticulum, Golgi apparatus, lysosomes, microbodies, vacuoles, mitochondria, and chloroplasts. The lipid bilayer membranes that surround organelles also regulate and partition the flow of material into and out of these compartments, just as the plasma membrane does for the cell and its exterior environment.

Nucleus

One of the largest organelles of the cell is the **nucleus**. The nucleus is the site in which the genes present in DNA are read to produce messenger RNA (the process of transcription). The DNA genome is replicated when the cell divides. Other activities like glycolysis and protein synthesis are excluded from the nucleus. The nucleus is surrounded by a two-layer **nuclear membrane** (or nuclear envelope) that maintains a nuclear environment distinct from that of the cytoplasm. Nuclear pores in this membrane allow a selective two-way exchange of materials between the nucleus and cytoplasm, importing some proteins into the nucleus that are involved in transcription, mRNA splicing, and DNA replication, while keeping out other factors like those involved in glycolysis and translation. The dense structure within the nucleus in which ribosomal RNA (rRNA) synthesis occurs is known as the **nucleolus**.

The nucleus also contains DNA genomes that have become complex with proteins called **histones,** which are involved in packaging DNA and regulating access to genes. The term **chromatin** is used to describe DNA that has been packaged with histones. Chromatin becomes condensed through several processes, leading to the development of **chromosomes**, which are the highest level of structure in the genome. Each chromosome contains a fully packaged and immensely long molecule of DNA containing many different genes. The activity of chromosomes during cell division and the role it plays in heredity will be discussed in Classical Genetics.

Ribosomes

Ribosomes are not membrane-bound organelles; rather they are relatively large, complex structures that are the sites of protein production and are synthesized by the nucleolus. They consist of two subunits, one large and one small; each subunit is composed of rRNA and many proteins. Free ribosomes are found in the cytoplasm, while bound ribosomes line the outer membrane of the endoplasmic reticulum. Prokaryotes have ribosomes that are similar in function to eukaryotic ribosomes, although they are smaller.

Endoplasmic Reticulum

The **endoplasmic reticulum** (ER) is a network of membrane-enclosed spaces connected with the nuclear membrane at various points. The network extends in sheets and tubes through cytoplasm. If this network has ribosomes lining its outer surface, it is termed **rough endoplasmic reticulum** (RER); without ribosomes, it is known as **smooth endoplasmic reticulum** (SER). The ER is involved in the transport of proteins in cells, especially proteins destined to be secreted from the cell. SER is involved in lipid synthesis and the detoxification of drugs and poisons, while RER is involved in protein synthesis.

KAPLAN

Proteins that are found in the cytoplasm are made by free ribosomes. Proteins that are secreted, found in the cell membrane, the ER, or the Golgi apparatus, are made by ribosomes on the RER. Proteins synthesized by bound ribosomes cross into the **cisternae** (the interior) of the RER. Small regions of ER membrane bud off to form small round membrane-bound vesicles that contain newly synthesized proteins. These cytoplasmic vesicles are then transported to the Golgi apparatus.

Golgi Apparatus

The **Golgi** is a stack of membrane-enclosed sacs. It receives intact vessels and their contents from the ER and modifies proteins (through glycosylation, the process of modifying proteins with carbohydrate chains, for example). Next, it repackages them into new vesicles and ships the vesicles to their next stop, such as lysosomes or the plasma membrane. In cells that are very active in the secretion of proteins, the Golgi is particularly active in the distribution of newly synthesized material to the cell surface. Secretory vesicles, produced by the Golgi, release their contents to the cell's exterior by the process of exocytosis.

Lysosomes

Lysosomes contain hydrolytic enzymes involved in intracellular digestion—the process in which proteins and structures that are worn out or not in use become degraded. Lysosomes fuse with endocytic vacuoles, breaking down material ingested by the cells. They also aid in renewing a cell's components by breaking them down and releasing their molecular building blocks into the cytosol for reuse.

Microbodies

Microbodies can be characterized as specialized containers for metabolic reactions. The two most common types of microbodies are **peroxisomes** and **glyoxysomes**. Peroxisomes break fats down into small molecules that can be used for fuel; they are also used in the liver to detoxify compounds, such as alcohol, that may be harmful to the body. Glyoxysomes, on the other hand, are usually found in the fat tissue of germinating seedlings. Until seedlings are mature enough to use photosynthesis to produce their own supply of sugars, they use glyoxysomes to convert fats into sugars.

Vacuoles

Vacuoles are membrane-enclosed sacs within the cell. Contractile vacuoles in freshwater protists pump excess water out of the cell. Plant cells have a large, central vacuole called the tonoplast, which is part of their endomembrane system. In plants, the tonoplast functions as a place to store organic compounds, such as proteins, and inorganic ions, such as potassium and chloride.

Mitochondria

Mitochondria are sites of aerobic respiration within the cell and are important suppliers of energy. Each mitochondrion has an outer and inner phospholipid bilayer membrane. The outer membrane has many pores and acts as a sieve, allowing molecules through on the basis of their size. The area between the inner and outer membranes is known as the intermembrane space. The inner membrane has many convolutions called **cristae**, as well as a high protein content that includes the proteins of the electron transport chain. The area bound by the inner membrane is known as the **mitochondrial matrix**, and is the site of many reactions that occur during cell respiration—including ATP production.

Mitochondria are somewhat unusual in that they are semiautonomous. They contain their own circular DNA and ribosomes, which enable them to produce some of their own proteins, and they self-replicate through binary fission. They are believed to have developed from early prokaryotic cells that evolved from a symbiotic relationship with the ancestors of eukaryotes and still retain vestiges of this earlier independent life.

Chloroplasts

Chloroplasts are found only in algal and plant cells. With the help of one of their primary components, chlorophyll, they function as the site where photosynthesis transpires. They contain their own DNA and ribosomes, exhibit the same semiautonomy as mitochondria, and are also believed to have evolved via symbiosis. For more information about chloroplasts, see the section titled Photosynthesis.

Cytoskeleton

Cells are not blobs of gelatin enclosed by a membrane bag. Cells have shape, and in some cases they move actively and change their shape. Cells gain mechanical support, maintain their shape, and carry out cell motility functions with the help of their **cytoskeleton**. This structure is composed of **microtubules**, **microfilaments**, and **intermediate fibers**, as well as chains and rods of proteins that all have distinct functions and activities.

Microtubules are hollow rods made of polymerized tubulin proteins. Microtubules radiate throughout cells, providing support and a framework for organelle movement within the cell.

Cilia and **flagella** are specialized arrangements of microtubules that extend from certain cells and are involved in cell motility.

Cell movement and support are maintained in part through the action of solid rods composed of actin subunits; these are termed **microfilaments**. Muscle contraction, for example, is based on the interaction of actin with myosin in muscle cells. Microfilaments move materials across the plasma membrane; they are active, for instance, in the contraction phase of cell division and in amoeboid movement.

Intermediate fibers are a collection of fibers involved in the maintenance of cytoskeletal integrity. Their diameters fall between those of microtubules and microfilaments.

Membrane Transport Across the Plasma

It is crucial for a cell to control what enters and exits it. In order to preserve this control, cells use the mechanisms described below.

Osmosis

Osmosis is the simple diffusion of water from a region of lower solute concentration to a region of higher solute concentration. Water flows to equalize the solute concentrations. If a membrane is impermeable to a particular solute, then water will flow across the membrane until the differences in the solute concentration have been equilibrated. Differences in the concentration of substances to which the membrane is impermeable affect the direction of osmosis. Water diffuses freely across the plasma membrane. When the cytoplasm of the cell has a lower solute concentration than the extracellular medium, the medium is said to be **hypertonic** to the cell; water will flow out, causing the cell to shrink. On the other hand, when the cytoplasm of a cell has a higher solute concentration than the extracellular medium, the medium is **hypotonic** to the cell, and water will flow in, causing the cell to swell. Finally, when solute concentrations are equal inside and outside, the cell and the medium are said to be **isotonic**. There is no net flow of water in either direction.

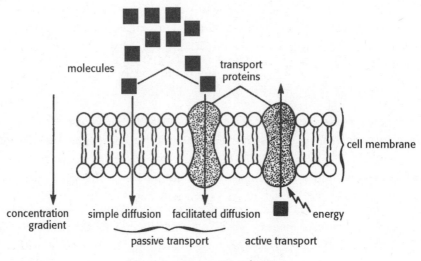

Movement Across Membranes

Permeability—Diffusion Through the Membrane

Traffic through the membrane is extensive, but the membrane is selectively permeable; substances do not cross its barrier indiscriminately. A cell is able to retain many small molecules and exclude others. The sum total of movement across the membrane is determined by the **passive diffusion** of material directly through the membrane and selective transport processes through the membrane that require proteins. Most molecules cannot passively diffuse through the plasma membrane. The hydrophobic core of the membrane impedes diffusion of charged and polar molecules. Hydrophobic molecules such as hydrocarbons can readily diffuse through the membrane, however. The ability of cells to get the oxygen needed to fuel electron transport depends on two factors: the ability of oxygen to diffuse through membranes *into* the cell and the passive diffusion *out of* the cell membrane and into the bloodstream. Although it is polar, water is also able to readily diffuse through the membrane. If two molecules are equally soluble, then the smaller molecule will diffuse through the plasma membrane faster. Small, polar, uncharged molecules can pass through easily, but the lipid bilayer is not permeable to large, uncharged polar molecules such as glucose.

Diffusion and Transport

Diffusion is the net movement of dissolved particles across concentration gradients, from a region of higher concentration to a region of lower concentration. **Passive diffusion** does not require proteins since it occurs directly through the membrane. Since molecules are moving down a concentration gradient, no external energy is required.

The net movement of dissolved particles across concentration gradients—with the help of carrier proteins in the membrane—is known as **facilitated diffusion**. This process does not require energy. Ion channels are one example of membrane proteins involved in facilitated diffusion. During this process, channels act as a passage for ions to flow through the membrane and into another concentration gradient. Ions will not flow through the membrane on their own. Some channels are always open for ions to flow through, while other ion channels open only in response to specific stimuli, such as a change in the voltage across the membrane or the presence of a molecule like a neurotransmitter.

Transport proteins aid in the process of **active transport,** which is the net movement of dissolved particles against their concentration gradient. This process requires energy and is necessary to maintain membrane potentials in specialized cells such as neurons. The most common forms of energy to drive active transport are ATP or a concentration gradient of another molecule. Active transport is used for uptake of nutrients against a gradient.

Transport Proteins

Molecules that do not diffuse through the membrane can often get in or out of the cell with the aid of proteins in the membrane. Hydrophilic substances that avoid contact with the lipid bilayer can still traverse the membrane by passing through transport proteins. There are three types of transport proteins: uniport, symport, and antiport. Uniport proteins carry a single solute across the membrane. Symport proteins translocate two different solutes simultaneously in the same direction; transport occurs only if both solutes bind to the proteins. Antiport proteins exchange two solutes by transporting one into the cell and the other out of the cell.

🇰 🇭 ORGANISMAL BIOLOGY

Living organisms must maintain constant interior conditions in a changing environment. The interior environment that cells must maintain includes water volume and salt concentration, as well as appropriate levels of oxygen, carbon dioxide, toxic metabolic waste products, and essential nutrients. Organisms must respond to their environment to avoid harm and seek out beneficial conditions; they must also reproduce. Single-cell organisms like prokaryotes or protists have relatively simple ways to meet these needs, while multicellular organisms have evolved more complex body plans that provide a variety of solutions to the common problems all organisms face. As multicellular organisms have over time evolved into larger and more complex forms, their cells have become removed from the external environment and specialized toward one specific function. These specialized cells form **tissues**, cells with a common function and often a similar form. Cells from different tissues come together to form **organs**, large anatomical structures made from several tissues working together toward a common goal. Organs, in turn, are part of organ systems that are the basis for digestion, respiration, circulation, immune reactions, excretion, and reproduction, among others.

Reproduction

One of the essential functions for all living things is the ability to reproduce, to produce offspring that will allow a species to continue. An individual organism can survive without reproducing, but if an entire species does not reproduce, it will not survive past a single generation. The reproduction of eukaryotes can occur either asexually or sexually. Prokaryotes have a different mechanism called **binary fission** for reproduction.

Cell Division

One of the inherent features in reproduction is cell division. Prokaryotic cells divide and reproduce through the relatively simple process of binary fission. Eukaryotic cells divide by one of two mechanisms: mitosis or meiosis. **Mitosis** is a process in which cells divide to produce two daughter cells with the same genomic complement as the parent cell; in the case of humans there are two copies of the genome in each cell. Mitotic cell division can be a means of asexual reproduction; it is also the mechanism for the growth, development, and replacement of tissues. **Meiosis** is a specialized form of cell division involved in sexual reproduction that produces male and female gametes (sperm and ova, respectively). Meiotic cell division creates cells with a single copy of the genome in preparation for sexual reproduction. During reproduction, gametes join to create a new organism with two copies of the genome, one from each parent.

Prokaryotic Cell Division and Reproduction

Prokaryotes are single-celled organisms and their mechanism for cell division, binary fission, is also their means of reproduction. As with all forms of cell division, one of the key steps is DNA replication. Prokaryotes have no organelles and only one chromosome in a single, long, circular DNA strand. The single prokaryotic chromosome is attached to the cell membrane and replicated as the cell grows. With two copies of the genome attached to the membrane after DNA replication, the DNAs are drawn apart from each other as the cell grows in size and adds more membrane between the DNAs.

When the cell grows to the size of multiple cells, the cell wall and membrane close off to create two independent cells. The simplicity of prokaryotic cells and the small size of their genome (in comparison to eukaryotes) may be a factor that assists in their rapid rate of reproduction. They are able to divide as rapidly as once every 30 minutes under ideal conditions. Bacteria and other prokaryotes do not reproduce sexually, but they do exchange genetic material with each other in some cases. **Conjugation** is one mechanism used by bacteria to move genes between cells by exchanging circular, extrachromosomal DNA with each other.

Mitosis

Eukaryotic cells use mitosis to divide into two new daughter cells with the same genome as the parent cell. During what is known as the **cell cycle**, cells grow and divide, creating new cells. The cell cycle is a highly regulated process, linked to the growth and differentiation of tissues. Growth factors can stimulate cells to move through the cell cycle more rapidly; there are also various other factors that can induce cells to differentiate and stop moving forward through the cell cycle. Failure to control the cell cycle properly can result in uncontrolled progression through the cell cycle, which can lead to cancer. Cancer cells contain mutations in genes that regulate the cell cycle. The four stages of the cell cycle are designated as G_1, S, G_2, and M. The first three stages of this cell cycle are interphase stages—that is, they occur between cell divisions. The fourth stage, mitosis, includes the actual division of the cell.

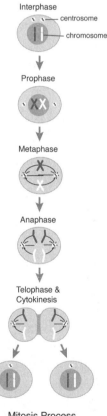

Mitosis Process

During mitosis and cytokinesis, the cell divides to create two similar but smaller daughter cells. Mitosis is further broken down into four stages: prophase, metaphase, anaphase, and telophase. Late prophase is often regarded as a separate step, prometaphase. Upon completion of mitosis, the cell completes its split into daughter cells through the process of cytokinesis.

Asexual Reproduction

Asexual reproduction is any method of producing new organisms in which fusion of nuclei from two individuals (fertilization) does not take place. In asexual reproduction, only one parent organism is involved. New organisms produced through asexual reproduction form daughter cells through mitotic cell division and are genetically identical clones of their parents. Asexual reproduction serves primarily as a mechanism for perpetuating primitive organisms and plants, especially in times of low population density. Asexual reproduction can allow more rapid population growth than sexual reproduction, but does not create the great genetic diversity that sexual reproduction does.

Sexual Reproduction

Most multicellular animals and plants reproduce sexually, as do many protists and fungi. **Sexual reproduction** involves the union of a **haploid cell** from two different parents, producing diploid offspring. These haploid cells are **gametes**—sex cells produced through meiosis in males and females. Haploid gametes have a single copy of the genome (one of each chromosome), and diploid cells have two copies of the genome (two of each chromosome). In humans, all of the cells of the body are diploid, with the exception of the gametes. When the male gamete (the sperm) and the female gamete (the egg) join, a **zygote** is formed that develops into a new organism genetically distinct from both its parents. The zygote is the diploid single-cell offspring, formed from the union of haploid gametes. Sexual reproduction ensures genetic diversity and variability in offspring. Since sexual reproduction is more costly in energy than asexual reproduction, the reason for its overwhelming prevalence must be that genetic diversity is worth the effort.

Sexual reproduction, however, does not create new alleles (different forms of a gene). Only mutation can do that. Sexual reproduction increases diversity in populations by creating new combinations of alleles in offspring and therefore new combinations of traits. Genetic diversity is not an advantage to an individual, but allows a population of organisms to adapt and survive in the face of a dynamic and unpredictable environment. The diversity created by sexual reproduction occurs in part during meiotic gamete production and in part through the random matching of gametes to make unique individuals.

Gamete Formation

Specialized organs called **gonads** produce gametes through meiotic cell division. Male gonads, **testes**, produce male gametes, **spermatozoa**, while female gonads, **ovaries**, produce **ova**. A cell that is committed to the production of gametes, which is not itself a gamete, is called a **germ cell**. The rest of the cells of the body are called **somatic cells**. Only the genomes of germ cells contribute to gametes and offspring. A mutation in a somatic cell, for example, may be harmful to that cell or the organism if it leads to cancer, but a mutation in a somatic cell will not affect offspring since the mutation will not be found in germ cell genomes. Germ cells are themselves diploid and divide to create more germ cells through the process of mitosis, but create the haploid gametes through meiosis. The production of both male and female gametes involves meiotic cell division. Meiosis during both spermatogenesis and oogenesis involves two rounds of cell division in which a single diploid cell first replicates its genome, and then divides into two cells, each with two copies of the genome. Without replicating their DNA, these two cells divide again to produce four haploid gametes. Meiosis in both cases also involves recombination between the homologous copies of chromosomes during the first round of meiotic cell division.

Meiosis

During asexual reproduction, a single diploid cell is used to create new identical copies of an organism. Two parents contributing to the genome of offspring characterize sexual reproduction, the end result being offspring that are genetically unique. This process requires that each parent contribute a cell with one copy of the genome. **Meiosis** is the process whereby these sex cells are produced.

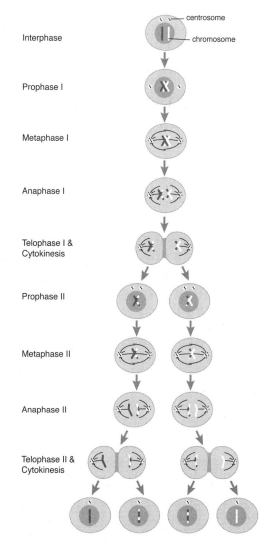

Meiosis Process

As in mitosis, the gametocyte's chromosomes are replicated during the **S phase** of the cell cycle. The first round of division (**meiosis I**) produces two intermediate daughter cells. The second round of division (**meiosis II**) involves the separation of the sister chromatids, resulting in four genetically distinct haploid gametes. In this way, a diploid cell produces haploid daughter cells. Since meiosis reduces the number of chromosomes in each cell from $2n$ to $1n$, it is sometimes called **reductive division**. Each meiotic division has the same four stages as mitosis, although it goes through each of them twice (except for DNA replication).

⒣ PLANTS

Plants are so distinct in their body form and so important to life on Earth that we present their physiology separately. Plants are multicellular autotrophs that use the energy of the sun, carbon dioxide, water, and minerals to manufacture carbohydrates through photosynthesis. The chemical energy plants produce is used for respiration by the plants themselves and is the source of all chemical energy in most ecosystems. The life cycle of vascular plants is distinct from that of animals, alternating between diploid and haploid forms in each generation.

Plant Organs

Although we may not usually think of plants as having organs, the fact is that roots, stems, and leaves each have a defined function and are composed of tissues that perform distinct functions, in the same manner as animal organs. Stems provide support against gravity and allow for the transport of fluid through vascular tissue. Water travels upward from the roots to the leaves and nutrients travel from the leaves down through the rest of the plant. The roots provide anchoring support, and also remove water and essential minerals from the soil. Another important plant tissue is the **phloem**. The phloem transports nutrients from the leaves to the rest of the plant. This nutrient liquid is commonly called sap. Cells present in the phloem are alive when they perform their transport function. The phloem cells are tube-shaped; liquid sap moves through the tube-shaped cells. Like terrestrial animals, plants need a protective coating. For plants, an external layer of epidermis cells provides this. Another plant tissue is the **ground tissue**, involved in storage and support.

Plant Cells

Plant cells have all of the same essential organelles as other eukaryotic cells, including mitochondria, ER, Golgi, and nucleus. A major distinction of plant cells is the presence of the photosynthetic organelle known as the **chloroplast**. Some plant cells contain large storage vacuoles not found in animal cells. Another distinct feature of plant cells is their cell wall. On the outside of its plasma membrane, each plant cell is surrounded by a stiff cell wall made of **cellulose**. The cellulose cell wall helps to provide structure and support for the plant. From grasses to trees, plants rely on the cellulose present in cell walls to help provide support against gravity.

Phyla

Within the plant kingdom there are several major phyla. One of the major distinctions for these plant groups is whether or not a plant has vascular tissue for the transport of fluids. Plants without vascular tissue are small, simple plants called **nontracheophytes**; mosses are an example of this group. The rest of plants—including pines, ferns, and flowering plants—are known as **tracheophytes**.

The evolution of vascular tissue was an important step in the colonization of land by plants, since it increases the support of plants against gravity, and increases their ability to survive dry conditions.

Asexual Reproduction in Plants

Many plants utilize asexual reproduction, such as **vegetative propagation**, to increase their numbers. Vegetative propagation offers a number of advantages to plants, including speed of reproduction, lack of genetic variation, and the ability to produce seedless fruit. This process can occur either naturally or artificially.

Sexual Reproduction in Plants

Most plants are able to reproduce both sexually and asexually; some do both in the course of their life cycles, while others do one or the other. Ferns are a phylum of tracheophytes that do not produce seeds for reproduction—they employ spores instead. In the life cycles of ferns and other vascular plants, there are two stages associated with life cycles: **diploid** and **haploid**.

Diploid and Haploid Generations

In the diploid or **sporophyte** generation, the asexual stage of a plant's life cycle, diploid nuclei divide meiotically to form haploid spores (not gametes) and the spores germinate to produce the haploid (or gametophyte) generation. The **gametophyte** generation is a separate haploid form of the plant concerned with the production of male and female gametes. Union of the gametes at fertilization restores the diploid sporophyte generation. Since there are two distinct generations, one haploid and the other diploid, this cycle is sometimes referred to as the **alternation of generations**. The relative lengths of the two stages vary with the plant type. In general, the evolutionary trend has been toward a reduction of the gametophyte generation and increasing importance of the sporophyte generation.

Sexual Reproduction in Flowering Plants

In flowering plants, also known as angiosperms, the evolutionary trend mentioned above continues; the gametophyte consists of only a few cells and survives for a very short time.

Flowers

The flower is the organ for sexual reproduction present in angiosperms; it consists of male and female organs. The flower's male organ is known as the **stamen**. It consists of a thin, stalk-like filament with a sac at the top. This structure is called the **anther**, and it produces

KAPLAN

haploid spores. The haploid spores develop into pollen grains. The haploid nuclei within the spores become sperm nuclei, which fertilize the ovum. Meanwhile, the flower's female organ is termed a **pistil**. It consists of three parts: the **stigma**, the **style**, and the **ovary**. The stigma is the sticky top part of the flower, protruding beyond the flower, which catches pollen. The tube-like structure connecting the stigma to the ovary at the base of the pistil is known as the style; this organ permits the sperm to reach the ovules. And the ovary, the enlarged base of the pistil, which is often the fruit of the plant, contains one or more ovules. Each ovule contains the monoploid egg nucleus.

Petals are specialized leaves that surround and protect the pistil. They attract insects with their characteristic colors and odors. This attraction is essential for cross-pollination—that is, the transfer of pollen from the anther of one flower to the stigma of another (introducing genetic variability). Note that some species of plants have flowers that contain only stamens (these plants are known as male plants) while others contain only pistils (these are known as female plants).

Male gametophytes (pollen grains) develop from the spores made by the sporophyte (for example, a rose bush). Pollen grains are transferred from the anther to the stigma. Agents of cross-pollination include insects, wind, and water. The flower's reproductive organ is brightly colored and fragrant in order to attract insects and birds, which help to spread male gametophytes. Pollen being carried directly from plant to plant is more efficient than relying on wind to do so; it also helps to prevent self-pollination, which does not create diversity. When the pollen grain reaches the stigma (pollination), it releases enzymes that enable it to absorb and utilize both food and water from the stigma, as well as to germinate a pollen tube. The pollen tube is what remains of the evolutionary gametophyte. The pollen's enzymes proceed to digest a path down the pistil to the ovary. Within the pollen tube are the haploid tube nucleus and two sperm nuclei. **Female gametophytes** develop in the ovule from one of four spores. This embryo sac contains nuclei, including the two polar (**endosperm**) nuclei and an egg nucleus.

The gametes involved in fertilization are nuclei, not complete cells. The sperm nucleus of the male gametophyte (pollen tube) enters the female gametophyte (embryo sac), and double fertilization occurs. One sperm nucleus fuses with the egg nucleus to form the diploid zygote, which develops into the embryo. The other sperm nucleus fuses with the two polar bodies to form the **endosperm** (**triploid** or **3n**). The endosperm provides food for the embryonic plant.

There is definitely more to know about flowers, but for now, this should cover the topics you might face on your nursing school entrance exam.

Ⓗ CLASSICAL GENETICS

The study of patterns and mechanisms in the transmission of inherited traits from one generation to another is known as classical genetics. The foundations for this field were laid by the monk Gregor Mendel, who in the mid-nineteenth century performed a series of experiments to determine the rules of inheritance in garden pea plants.

The study of classical genetics requires an understanding of meiosis, the mechanism of gamete formation. Mendel knew that alleles are inherited from each parent, and that these alleles were somehow linked to the various characteristics he studied in peas, but it was not until meiosis was truly elucidated that the mechanisms behind heredity were understood.

Mendelian Genetics

Around 1865, based on his observations of seven characteristics of the garden pea, Mendel developed the basic principles of genetics—**dominance**, **segregation**, and **independent assortment**. Although Mendel formulated these principles, he was unable to propose any mechanism for hereditary patterns, since he knew nothing about chromosomes or genes. Hence his work was largely ignored until the early 1900s.

After Mendel's work was rediscovered, Thomas H. Morgan tied the principles of genetics to the chromosome theory. He linked particular traits to regions of specific chromosomes visible in the salivary glands of the fruit fly *Drosophila melanogaster*. Morgan brought to light the giant chromosomes that are found in the fruit fly's salivary glands—they are at least 100 times the size of normal chromosomes. These chromosomes are banded, and the bands coincide with gene locations, allowing geneticists to see major changes in the fly genome. Morgan also described sex-linked genes. The fruit fly is a highly suitable organism for genetic research. With its short life cycle, it reproduces often and in large numbers, providing large sample sizes. It is easy to breed in a laboratory, and has a fairly complex body structure. Its chromosomes are large and easily recognizable in both size and shape, but few in number (eight chromosomes and four pairs of chromosomes). Finally, mutations occur relatively frequently in this organism, allowing genes of affected traits to be studied.

There are several basic rules of gene transmission and expression.

- **Genes** are elements of DNA that are responsible for observed traits.
- In eukaryotes, genes are found in large, linear chromosomes, and each chromosome is a very long, continuous DNA double helix.
- Humans have 23 different chromosomes, with two copies of each chromosome in most cells.
- Each chromosome contains a specific sequence and arrangement of genes.
- Each gene has a specific location on a chromosome.
- Diploid organisms have two copies of each chromosome and therefore two copies of each gene (except for the **X** and **Y** chromosomes in males).
- The two copies of each gene can have a different sequence in an organism and a gene can have several different sequences in a population. These different versions of a gene are called **alleles**.
- The type of alleles an organism has—that is, its genetic composition—is called the **genotype**.
- The appearance and physical expression of genes in an organism are called the **phenotype**.

- Types of alleles include dominant and recessive alleles. A dominant allele is expressed in an organism regardless of the second allele in the organism. A recessive allele will not be expressed if the other allele an organism carries is a dominant one.
- A **homozygous** individual has two copies (two alleles) of a gene that are identical and a **heterozygous** individual has two different alleles for a gene.
- The phenotype of an individual is determined by the genotype.

Dominant Versus Recessive

If two members of a pure-breeding strain are mated, their offspring will always have the same phenotype as their parents because they are all homozygous for the same allele. What happens if two different pure-breeding strains that are homozygous for two different alleles are crossed? A good example is a flower that has its color determined by two different alleles. All of the offspring of the cross-match utilize the phenotype of one parent and not the other. For example, if a pure-breeding red strain is crossed with a pure-breeding white one, the offspring may all be red. Where did the allele coding for the white trait go? Did it disappear from the offspring? If it is true that both parents contribute one copy of a gene to each of their offspring, then the allele cannot disappear. The offspring must all contain both a white allele and a red allele. Despite having both alleles, they only express one. To continue the example, the red allele would be considered the dominant allele and white a recessive allele.

Every human has two copies of each of their 23 chromosomes, with the exception of the **X** and **Y** chromosome in men. Thus, each gene is present in two copies that can either be the same or different. For example, a gene for eye color could have two alleles: **B** or **b**. **B** is a **dominant allele** for brown eye color and **b** is a **recessive allele** for blue eye color. There are three potential genotypes: **BB**, **Bb**, or **bb**. Individuals with the BB or Bb genotype have brown eyes. Because the **B** allele is dominant and the recessive **b** allele is not expressed in the heterozygote, only people with the homozygous **bb** genotype have blue eyes.

Test Crosses

Often, a geneticist will study the transmission of a trait in a species by performing crosses (matings) between organisms with defined traits. For example, an investigator may identify two possible phenotypes for flower color in pea plants: pink and white. Pink plants bred together always produce pink offspring and white plants bred together always produce offspring with white flowers. It is likely that the differences in flower color are caused by different alleles in a gene that controls flower color. Which of these traits is determined by a recessive or dominant allele? You cannot tell based on the color alone which trait will be dominant or recessive. Either pink or white could be dominant—or neither. The way to determine the dominant or recessive nature of each allele is by performing a test cross. Since the pink plants always produce pink plants and the white plants always produce white plants, these are both termed **pure-breeding** plants and are each homozygous for either the **P** allele (**PP** genotype has a pink phenotype) or for the **p** allele (**pp** genotype has a white phenotype). What will be the phenotype of a plant with the **Pp** genotype?

Punnett Square

When performing a test cross, a useful tool is called a **Punnett square**. To perform a Punnett square, first determine the possible gametes each parent in the cross can produce. In the example above, a **PP** parent can only make gametes with the **P** allele and the **pp** parent can only make gametes with the **p** allele:

- **PP** parent: Gametes have either one **P** allele or the other **P** allele.
- **pp** parent: Gametes have either one **p** allele or the other **p** allele.

The next step is to examine all of the ways these gametes could combine if these two parents were mated together in a test cross. This is where the Punnett square comes in. On one side of the square, align the gametes from one parent, and across the top of the square, align the gametes from the other parent. At the intersection of each potential gamete pairing, fill in the square with the diploid zygote produced by matching the alleles. In this example, all of the offspring of this cross are going to be heterozygous.

If all of the offspring are pink, what does this reveal about the nature of these alleles? If the heterozygous **Pp** plant has the same phenotype as the homozygous **PP** plant, then the **P** allele is dominant over the **p** allele. The offspring of this cross (shown within the box) can be called the F_1 generation.

A cross between two pure-breeding strains (F_1 generation):

	P	*P*
p	*Pp*	*Pp*
p	*Pp*	*Pp*

The F_1 offspring all have the **Pp** genotype and the pink phenotype. What will occur if two of these F_1 plants are crossed? A Punnett square can be used again to predict the genotypes in the F_2 generation.

- Parent 1: **P** and **p** gametes are produced.
- Parent 2: **P** and **p** gametes are produced.

F_2 generation Punnett square:

	P	*p*
P	*PP*	*Pp*
p	*Pp*	*pp*

Since we know the **P** allele for pink is dominant, we can use the genotypes to predict phenotypes of the F_2 generation. **PP** homozygotes will be pink, and **Pp** heterozygotes will also be pink since **P** is dominant. Like the original pure-breeding white plants, **pp** plants will be white.

KAPLAN

	P	*p*
P	*PP* (pink)	*Pp* (pink)
p	*Pp* (pink)	*pp* (white)

The ratios of the different genotypes and phenotypes in the Punnett square should match the statistical probability of what would be produced by such a cross. For example, if two heterozygous **Pp** plants are crossed, 75% of the offspring will be pink and 25% white. This prediction from the Punnett square is based on the ratio of 3:1 for phenotypes that will produce pink (3) to white (1).

The different pea plant traits helped Mendel formulate the two fundamental rules of Mendelian genetics, the Law of Segregation and the Law of Independent Assortment. Mendel derived these rules based purely on his knowledge of the transmission of traits, without knowing anything about the molecular basis for his observations or the mechanisms of meiosis.

Law of Segregation

The Law of Segregation states that if there are two alleles in an individual that determine a trait, these two alleles will separate during gamete formation and act independently. For example, when a heterozygous **Pp** plant is forming gametes, the **P** and the **p** alleles can separate into different gametes and act independently during a cross. If this were not the case, and the **P** and **p** alleles could not separate, then all of the offspring would remain **Pp** and all of the F_2 would be pink. The fact that white offspring are produced indicates that alleles do indeed segregate into gametes independently. The molecular basis for this observation is that during meiosis, each homologous chromosome carrying two different alleles will end up in a different haploid gamete.

Law of Independent Assortment

The Law of Independent Assortment describes the relationship between different genes. If the gene that determines plant height is on a different chromosome than the gene for flower color, then these traits will act independently during test crosses.

Linkage

There is a significant exception to the Law of Independent Assortment. For genes to assort independently into gametes during meiosis, they must be on different chromosomes. If two genes are located near each other on the same chromosome, then the alleles for these genes will stay together during meiosis. The phenomenon in which alleles fail to assort independently because they are on the same chromosome is called **linkage**.

Inheritance Patterns

Ethical restraints forbid geneticists from performing test crosses in human populations. Instead, they must rely on examining matings that have already occurred, using tools such as pedigrees. A **pedigree** is a family tree depicting the inheritance of a particular genetic trait over several generations. By convention, males are indicated by squares and females by circles. Matings are indicated by horizontal lines, and descendants are listed below matings, connected by a vertical line. Individuals affected by a particular trait are generally shaded, while the symbols for unaffected individuals are left unshaded. When carriers of sex-linked traits have been identified (typically, female heterozygotes), they are usually half shaded.

The sample pedigrees illustrate two types of heritable traits: recessive disorders and sex-linked disorders. When analyzing a pedigree, look for individuals with the recessive phenotype. Such individuals have only one possible genotype—homozygous recessive. Matings between them and the dominant phenotype behave as test crosses; the ratio of phenotypes among the offspring allows deduction of the dominant genotype. In any case where only males are affected, sex linkage should be suspected.

Recessive Disorders

Note how the autosomal recessive disorder presented in the following figure has skipped a generation. Albinism is an example of this form of disorder.

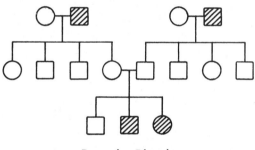

Recessive Disorder

Sex-Linked Disorders

Gender skewing is evident in this type of disorder, which includes traits such as hemophilia. Sex-linked recessive alleles are almost always expressed only by males and transmitted from one generation to another by female carriers.

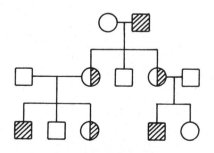

Sex-Linked Disorder

Non-Mendelian Inheritance Patterns

While Mendel's laws hold true in many cases, these laws cannot explain the results of certain crosses. Sometimes an allele is only incompletely dominant or, perhaps, codominant. The genetics that enable the human species to have two genders would also not be possible under Mendel's laws.

Incomplete Dominance

Incomplete dominance is a blending of the effects of contrasting alleles. Both alleles are expressed partially, neither dominating the other. An example of incomplete dominance is found in the four o'clock plant and the snapdragon flower. When a red flower (**RR**) is crossed with a white flower (**WW**), a pink blend (**RW**) is created. When two pink flowers are crossed, the yield is 25% red, 50% pink, and 25% white (phenotypic and genotypic ratio 1:2:1).

Codominance

In a pattern of codominance, both alleles are fully expressed without one allele being dominant over the other. An example is blood types. Blood type is determined by the expression of antigen proteins on the surface of red blood cells. The **A** allele and the **B** allele are codominant if both are present, combining to produce AB blood.

Sex Determination

Most organisms have two types of chromosomes: **autosomes**, which determine most of an organism's body characteristics, and **sex chromosomes**, which determine the sex of an organism. Humans have 22 pairs of autosomes and one pair of sex chromosomes. The sex chromosomes are known as **X** and **Y**. In humans, **XX** is present in females and **XY** in males. The Y chromosome carries very few genes. As all eggs contain X chromosomes only, sex is determined at the time of fertilization by the type of sperm fertilizing the egg. If the sperm carries an X chromosome, the offspring will be female (**XX**); if the sperm carries a Y chromosome, the offspring will be male (**XY**).

This process is illustrated in the Punnett square that follows.

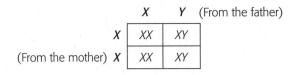

The ratio of the sex of the offspring is 1:1.

Sex Linkage

Genes for certain traits, such as color blindness or hemophilia, are located on the X chromosomes. Hence these genes are linked with the genes controlling sex determination. These genes seem to have no corresponding allele on the Y chromosome, with the result that the X chromosome contributed by the mother is the sole determinant of these traits in males.

Mutations

Mutations can create new alleles, the raw material that drives evolution via natural selection. Mutations are changes in the genes that are inherited. To be transmitted to the succeeding generation, mutations must occur in sex cells—eggs and sperm—rather than somatic cells (body cells). Mutations in non-sex cells are called somatic cell mutations and affect only the individual involved, not subsequent generations. A somatic mutation can cause cancer, but will have no affect on offspring since it is not present in gametes. Many mutations are recessive and harmful. Because they are recessive, these mutations can be masked or hidden by the dominant normal genes.

Chromosomal Mutations

These mutations result in changes in chromosomal structure or abnormal chromosome duplication. In crossing over, segments of chromosomes switch positions during meiotic synapsis. This process breaks linkage patterns normally observed when the genes are on the same chromosome. A translocation is an event in which a piece of a chromosome breaks off and rejoins a different chromosome.

Ⓗ EVOLUTION AND DIVERSITY

In this section, we'll be covering topics ranging from types of evidence for evolution to the taxonomic classification of various common species.

Evidence of Evolution

Evolution provides a sweeping framework for the understanding of the diversity of life on Earth. Living systems—which include cells, organisms, and ecosystems—arose over geologic time, selected out of diverse possibilities. What is the evidence that supports the evolutionary view of life? The evidence takes several forms.

The Fossil Record

Fossils are preserved impressions or remains in rocks of living organisms from the past. Fossils provide some of the most direct and compelling evidence of evolutionary change and are generally found in sedimentary rock. After death, animals' remains can be embedded in the sediment. These sediments then might be covered over with additional layers of sediment that turn to rock through exposure to heat and pressure over many millions of years. The embedded remains turn to stone, replaced with minerals that preserve an impression of the form of the organism, often in a quite detailed state. Most fossils are of the hard, bony parts of animals, since these are preserved the most easily. Fossils of soft body parts or of invertebrates are much more unusual, more than likely because these parts usually decay before fossil formation can occur. In some cases, however, animals that died in anaerobic sediments have resisted decay and have provided soft-body fossils.

When a fossil is discovered, its age must be determined in order to place it correctly in the timeline of life on Earth. One way to place the date is to compare the location of the fossil sediment to other sedimentary rock formations in which the age is already known. Dating using **radioactive decay** (carbon dating) is also very useful. Carbon dating is frequently used for material that is only a few thousand years old, but cannot be used for older material since the decay rate of carbon is too rapid.

The conditions for fossil formation are relatively particular, especially for the preservation of invertebrates or soft body parts. Scientists locate fossils by luck, and can only look at a tiny percentage of possible fossil locations. A great variety of fossils have been located, including fossils that provide a clear story of the evolution of modern species.

Fossils have revealed that the archaeopteryx is an example of a feathered dinosaur that was probably an intermediate species in the evolution of birds. Changes that have appeared in fossils created during various frames of time have provided a great deal of insight into the evolutionary paths that resulted in modern species including horses, whales, and humans. Any of the so-called "gaps" in the fossil record are probably the result of the scarcity of fossils and difficulty in finding them, and is not evidence that evolution did not occur.

Comparative Anatomy

One way to find an evolutionary relationship between organisms is by examining their external and internal anatomy. Animals that evolved from a common ancestor might share anatomical features with that common ancestor. Alternatively, two organisms might share features that look the same but evolved from different ancestors and resulted in similar structures as a result of similar functions. When we compare the anatomies of two or more living organisms, not only can we form hypotheses about their common ancestors, but we can also glean clues that shed light upon the selective pressures that led to the development of certain adaptations, such as the ability to fly. Comparative anatomists study **homologous** and **analogous structures** in organisms.

Homologous Structures

Homologous structures have the same basic anatomical features and evolutionary origins. They demonstrate similar evolutionary patterns with late divergence of form due to differences in exposure to evolutionary forces. Examples of homologous structures include the wings of bats, the flippers of whales, the forelegs of horses, and the arms of humans. These structures were all derived from a common ancestor but diverged to perform different functions in what is termed **divergent evolution**.

Analogous Structures

Analogous structures have similar functions but may have different evolutionary origins and entirely different patterns of development. The wings of a fly (membranous) and the wings of a bird (bony and covered in feathers) are analogous structures that have evolved to perform a similar function—to fly. The wings of flies and birds might look the same but this does not indicate that they share a winged ancestor. When structures look the same and share a common function but are not derived from a common ancestor, it is called **convergent evolution**. Analogous organs demonstrate superficial resemblances that cannot be used as a basis for classification.

Comparative Embryology

Comparison of embryonic structures and routes of embryo development is another way to derive evolutionary relationships. The development of the human embryo is very similar to the development of other vertebrate embryos. Adult tunicates (sea squirts) and amphibians lack a notochord (a stiff, solid dorsal rod), one of the key traits of the chordate phylum, but their embryos both possess notochords during development. This indicates these animals are in fact vertebrates with a common evolutionary ancestor even though the adults do not resemble each other. The earlier that embryonic development diverges, the more dissimilar the mature organisms are. Thus, it is difficult to differentiate between the embryo of a human and that of an ape until relatively late in the development of each embryo, while human and sea-urchin embryos diverge much earlier.

Other embryonic evidence of evolution includes characteristics such as the teeth that appear in an avian embryo (recalling the reptile stage); the resemblance of larval mollusks (shellfish) to annelids (segmented worms); and the tail that is present on the human embryo for a period of time (indicating relationships to other mammals).

Molecular Evolution

If organisms are derived from a common ancestor, this should be evident not just at the anatomical level but also the molecular level. The traits that distinguish one organism from another are ultimately derived from differences in genes. With the advent of molecular biology, the genes and proteins of organisms can be compared to determine their evolutionary relationship. The closer the genetic sequences of organisms are to each other, the more closely their evolutionary progression has been related and the more recently they diverged from a common ancestor. Some genes change rapidly during evolution, while others have changed extremely slowly. The rate of change in a gene over time is called the **molecular clock**. The rate of change in a gene's sequence is probably a function of the level of resistance a gene has to changes.

Genes that change very slowly over extremely long periods of time do not tolerate change very well and play key roles in the life of cells and organisms. Ribosomal RNA has changed slowly enough that it can be used to compare organisms all the way back to the divergence of eukaryotes, bacteria, and archaebacteria. The enzymes involved in glycolysis play an essential role in energy production for all life; they also evolve very slowly, allowing comparison of their genetic sequences and illuminating evolutionary relationships over billions of years. Computers can be used to compare the gene sequences of many organisms, allowing researchers to determine how long ago organisms evolved from a common ancestor. Genes that have evolved over a more recent period of time and genes that evolve more rapidly can be used to analyze recent evolutionary events.

Vestigial Structures

Vestigial structures are structures that appear to be useless in the context of a particular modern-day organism's behavior and environment. It is apparent, however, that these structures had some function in an earlier stage of a particular organism's evolution. They serve as evidence of an organism's evolution over time, and can help scientists to trace its evolutionary path. There are many examples of vestigial structures in humans, other animals, and plants. The appendix—small and seemingly useless in humans—assists digestion of cellulose in herbivores, indicating a vegetarian ancestry in humans.

Mechanisms of Evolution

The Population as the Basic Unit of Evolution

Evolution is the change a species undergoes over time. These changes are the result of modifications in the gene pool of a population of organisms. Evolution does not happen in one individual, but in a population of organisms. What is a population? A **population** is a group of individuals in a particular species that interbreed.

In classical genetics, it is observed that a genotype of organisms produces their phenotype, the physical expression of inherited traits. A population of organisms includes individuals with a range of phenotypes and genotypes. However, it is possible to describe a population by certain traits exhibited by the group as a whole, such as the abundance of particular alleles. The sum total of all alleles in a population is called the **gene pool**, and the frequency with which a specific allele appears in a gene pool is called the **allele frequency**. Each individual receives its specific set of alleles from the gene pool, and not every individual receives the same alleles, leading to individual variation in genotypes and phenotypes. All of these allow for mixing of alleles in a population to create variation in individual genotypes and phenotypes. Mutation in a population can create new alleles. Evolution is caused by changes in the gene pool of a population over time, as a result of changes to individuals in a population caused by the alleles they carry.

Speciation

A **species** is a group of organisms that is able to successfully interbreed with each other to produce fertile offspring. They cannot successfully interbreed with other organisms. The key to defining a species is not external appearance. Within a species, there can be great phenotypic variation, as in domesticated dogs. What defines a biological species is reproductive isolation, an inability to interbreed and create fertile offspring. Horses and donkeys can interbreed and create offspring, mules. However, mules are sterile, meaning the horses and donkeys are two different species.

Classification and Taxonomy

Evolution has created a great diversity of organisms on Earth, but these organisms are related to each other through common ancestors they shared in the history of life. By examining organisms for common features and common ancestors, it should be possible to make sense of the diversity of life by grouping organisms into categories. The science of classifying living things and using a system of nomenclature to name them is called **taxonomy**. Carolus Linnaeus invented modern taxonomy in the 1700s, grouping organisms by physical and structural similarities and naming them according to a hierarchical system.

Modern classification systems seek to build on Linnaeus' system and also group organisms on the basis of evolutionary relationships. The bat, whale, horse, and human are placed in the same class of animals (mammals) because they are believed to have descended from a common ancestor. The taxonomist classifies all species known to have descended from the same common ancestor within the same broad taxonomic group.

Since much about early evolutionary history is not understood, there is some disagreement among biologists as to the best classification system to employ, particularly with regard to groups of unicellular organisms. Taxonomic organization proceeds from the largest, broadest group to the smaller, more specific subgroups. The largest group, known as a domain, contains the six kingdoms. Each kingdom is broken down into smaller and smaller subdivisions. Members of each smaller group have more specific characteristics in common. Furthermore, each subgroup is distinguishable from the next. The names used to classify these systems are subject to discussion and revision as time and research yields new insights into the relationships between organisms.

Some classifications are clearer than others. Viruses are obligate intracellular parasites that cannot conduct metabolic activities or replicate on their own. As such, they are not generally considered living, although they are certainly important to living systems. They are not classified within taxonomic systems, however.

Classification and Subdivisions

All life on Earth is classified into three **domains**—Bacteria, Archaea, and Eukarya. Typically, living organisms have been separated into prokaryotes and eukaryotes. The prokaryotes include bacteria and archaebacteria. Like the bacteria, archaebacteria have no organelles and have a simple circular DNA genome. Archaebacteria were relatively unknown until recently because they tend to inhabit harsh environments like hot springs and thermal ocean vents, which may resemble the early Earth. Archaebacteria are distinct from bacteria in many ways and appear to be more closely related to eukaryotes than prokaryotes. For this reason, bacteria and archaebacteria are classified separately.

These three domains are divided into six kingdoms:

Domain	Kingdom(s)
Archaea	Archaebacteria
Bacteria	Eubacteria
Eukarya	Protista Fungi Plantae Animalia

Each **kingdom** has several major divisions known as phyla. A **phylum** has several **subphyla**, which are further divided into **classes**. Each class consists of many **orders**, and these orders are subdivided into **families**. Each family is made up of a **genus** or many **genera**. Finally, the **species** is the smallest subdivision.

The Kingdoms	
Archaebacteria	Live in extreme environments such as swamp, hydrothermal deep-ocean vents, and sea water evaporating ponds. Several hundred species have been identified since their discovery. Archaebacteria differ from bacteria in the composition of their membrane lipids and cell walls and the sequence of nucleic acids in their ribosomal RNA.
Eubacteria	Considered "true" bacteria. Represents all other prokaryotes including blue-green algae and primitive pathogens.
Protista	The simplest eukaryotes (cells have nuclei). Includes protozoa, unicellular and multicellular algae, and slime molds. Ancestor organisms to plants, animals, and fungi; most can move around by means of flagella.
Fungi	Includes mushrooms, bread molds, and yeasts. Fungi lack the ability to photosynthesize, so they are called decomposers, breaking down and feeding on dead protoplasm.
Plantae	Have the ability to photosynthesize, so they are called producers. There are two major phyla, Bryophyta, or mosses, and Tracheophyta, which have vascular systems and include most of the plants you know.
Animalia	Produce energy by consuming other organisms, so they are called consumers. Can be either vertebrates—phylum Chordata—or invertebrates such as mollusks, arthropods, sponges, coelenterates, worms, etc.

Hence, the order of classificatory divisions is as follows:

DOMAIN → KINGDOM → PHYLUM → SUBPHYLUM → CLASS → ORDER → FAMILY → GENUS → SPECIES

The complete classification of humans is:

Domain: *Eukarya*

Kingdom: *Animalia*

Phylum: *Chordata*

Subphylum: *Vertebrata*

Class: *Mammalia*

Order: *Primates*

Family: *Hominidae*

Genus: *Homo*

Species: *Sapiens*

Assignment of Scientific Names

All organisms are assigned a scientific name consisting of the genus and species names of that organism. Thus, a human is a *Homo sapiens*, and the common house cat is *Felis domestica*.

Kingdom Eubacteria

The ubiquitous bacteria are single-celled, lack true nuclei, lack a cytoskeleton, and contain double-stranded circular chromosomal DNA that is not enclosed by a nuclear membrane. These creatures nourish themselves heterotrophically—either saprophytically or parasitically—or autotrophically, depending upon the species. Bacteria are classified by their morphological appearance: cocci (round), bacilli (rods), and spirilla (spiral). Some forms are duplexes (diplococci), clusters (staphylococci), or chains (streptococci).

Kingdom Protista

The simplest eukaryotic organisms are the **protists**. Protists probably represent the evolution between prokaryotes and the rest of the eukaryotic kingdoms, including fungi, plants, and animals. Most, but not all, protists are unicellular eukaryotes. One way to define the protists is that the group includes organisms that are eukaryotes but are not plants, animals, or fungi. Protists include heterotrophs like **amoebas** and **paramecia**, photosynthetic autotrophs like **euglenas** and **algae**, and fungi-like organisms like **slime molds**. Some protists are mobile through the use of flagella, cilia, or amoeboid motion. Protists use sexual reproduction in some cases and asexual reproduction in others.

One of the best-known protists are the **amoebas**. Amoebas are large, single-celled organisms that do not have a specific body shape. They move and change their shape through changes in their cytoskeleton and streaming of cytoplasm within the cell into extensions called pseudopods.

Algae are an important group of photosynthetic protists that are mostly unicellular. Algae include diatoms, single-celled organisms with intricate silica shells; dinoflagellates with flagella; and brown algae. Algae include large multicellular forms like giant kelp that might be grouped with the protists since they are an algae, but are also grouped with plants by others. It is likely that the plants evolved from one group of algae, the green algae.

Kingdom Fungi

Fungi are heterotrophs that absorb nutrients from their environment. Fungi are often saprophytic, feeding off of dead material, which is their nutrition source; because of this, along with bacteria, they are fundamental components of balanced ecosystems. Without fungi and bacteria, there would be an abundance of decaying material that would hinder ecosystems. Absorptive nutrition involves the secretion of enzymes that digest material in an extracellular environment, followed by cells absorbing the digested material. One of the distinguishing features of fungi is their cell wall made of chitin, unlike the cellulose found in plants. Fungi often form long, slender filaments called hyphae. Mushrooms, molds, and yeasts are all examples of fungi.

KAPLAN

Kingdom Plantae

Plants are multicellular eukaryotes that produce energy in their chloroplasts through photosynthesis, using the energy of the sun to drive the production of glucose. Plants are distinct from animals in several ways. First, plants are usually nonmotile, while most animals move. Plants are autotrophic, while animals are heterotrophic. With its ability to branch out extensively, the plant structure is adapted for maximum exposure to light, air, and soil; animals, on the other hand, have adapted to compact structures to ensure minimum surface exposure and maximum motility. Animals have much more centralization in their physiology, while plants often exhibit delocalized control of processes and growth.

The evolution of plants has included an ongoing increase in their ability to conquer land due to modifications that allow them to resist gravity and tolerate drier conditions. The first plants probably evolved from green algae in or near shallow water.

The evolution of vascular systems was a major adaptation in plants. The first vascular plants, tracheophytes, that did not produce seeds included ferns and horsetails—plants with cells called tracheids that form tubes that enable the movement of fluid in the plant tissue called xylem. This vascular system also helps to provide rigid stems that plants need to live on land. These plants colonized land about 400 million years ago, making it possible for animals like arthropods to colonize land soon after.

The evolution of the seed was the next major event in plant evolution, found first in gymnosperms and later in flowering plants, known as angiosperms. The seed is a young sporophyte that becomes dormant early in development. The embryo is usually well protected in the seed and able to survive unfavorable conditions by remaining dormant until conditions become more favorable again. Once those conditions arise, the embryo begins to grow again, sprouting. In some cases seeds can remain viable for many years, waiting for the right conditions for the sporophyte to grow. This increases the ability of plants to deal with the variable conditions found on land.

Following the evolution of the seed, the next big innovation in plant evolution was the flower. Angiosperms represent the flowering plants and are today the predominant plant group in many ecosystems.

Kingdom Animalia

Animals are fairly easy to recognize, as they are all multicellular heterotrophs. The evolution of animals has included many evolutionary modifications to body plans that aid in fundamental necessities such as getting food, avoiding predators, and reproducing. Members of the animal kingdom have evolved increasingly complex nervous systems that enable complex behaviors in response to the environment. Over time, animals have tended to become larger in size, and more complex, with greater specialization of tissues. Different groups of animals have evolved different body shapes, reflecting their different lifestyles. The body of an animal with **radial symmetry** is organized in a circular shape radiating outward. The echinoderms, such as sea stars and cnidarians like jellyfish, are examples of animals with radial symmetry. Another common body plan is **bilateral symmetry**, in which the body has a left side and a right side that are mirror images of each other.

The human body is a good example of bilateral symmetry. If a plane is drawn vertically through the body, it splits the body into left and right sides that look the same. The front of the body, where the head is located, is the anterior, and the rear of the animal is the posterior. The back of the animal, where the backbone is located in vertebrates, is the dorsal side (like the dorsal fin), and the front of the animal is the ventral side.

Phylum Chordata

At some stage of their embryologic development, chordates have a stiff, solid dorsal rod called the **notochord,** and paired gill slits. Chordata have hollow dorsal nerve cords, tails extending beyond the anus (at some point in their development), and ventral hearts. These adaptations may not sound impressive but they paved the way for the evolution of vertebrates, a major subphylum of chordates. The chordates probably originated from animals like tunicates, commonly called sea squirts. Adult tunicates are sessile filter feeders that do not resemble vertebrates at all. Tunicate larvae, however, are free-swimming, resemble tadpoles, and have both a notochord and a dorsal nerve cord. Vertebrates are a subphylum of the chordates that includes fish, amphibians, reptiles, birds, and mammals. In vertebrates the notochord is present during embryogenesis but is replaced during development by a bony, segmented vertebral column that protects the dorsal spinal cord and provides anchorage for muscles. Vertebrates have bony or cartilaginous endoskeletons, chambered hearts for circulation, and increasingly complex nervous systems. The vertebrate internal organs are contained in a coelomic body cavity.

The first vertebrates were probably filter-feeding organisms that evolved into swimming, jawless fishes that were still filter feeders. Jawless fish such as lampreys still exist. The evolution of fish with jaws led to the development of the cartilaginous and bony fishes that are dominant today. The jaw allows fish to adopt new life styles other than filter feeding, grabbing food with their jaws. The majority of fish use gills for respiration. The water from which fish extract the oxygen they need to survive moves over their gills through paired gill slits. Cartilaginous fish (class Chondrichthyes) like sharks and rays have an endoskeleton that is made entirely of cartilage rather than hard, calcified bone. Bony fishes (class Osteichthyes) have swim bladders to regulate their buoyancy in water.

Two adaptations were important to set the stage for vertebrates to colonize land. One was the presence of air sacs that allowed some fish in shallow water to absorb oxygen from air for brief periods. The other adaptation was a structural change in fins; fin lobes allowed some degree of movement on land. Fish with these features evolved into **amphibians** about 350 million years ago. Most amphibians, such as frogs and salamanders, still live in close association with water and have only simple lungs or gills. Their intake of oxygen is supplemented by the ability to absorb it through the skin. Another reason that amphibians are mostly associated with water is that amphibian eggs lack hard shells and dry out on land. Amphibian larvae often live in water and then metamorphose into an adult form that lives primarily on land.

KAPLAN

Reptiles, on the other hand, have evolved to produce hard-shelled eggs that do not dry out on land. The eggshell protects the developing embryo but still allows a gas exchange with the environment. The heart and lungs of reptiles also evolved to be more effective, particularly for the climates and environments in which they live. Their thick, dry skin allows them greater metabolic activity than amphibians and the ability to survive on land.

The development of wings, feathers, and light bones that allowed for flight distinguished **birds** from their reptilian relatives—dinosaurs. Birds also have four-chambered hearts and uniquely adapted lungs to supply the intense metabolic needs of flight. Birds produce hard-shelled eggs and usually provide a great deal of parental care during embryonic development and the maturation that takes place after hatching.

Mammals are the major class of vertebrates. Mammals have hair, sweat glands, mammary glands, and four-chambered hearts. The fossil record indicates that mammals evolved 200 million years ago and coexisted with dinosaurs up until dinosaurs became extinct 65 million years ago. When mammals no longer had to compete with dinosaurs for dominance, they diversified and occupied many environmental niches, becoming the dominant terrestrial vertebrate present in many ecosystems. Mammals have highly effective regulation systems to control their body temperature, and most mammals provide extensive care for their young. One small group of mammals, the Monotremes (for example, the duck-billed platypus), lays eggs. The embryos of most other mammals undergo internal gestation and are then birthed. **Marsupial** mammals give birth after a short time and complete development of young in an external pouch. **Placental** mammals gestate their young to a more mature state, providing nutrition to the embryo with the exchange of material in the placenta. Marsupial mammals were once widespread across the globe, but were replaced in most cases by placental mammals. As Australia is isolated, it was a haven for marsupial mammals, and continues to be in the present day.

Among mammals, the primates have opposable thumbs and stereoscopic vision for depth perception, adaptations that evolved to support their existence in their preferred environment: trees. Adaptations displayed by primates are traits that have been important factors in the evolution of humans. Many primates also have complex social structures.

Ancestors of humans include **australopithecines**. Fossils indicate these ancestors were able to walk upright on two legs. Fossil remains of hominids such as *Homo habilis*, which lived 2–3 million years ago, show that this human ancestor had a cerebral cortex that had greatly increased in size. *Homo habilis* probably used tools, setting the stage for modern humans, *Homo sapiens*.

Now that you have reviewed the basics of biology, you can review strategies for this part of the test. After reviewing the strategies and completing the questions at the end of this chapter, you are ready to study anatomy and physiology.

Ⓚ Ⓗ BIOLOGY STRATEGIES

It's important to know that the science portions of the nursing school entrance exams contain knowledge-based questions. What that means is you can't always reason your way to the correct answer—most likely, you will either know the answer or you will not.

Don't panic! That doesn't mean that there are no strategies to use on Test Day. It just means the strategies for this part of the test are slightly different from those for other sections. Here are Kaplan's favorite strategies for knowledge-based test questions.

- Mnemonic devices
- Review of terms and concepts commonly confused with each other
- Building blocks of words
- Organizing concepts
- Quiz yourself
- General test-taking strategies

Keep reading to find out how each one of these works for the Life Science section of the test.

Mnemonic Devices

A mnemonic device is a way to remember something. You may remember the mnemonic tool PEMDAS (Please Excuse My Dear Aunt Sally) that was presented in Chapter Six, Mathematics Review. This phrase could help you remember the order of operations: Parentheses, Exponents, Multiplication, Division, Addition, Subtraction. This same approach can be applied to concepts that might be presented in the Biology section of the test. Try to come up with mnemonic tools for lists of terms or concepts that are difficult to remember on their own. In the following section we present several examples of how this method could help you tackle science.

> **Concept: The correct order of taxonomic classifications.**
>
> The order is: **D**omain, **K**ingdom, **P**hylum, **S**ubphylum, **C**lass, **O**rder, **F**amily, **G**enus, **S**pecies.

Again, make a list of the first letters of each group. You are left with D-K-P-S-C-O-F-G-S. Unlike the last example, when this combination of letters is sounded out, it doesn't mean anything. The easiest thing to do is to build a sentence around the letters you need to remember.

> **Mnemonic device:** Didn't King Phillip Swiftly Come Over For Good Sushi?

This sentence may act as a tool to help you remember the correct order of classification. If this sentence is hard for you to remember because you do not have mental associations with the words we chose, try building your own sentence.

Terms That Are Commonly Confused with Each Other

After long hours of study, you might not even care what the difference between mitosis and meiosis is. However, you would care if that were something you were facing on Test Day. Here are a few biology terms that are commonly misidentified and confused with one another.

Don't Mix These Up on Test Day

- **Stomata** are pores in the surface of a leaf through which carbon dioxide enters and oxygen exits the plant.
- **Stroma** is the dense fluid within the chloroplast in which carbon dioxide is converted into sugars.

- **mRNA**, or messenger RNA, carries messages that encode proteins.
- **tRNA**, or transfer RNA, carries amino acids to make proteins.
- **rRNA**, or ribosomal RNA, is a structural component of ribosomes.

- **Transcription** involves DNA being read and that information being transcribed or transferred to RNA.
- **Translation** is when RNA is read, leading to the process of protein synthesis.

- **Prokaryotes** have no nucleus and no membrane-bound organelles, but do have ribosomes and cell walls made up of peptidoglycans.
- **Eukaryotes** have a nucleus, membrane-bound organelles, and ribosomes. Examples include protists, fungi, plants, and animals. Fungi and plant eukaryotic cells have cell walls made of cellulose.

- **Mitosis** has the following characteristics and functions:
  - *Produces diploid cells from diploid cells.*
  - *Occurs in all dividing cells.*
  - *Does not involve the pairing up of homologous chromosomes.*
  - *Does not involve crossing over (recombination).*

- **Meiosis** has the following characteristics and functions:
  - *Produces haploid cells from diploid cells.*
  - *Occurs only in sex cells (gametocytes).*
  - *Involves the pairing up of homologous chromosomes at the metaphase plate, forming tetrads.*
  - *Involves crossing over.*

- **Incomplete dominance** is when two traits are blended together; both are partially expressed, and neither dominates.
- **Codominance** is when both traits are fully expressed and neither dominates.

- **Homologous** structures share a common ancestry.
- **Analogous** structures are not inherited from a common ancestor but perform similar functions.

Building Blocks of Words

Many new vocabulary words that you will encounter when studying life science sound or look like other words you might be familiar with. For example, biology contains the prefix "bio," meaning "life," which can be found in biography, biotechnology, and biodegradable. Knowing the meaning of "bio" can help you decipher many terms in the study of life science such as **bio**tic, a**bio**tic, **bio**sphere, and sym**bio**tic. Learning common prefixes, suffixes, and root words can be a useful tool when you are responsible for a large amount of content. Use the table below as a starting place for your studies.

Word part (prefix, suffix, root)	Meaning	Examples
a-/an-	Without	Anaerobic, abiotic
aero-	Oxygen	Aerobic
-ase	Related to enzyme	Amylase, lactase
auto-	Self	Autosome, autotrophic
bio-	Life	Biology, biosphere, biotic
chloro-	Color	Chloroplast, chlorophyll
cyto-/kary-	Cell	Cytoplasm, cytotoxic, eukaryotic, karyotype
di-/dipl-	Two, double	Diploid, dichotomy
eco-	Environment	Ecology, ecosystem
endo-	Internal, within	Endometrium, endoderm
exo-	Outside	Exoskeleton, exocytosis
-gen/gen-	That which produces	Genotype, genetics, hydrogen
hapl-	Half	Haploid
heter-	Different, other	Heterogeneous, heterotrophic
hom-	Same	Homologous, homogeneous, homeostasis
hydro-	Water	Hydrogen, hydrosphere, hydrophobic
kine-	Energy, movement	Kinetics, kinesthesiology
meta-	Among, changed	Metaphase, metastasis
-morph-	Form, shape	Morphology, anthropomorphic
-neuro-	Nerve	Neuroscience, neuron
-ology	Study of	Biology, geology, ecology
-path/path-	Feeling, suffering	Pathology
-phase	Stage	Anaphase, metaphase, prophase
phen-	Appearing, seeming	Phenotype
phob-	Fear of	Hydrophobic
pro-/proto-	First, before	Prophase, prokaryotic, protoplasm
-sis	State or condition of	Homeostasis, metastasis, phagocytosis
sym-/syn-	With, together	Symbiotic, synthesis
tele-	Distance	Telephase
therm-	Heat	Thermometer, exotherm
trans-	Across	Transpiration, translation, transcription
-vac/vac-	Empty	Vacuole, evacuate, vaccine

KAPLAN

Organizing Concepts

The study of biology is full of processes, systems, and complex concepts. Beyond understanding the terms that make up these processes, it is also important to know how these are connected. Unlike on the reading or math sections, you will be tested mostly on your general knowledge of science content rather than on specific skills. To prepare yourself for this type of test, you need to develop a study strategy. Graphic organizers such as sequencing maps or concept maps can help you to organize this information in a visual way. Sequencing maps can be made for photosynthesis and ATP production. Concept maps can be created for the six-kingdom classification system. A template and a sample of each type of map are shown below.

Sequencing Map Template

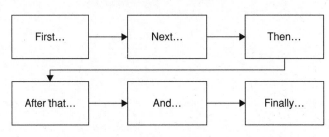

Sample Sequencing Map

How Nutrients Are Absorbed into Blood

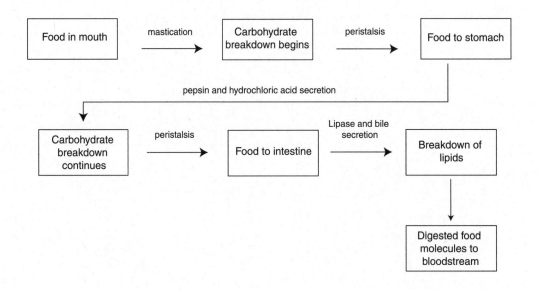

Concept Map Template

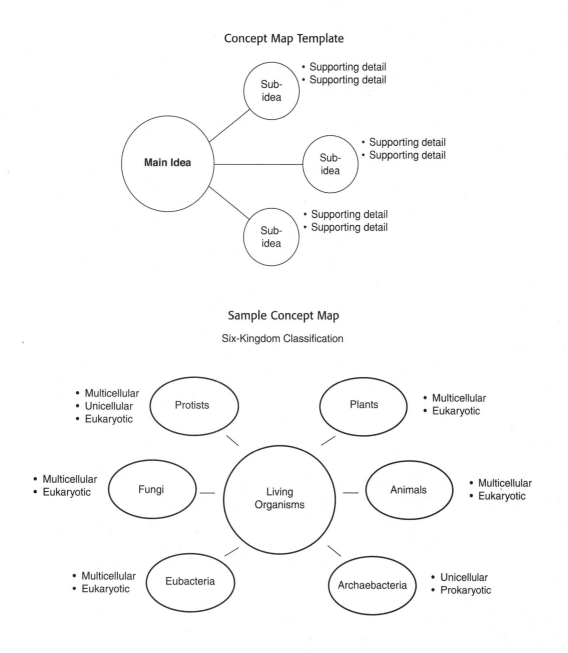

Sample Concept Map

Six-Kingdom Classification

REVIEW QUESTIONS

The following questions are not meant to mimic actual test questions. Instead, these questions will help you review the concepts and terms covered in this chapter.

1. List five biological molecules.

_____

_____

_____

_____

_____

2. Which of the following is NOT a biochemical reaction that makes ATP?

   (A) Krebs cycle

   (B) Glycolysis

   (C) Transcription

   (D) Electron transport

3. Fill in the blank. In plants, photosynthesis occurs in the _____, an organelle that is specific to plants.

4. Which of the following is NOT a part of the Central Dogma?

   (A) RNA is produced when DNA is read during a process called transcription.

   (B) DNA contains the genes that are responsible for the physical traits (phenotype) observed in all living organisms.

   (C) RNA serves as the key used to decode and transmit the genetic information, as well as synthesize proteins according to the encoded information. This process of protein synthesis is called translation.

   (D) The structure of DNA was elucidated by Watson and Crick in 1953 and it became clear how DNA could play a role as the source of genetic material.

   (E) DNA is replicated from existing DNA to produce new genomes.

5. Name the four types of nucleotides that make up DNA.

_____

_____

_____

_____

6. Match each type of RNA with its description.

   _____ mRNA

   _____ rRNA

   _____ tRNA

   (A) Plays a role in protein synthesis.

   (B) Part of the structure of ribosomes and is involved in translation (protein synthesis).

   (C) Encodes gene messages that are to be decoded during protein synthesis to form proteins.

7. True or False? Humans are composed of prokaryotic cells.

8. Explain what purpose the organelle mitochondria serves.

   _____

   _____

9. Fill in the blank. _____ is the simple diffusion of water from a region of lower solute concentration to a region of higher solute concentration.

10. Which of the following is NOT one of the four stages of mitosis?

    (A) Cytokinesis

    (B) Prophase

    (C) Metaphase

    (D) Anaphase

    (E) Telophase

11. Which of the following is NOT one of the three basic principles of genetics developed by Gregor Mendel?

    (A) Dominance

    (B) Phenotype

    (C) Segregation

    (D) Independent assortment

12. Write out the Law of Segregation.

    _____

    _____

    _____

13. True or False? The populations within a community interact with each other in a variety of ways, including predation, competition, or symbiosis.

14. Fill in the blank. A _____ is a group of organisms that is able to successfully interbreed with each other and not with other organisms.

15. Write the taxonomic classifications in order, from least specific to most specific.

    _____

    _____

    _____

    _____

    _____

    _____

    _____

    _____

16. List at least two characteristics of mammals.

    _____

    _____

    _____

REVIEW ANSWERS

1. Carbohydrates
   Lipids
   Proteins
   Enzymes
   Nucleic acids

2. **C**   Transcription is not a biochemical reaction that makes ATP. Transcription occurs when DNA is read in order to produce RNA.

3. Photosynthesis occurs in the **chloroplast**, an organelle that is specific to plants.

4. Although (D) is true, it is not a part of the Central Dogma.

5. Adenine (A)
   Guanine (G)
   Thymine (T)
   Cytosine (C)

6. **C**   mRNA encodes gene messages that are to be decoded in protein synthesis to form proteins.

   B   rRNA is a part of the structure of ribosomes and is involved in translation (protein synthesis).

   A   tRNA also plays a role in protein synthesis.

7. False. Humans are composed of eukaryotic cells.

8. Mitochondria are sites of aerobic respiration within the cell and are important suppliers of energy.

9. Osmosis is the simple diffusion of water from a region of lower solute concentration to a region of higher solute concentration.

10. **A**   Cytokinesis is not one of the four stages of mitosis. During cytokinesis, the cytoplasm and all the organelles of the cell are divided as the plasma membrane pinches inward and seals off to complete the separation of the two newly formed daughter cells from each other.

11. **B**   A phenotype is the appearance and physical expression of genes in an organism.

12. The Law of Segregation states that if there are two alleles in an individual that determine a trait, these two alleles will separate during gamete formation and act independently.

13. True. The populations within a community interact with each other in a variety of ways, including predation (the consumption of one organism by another, usually resulting in the death of the organism that is eaten); competition (a competitive relationship between populations in a community existing when different populations in the same location use a limited resource); and symbiosis (symbionts live together in an intimate, often permanent, association that may or may not be beneficial to them).

14. A species is a group of organisms that is able to successfully interbreed with each other and not with other organisms.

15. Domain
    Kingdom
    Phylum
    Subphylum
    Class
    Order
    Family
    Genus
    Species

16. Mammals have hair, sweat glands, mammary glands, and four-chambered hearts.

Chapter Eight: **Anatomy and Physiology Review**

Anatomy and physiology is the most thoroughly covered aspect of biology on both the Kaplan and HESI exams. You will be asked detailed questions regarding organ systems and body functions. You will have to remember not only the names of many different anatomical features, but also what they do and how they fit within larger systems and processes.

Be aware that physiology concepts are heavily tested on the Kaplan Nursing School Admission Test. Many exam candidates find the Kaplan exam questions on these topics more difficult than they expected. Don't be surprised on Test Day! Master the content in this chapter, and if needed, solidify your knowledge with a review of fundamentals from your physiology textbook.

K H ANATOMY LESSON

Body Planes and Directions

When referring to parts of the body, it is important to remember the many terms used in the medical field to indicate locations and directions relative to the body. Visualize an upright human body, arms straight at the sides, palms forward. This is known as the anatomical position. Now visualize three imaginary planes cutting through that body:

- A vertical plane extending through the center of the body from the feet to the head, front to back, dividing the two sides into equal halves; this is the median or sagittal plane.
- Another vertical plane extending through the body from side to side, dividing the front half from the back half; this is the coronal or frontal plane.
- A horizontal plane extending through the midsection of the torso, dividing the top half of the body from the bottom half; this is the transverse or cross-sectional plane.

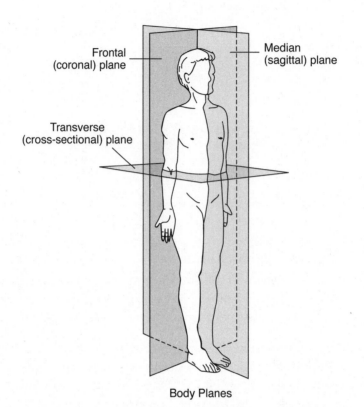

Frontal (coronal) plane

Median (sagittal) plane

Transverse (cross-sectional) plane

Body Planes

A body lying face-down is in the prone position. A body lying face-up is in the supine position.

A number of different terms are used to indicate direction and location on the human body. Here is a list of the most important directional terms:

Term	What It Means
Anterior	At or toward the front of the body
Posterior	At or toward the back of the body
Superior	At or toward the top of the body or head
Inferior	Away from the top of the body or head
Medial	Toward the center of the body
Lateral	Away from the center of the body
Proximal	Close to or toward the point of attachment (as in limbs)
Distal	Far or away from the point of attachment
Superficial	Near or on the outer surface of the body
Deep	Away from the outer surface of the body

Types of Tissue

Tissue is a collection of similar cells that work together to perform a specific function. The study of body tissues and cells is known as histology.

There are four basic types of tissue in the human body:

- Connective tissue serves as the foundation and structure for organs. This is the most abundant of the body tissues.
- Epithelial tissue forms the outer layer of the body and provides a protective layer for cavities and organs.
- Muscle tissue can contract, allowing for a wide array of movements, ranging from waving a hand in the air to the beating of a heart.
- Nerve tissue makes up most of the nervous system. It consists of cells called neurons and neuroglia (also known as glial cells).

(K) THE ROLE OF ELECTROLYTES IN THE BODY

Chemically, electrolytes are substances that become ions in solution and have the capacity to conduct electricity. Electrolytes are present in the human body, and the balance of these electrolytes is essential for the normal function of cells and organs. Electrolytes are critical for cells to generate energy, to maintain the stability of cell walls, and to function in general. They generate electricity, contract muscles, move water and fluids within the body, and participate in myriad other activities.

The concentration of electrolytes in the body is controlled by a variety of hormones, most of which are manufactured in the kidney and the adrenal glands. Keeping electrolyte concentrations in balance also includes stimulating the thirst mechanism when the body gets dehydrated.

The key electrolytes are sodium, potassium, chloride, bicarbonate, and magnesium. Sodium regulates the amount of water in the body and is critical to the production of electric signals needed for body system communication. Potassium is essential for normal cell function. Among its many functions are regulation of the heartbeat and the function of the muscles. Chloride aids in maintaining a normal balance of bodily fluids. Bicarbonate acts as a buffer to maintain the normal levels of acidity (pH) in blood and other fluids in the body. Magnesium is involved in a variety of metabolic activities in the body, including relaxation of the smooth muscles. Magnesium is also a factor in many of the body's enzyme-regulated activities.

K H SYSTEMS OF THE HUMAN BODY

Digestive System

The human digestive system consists of the **alimentary canal** and the associated glands that contribute secretions into this canal. The alimentary canal is the entire path food follows through the body: the **oral cavity**, **pharynx**, **esophagus**, **stomach**, **small intestine**, **large intestine**, and **rectum**. Many glands line this canal, such as the gastric glands in the wall of the stomach and intestinal glands in the small intestine. Other glands, such as the pancreas and liver, are outside the canal proper, and deliver their secretions into the canal via ducts. For example, the liver works with the gall bladder to regulate the secretion of bile.

Mechanical Digestion

Food is crushed and liquefied by the teeth, tongue, and peristaltic contractions of the stomach and small intestine, increasing the surface area for the digestive enzymes to work upon. **Peristalsis** is a wave-like muscular action conducted by smooth muscle that lines the gut in the esophagus, stomach, small intestine, and large intestine. During this process, rings of muscle encircling the gut contract, which moves food through the gut.

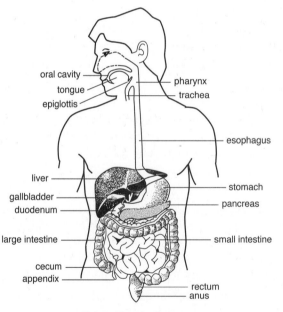

Human Digestive System

Chemical Digestion

Several exocrine glands associated with the digestive system produce secretions involved in breaking food molecules into simple molecules that can be absorbed. Polysaccharides are broken down into glucose, triglycerides are hydrolyzed into fatty acids and glycerol, and proteins are broken down into amino acids.

Chemical digestion begins in the mouth. In the mouth, the **salivary glands** produce saliva, which lubricates food and begins starch digestion. **Saliva** contains **salivary amylase** (ptyalin), an enzyme that breaks the complex starch polysaccharide into maltose (a disaccharide). As food leaves the mouth, the **esophagus** conducts it to the stomach by means of peristaltic waves of smooth-muscle contraction.

There are several more detailed steps involved in the human digestive system, but for now it should suffice to know the basics of mechanical and chemical digestion.

Circulatory System

Through ingestion and digestion, organisms make nutrients available to cells through absorption. These nutrients, along with gases and wastes, must also be transported throughout the body to be used. The system involved in transport of these materials to different parts of the body is called the **circulatory system**. Small animals have their cells either directly in contact with the environment or in close enough proximity that diffusion alone provides for the movement of gases, wastes, and nutrients making a specialized system for circulation unnecessary. Larger, more complex organisms require circulatory systems to move material within the body.

Circulation in Vertebrates

Vertebrates have closed circulatory systems, with a chambered heart that pumps blood through arteries into tiny capillaries in the tissues. Blood passing through capillaries is led into veins that connect to the heart. The chambers of vertebrate hearts include atria and ventricles. **Atria** are chambers where blood from veins collects and is pumped into ventricles, while **ventricles** are larger, more muscular chambers that pump blood through the body.

Birds and mammals have four-chambered hearts, with two atria and two ventricles. The right ventricle pumps deoxygenated blood to the lungs through the pulmonary artery. Oxygenated blood returns through the pulmonary vein to the left atrium. From there it passes to the left ventricle and is pumped through the aorta and arteries to the rest of the body. Valves in the chambers of the heart keep blood from moving backward. There are two separate circulatory systems: one for the lungs, called pulmonary circulation, and systemic circulation for the rest of the body. A four-chambered heart splits the blood that is pumped through the lungs and the blood that travels through the rest of the body, which allows much greater pressure in the systemic circulatory system than is possible with a two-chambered heart.

The heartbeat a doctor hears through a stethoscope is the sound of the chambers of the heart contracting in a regular pattern called the **cardiac cycle**. The heart is composed of specialized muscle tissue called **cardiac muscle**. Cardiac muscle cells are connected together in an electrical network that transmits nervous impulses throughout the muscle to stimulate contraction.

The transmission and spreading of the signal is highly controlled to coordinate the beating of the chambers. During each cardiac cycle, the signal to contract initiates on its own in a special part of the heart called the **sinoatrial node**, or the pacemaker region. Cells from this region fire impulses in regular intervals all on their own, without stimulation from the nervous system. Once the signals start, they spread through both atria, which then contract, forcing blood into the ventricles. The signal then passes into the ventricles and spreads throughout their walls, causing the ventricles to contract and move blood into the major arteries. Ventricular contraction occurs during the **systole** part of the cardiac cycle, and the atria contract during the **diastole** part of the cardiac cycle. The signal that causes the beating of the heart originates spontaneously within the heart without nervous stimulation, but the heart rate can be altered by nervous stimulation. The most important nervous stimulation of the heart is induced by the vagus nerve of the parasympathetic nervous system, which acts to slow the heart rate. The vagus nerve is more or less always stimulating the heart, and can increase the heart rate simply by stimulating the heart less than usual. Normal aging also decreases the strength of the heartbeat. The sympathetic nervous system and epinephrine increase the heart rate.

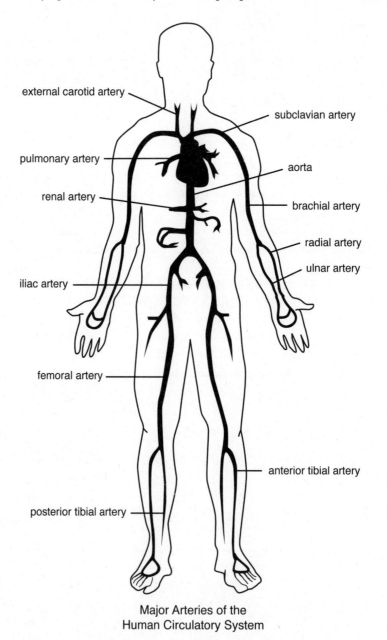

Major Arteries of the
Human Circulatory System

Arteries

The **arteries** carry blood from the heart to the tissue of the body. They repeatedly branch into smaller arteries (arterioles) until they reach capillaries, where exchange with tissues occurs. Arteries are thick-walled, muscular, and elastic; they conduct blood at high pressure and have a pulse caused by periodic surges of blood from the heart. Arterial blood is oxygenated; however, blood in the pulmonary artery is not, as it carries deoxygenated blood from the heart to the lungs to renew the oxygen supply.

Veins

Veins carry blood back to the heart from the capillaries. Veins are relatively thin-walled, conduct at low pressure because they are at some distance from the pumping heart, and contain many valves to prevent backflow. Veins have no pulse; they usually carry dark red, deoxygenated blood (except for the pulmonary vein, which carries recently oxygenated blood from the lungs). The movement of blood through veins is assisted by the contraction of skeletal muscle around the veins, squeezing blood forward. Once it moves forward in this way, valves keep the blood from going back.

Capillaries

Capillaries are thin-walled vessels that are very small in diameter. In fact, their walls are made of only one layer of endothelial cell; as such, red blood cells must pass through capillaries in a single file. Capillaries, not arteries or veins, permit the exchange of materials between the blood and the body's cells. Their small size and thinness of the endothelium assist in the diffusion of material through the walls. Also, some of the liquid component of blood seeps from capillaries, bathing cells with nutrients. Proteins and cells are too large to pass into tissue and stay in the blood within the capillary walls. Some of the fluid that enters tissues passes directly into the blood at the other end of the capillary, and the rest circulates in the lymphatic system. If the capillaries are too permeable or too much liquid stays in the tissues, swelling results.

At times, diverse tissues require differing blood flow. The body regulates much blood flow in tissues locally. Arterioles that feed capillaries in tissue have smooth muscle in their walls that can relax or constrict to allow more or less blood into a specific area. Factors like the level of oxygen and carbon dioxide in blood that are affected by metabolic activity also act on the arteriole smooth muscle, matching blood flow to the metabolic needs of the tissue.

Lymphatic System

Lymph vessels are the foundation for the lymphatic system, which is independent of the circulatory system. This system carries extracellular fluid (at this stage known as **lymph**) at very low pressure, without cells. The **lymph nodes** are responsible for filtering lymph to rid it of foreign particles, maintaining the proper balance of fluids in tissues of the body, and transporting chylomicrons as part of fat metabolism. The system ultimately returns lymph to the blood system via the largest lymph vessel, the thoracic duct, which empties lymph back into circulation shortly before it enters the heart.

Blood

The fluid moved through the body by the circulatory system is blood, which is composed of a liquid component, plasma, and cells. The cells include red blood cells (**erythrocytes**), **platelets**, and white blood cells (**lymphocytes**). Each of these types of cells has specific functions. **Plasma** is composed of water, salts, proteins, glucose, hormones, lipids, and other soluble factors. The main salts in plasma are sodium chloride and potassium chloride; because of this, it has been noted that plasma is similar in composition to seawater, our evolutionary origin. Calcium is another important element in extracellular fluid, including blood. The body regulates the blood volume and salt content through water intake and through excretion of urine.

Oxygen is dissolved as a gas to a small extent in blood, although most oxygen is transported bound to hemoglobin in red blood cells. Carbon dioxide is converted to carbonic acid in the blood. Glucose present in blood is transported as dissolved sugar for cells to uptake as needed. Hormones are transported through blood from the tissue from which they are secreted to the tissues where they exert their actions. The protein component of plasma consists of antibodies for immune responses, fibrinogen for clotting, and serum albumin. The protein component of blood helps draw water into blood in the capillaries, preventing loss of fluid from the blood into the tissues, which would cause swelling.

Red blood cells are the most abundant cells present in blood, and their primary function is to transport oxygen. After they are formed in the bone marrow, mature red blood cells lose their nuclei and become biconcave discs. They live for about four months in the circulatory system before they are worn out and destroyed, along with the foreign particles from the lymphatic system, in the spleen. Without a nucleus, mature red blood cells cannot make new proteins to repair themselves. Red blood cells also lose mitochondria, which renders them incapable of performing aerobic respiration. If they were able to carry on this form of respiration, they would use up the oxygen they carry to the tissues of the body. Instead, they produce energy in the form of ATP without using oxygen, through the process of glycolysis.

The oxygen-carrying component of red blood cells is the protein **hemoglobin**. In the lungs, where the partial pressure of oxygen is high, hemoglobin readily picks up oxygen. In the tissues, where the partial pressure of oxygen is low, oxygen leaves hemoglobin to diffuse into tissues. The hemoglobin molecule has evolved to deliver oxygen more efficiently in response to changes in tissues. During periods of great metabolic activity in muscle, the pH of the blood can decrease and carbon dioxide increase, both of which tend to reduce the affinity of hemoglobin for oxygen and cause it to leave more oxygen in the tissue.

Blood Types

Red blood cells manufacture two prominent types of antigens, antigen A (associated with blood type A) and antigen B (blood type B). In any given individual, one, both, or neither antigen may be present.

The plasma of every individual also contains antibodies for the antigens that are not present in the individual's red blood cells (if an individual were to produce antibodies against his or her own red cells, they would agglutinate and the blood would clump). People with type A blood have anti-B antibodies, and individuals with type B blood produce anti-A antibodies. Those with type O blood have neither A nor B antigens; rather, they have both anti-A and anti-B antibodies. People with type AB blood have neither type of antibody.

Another component of blood is an antigen called the Rh or Rhesus factor. Individuals can be either Rh positive or Rh negative, meaning that they have an Rh antigen or they do not, respectively. This is why you often hear a person's blood type described as "A-positive" or "AB-negative."

Immune System

The interior of the body is an ideal growth medium for some pathogenic organisms, such as disease-causing bacteria and viruses. To prevent this, the body has defenses that either prevent organisms from getting into the interior of the body or stop them from proliferating if they are within the body. The system that plays this protective role is called the **immune system**. The trick for the immune system is to be able to mount aggressive defenses, and, at the same time, to distinguish foreign bodies to avoid attacking one's own tissues and causing disease. Autoimmune disorders cause the body's immune system to assault its own tissue as if it were a foreign invader.

Passive immune defenses are barriers to entry. These include the skin, and the lining of the lungs, the mouth, and stomach. The skin is a very effective barrier to most potential pathogens, but if wounded, the barrier function of skin is lost. This is why burn patients are very susceptible to infection. The lungs are a potential route of entry but are patrolled by immune cells and have mucus to trap invaders; the cilia lining the respiratory tract can remove trapped invaders.

Active immunity is conferred by the cellular part of the immune system. White blood cells are composed of several different cell types that are involved in the defense of the body against foreign organisms in different ways. White blood cells include **phagocytes**, which engulf bacteria with amoeboid motion, and **lymphocytes**. There are several types of lymphocytes, but the most abundant are B and T cells, which are involved in immune responses. B cells produce **antibodies**, or **immunoglobulins**, which are secreted proteins specific to foreign molecules such as viral or bacterial proteins. "Helper" T cells coordinate immune responses, while "killer" T cells directly attack and dispose of cells that are infected with intracellular pathogens, such as viruses, or cells that are aberrant, such as malignant cells. These lymphocytes respond to a specific antigen. Since the body does not know what antigens or pathogens may attack it, the immune system creates a varied population of B and T cells in which each cell recognizes only one antigen, but the population of cells contains a huge range of specificities. If a B cell or T cell encounters an antigen that matches its specificity, then it is stimulated to proliferate and create more cells with the same specificity. This amplification of a clone of cells that respond to the invading antigen helps the body respond and remain immune from future infections by the same pathogen. When a B cell encounters an antigen it recognizes, it proliferates to make more B cells that produce antibody. The stimulated B cells also produce memory cells that do not make antibody, but have the same specificity and will lie dormant for many years, ready to respond if the body is challenged again with the same antigen.

Respiratory System

Cells performing aerobic respiration require oxygen and need to eliminate carbon dioxide. To do this, organisms must exchange gases with the environment. The respiratory system provides oxygen and removes CO_2. The oxygen is used to drive electron transport and ATP production, and CO_2 is produced from burning glucose. No human can live without breathing for more than a few minutes.

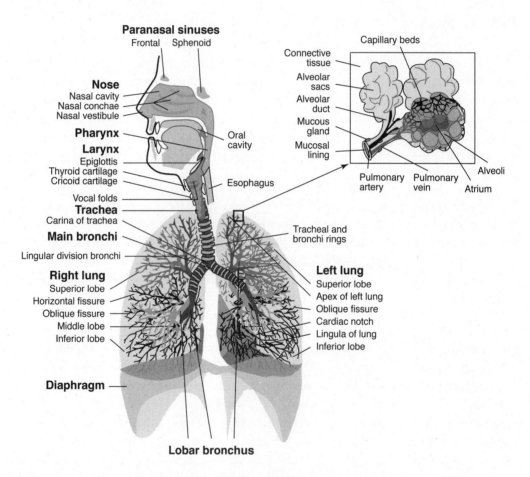

Humans have developed a complex system of respiration to transport oxygen to their cells and rid their bodies of waste products like carbon dioxide. The **lungs** are designed to move air between the exterior atmosphere and an interior air space that is in close contact with capillaries. Here, oxygen and carbon dioxide diffuse between the blood and air; blood circulates through the body to exchange gases with the tissues, and then returns to the lungs. The lungs are found in a sealed cavity in the chest, bound by the ribs, chest wall, and the muscular **diaphragm** on the bottom. The diaphragm is curved upward when released, and flattens when contracted, expanding the chest cavity. During inhalation, chest muscles move the ribs up and out as the diaphragm moves down; this creates both a larger chest cavity and a vacuum that draws air into the respiratory passages. The reverse process decreases the size of the chest cavity and forces air out of the lungs (exhalation). Exhalation is largely a passive process that does not require muscle contraction. During exhalation the elasticity of the lungs draws the chest and diaphragm inward when the muscles relax, decreasing the volume of the lungs and causing air to be forced out. The breathing rate is controlled by the **medulla oblongata**, the part of the brain that monitors carbon dioxide content in the blood. Excess CO_2 in the blood stimulates the medulla to send messages to the rib muscles and the diaphragm to increase the frequency of respiration.

The air passages involved in respiration consist of the **nose, pharynx, larynx, trachea, bronchi, bronchioles,** and the **alveoli**. The **nose** adds moisture and warmth to inhaled air, and helps to filter it, removing particulates and organisms before the air passes to the next air passage. The **pharynx** is involved in diverting ingested material into the esophagus and away from the lungs to prevent choking. The **larynx** contains a membrane that vibrates in a controlled manner with the passage of air to create the voice. The **trachea** carries air through the vulnerable throat protected by flexible but strong rings of cartilage. At the end of the trachea the respiratory passage splits into the two lungs and into smaller and smaller passages that terminate in the **alveoli**, tiny air sacs that are the site of gas exchange in the lungs.

The alveoli have thin, moist walls and are surrounded by thin-walled capillaries. Oxygen passes into the blood by diffusion through the alveolar and capillary walls; CO_2 and H_2O pass out in the same manner. Note that all exchanges at the alveoli involve passive diffusion. Since passive diffusion drives gas exchange, both in the lungs as well as the tissues, gases always diffuse from higher to lower concentration. In the tissues, O_2 diffuses into tissues and CO_2 leaves, while in the lungs this is reversed due to high oxygen pressure and low CO_2 levels. CO_2 is carried in blood mainly as dissolved carbonate ions.

Thermoregulation and the Skin

In humans, the **skin** protects the body from microbial invasion and environmental stresses like dry weather and wind. Specialized epidermal cells called **melanocytes** synthesize the pigment **melanin**, which protects the body from ultraviolet light. The skin is a receptor of stimuli (such as pressure and temperature), an excretory organ (removing excess water and salts from the body), and also a thermoregulatory organ (helping control both the conservation and release of heat). **Sweat glands** secrete a mixture of water, dissolved salts, and urea via sweat pores. As sweat evaporates, the skin is cooled. Thus, sweating has both an excretory and thermoregulatory function. Sweating is under autonomic (involuntary) nervous control.

The epidermis is made up of several different layers, or strata, of skin cells. The outermost layer is the stratum corneum, which is made up of dead skin cells that protect the layers of live skin cells beneath. In the palms of the hands and soles of the feet, the next layer is the stratum lucidum, which provides an additional thick layer of dead skin cells for protection. Below the layers of dead skin cells is the stratum granulosum. The next layer down is the stratum spinosum, where epithelial cells begin to become keratinized before migrating through the layers toward the outer surface; keratinization makes the cells more durable and water-resistant, to better serve as a protective layer. The bottom-most layer of the epidermis is the stratum basale, also known as the stratum germinativum. It is a very thin layer of cells that marks the boundary between the epidermis and the dermis.

Subcutaneous fat in the **hypodermis** insulates the body. Hair entraps and retains warm air at the skin's surface. Hormones such as epinephrine can increase the metabolic rate, thereby increasing heat production. In addition, muscles can generate heat by contracting rapidly (shivering). Heat loss can be inhibited through the constriction of blood vessels (**vasoconstriction**) in the **dermis**, moving blood away from the cooling atmosphere. Likewise, dilation of these same blood vessels (**vasodilation**) dissipates heat.

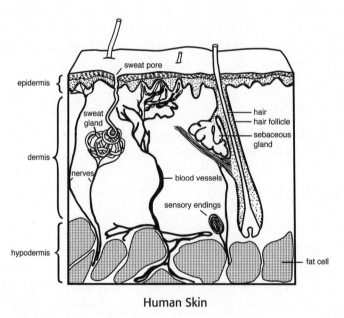

Human Skin

Excretory System

Excretion is the term given to the removal of metabolic wastes produced in the body. (Note that it is to be distinguished from elimination, which is the removal of indigestible materials.) Sources of metabolic waste are listed in the following table.

Waste	Metabolic Activity Producing the Waste
Carbon dioxide	Aerobic respiration
Water	Aerobic respiration, dehydration synthesis
Nitrogenous wastes (urea, ammonia, uric acid)	Deamination of amino acids
Mineral salts	All metabolic processes

The principal organs of excretion in humans are the **kidneys**. The kidneys form urine to remove nitrogenous wastes in the form of urea; they also regulate the volume and salt content of the extracellular fluids. The key structures that remove waste in the kidneys are small filtration tubes known as nephrons. From the kidney, the urine passes into a **ureter tube** leading to the **urinary bladder**, where urine is stored until urination occurs. During urination, the urine leaves the bladder through the **urethra**.

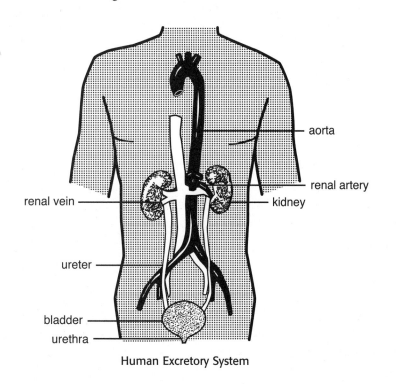

Human Excretory System

Endocrine System

The body has two communication systems to coordinate the activities of different tissues and organs, the nervous system and the **endocrine system**. The endocrine system is the network of glands and tissues that secrete **hormones**, chemical messengers produced in one tissue and carried by the blood to act on other parts of the body. Compared with the nervous system, the signals conveyed by the endocrine system take much more time to take effect. A nervous impulse is produced in a millisecond and travels anywhere in the body in less than a second. Hormones require time to be synthesized, can travel no more quickly than the blood can carry them, and often cause actions through inducing protein synthesis or transcription, activities that require time. However, hormone signals tend to be more long-lasting than nerve impulses. When the nerve impulse ends, a target such as skeletal muscle usually returns quickly to its starting state. When a hormone induces protein synthesis, the proteins remain long after the hormone is gone. Often the two systems work together. The **endocrine glands**, such as the pancreas or the adrenal cortex, can be the direct targets (effectors) of the autonomic nervous system. The hormone adrenaline acts in concert with the sympathetic nervous system to produce a set of results similar to those produced by sympathetic neurons.

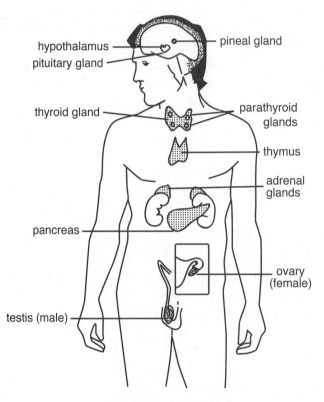

Human Endocrine System

Endocrine glands secrete hormones directly into the bloodstream. This is in contrast to **exocrine secretions** that do not contain hormones and are released through ducts into a body compartment. An example of exocrine secretion is the release of digestive enzymes by the pancreas into the small intestine through the pancreatic duct. Both endocrine and exocrine functions can be found in the same organ. The pancreas simultaneously produces exocrine secretions, such as digestive enzymes, and endocrine secretions, such as insulin and glucagon, which are released into the blood to exert their effects throughout the body.

Hormones are secreted by a variety of tissues, including the **hypothalamus**, **pituitary**, **thyroid**, **parathyroids**, **adrenals**, **pancreas**, **testes**, **ovaries**, **pineal**, **kidneys**, **heart**, and **thymus**. It is likely that additional tissues like skin and fat, though not traditionally considered glands, also have endocrine functions. Some hormones regulate a single type of cell or organ, while others have more widespread actions. The specificity of hormonal action is determined by the presence of specific receptors on or in the target cells. A common principle that regulates the production and secretion of many hormones is the **feedback loop**, in which several hormones regulate each other in a chain.

Hypothalamus

The **hypothalamus**, a section of the posterior forebrain, is located above the pituitary gland and is intimately associated with it via a portal circulatory system that carries blood directly from the hypothalamus to the pituitary. In most parts of the circulatory system, blood flows directly back to the heart from capillaries, but in a portal system, blood flows from capillaries in one organ to capillaries in another. The hypothalamus connects the nervous system with the endocrine system. When the hypothalamus is stimulated (by feedback from endocrine glands or by neurons innervating it), it releases hormone-like substances called **releasing factors** into the anterior pituitary-hypothalamic portal circulatory system. These hormones are carried directly to the pituitary by the portal system. In their turn, these releasing factors stimulate cells of the anterior pituitary to secrete the hormone indicated by the releasing factor.

Pituitary

The **pituitary gland** is a small gland with two lobes lying at the base of the brain. The two lobes, anterior and posterior, function as independent glands. The anterior pituitary secretes several hormones.

- **Growth hormone** (GH) fosters growth in a variety of body tissues.
- **Thyroid-stimulating hormone** (TSH) stimulates the thyroid gland to secrete its own hormone, thyroxine.
- **Adrenocorticotropic hormone** (ACTH) stimulates the adrenal cortex to secrete its corticoids.
- **Prolactin** is responsible for milk production by the female mammary glands.
- **Follicle-stimulating hormone** (FSH) spurs maturation of seminiferous tubules in males and causes maturation of ovaries in females. It also encourages maturation of follicles in the ovaries.
- **Luteinizing hormone** (LH) induces interstitial cells of the testes to mature by beginning to secrete the male sex hormone testosterone. In females, a surge of LH stimulates ovulation of the primary oocyte from the follicle. LH then induces changes in the follicular cells and converts an old follicle into a yellowish mass of cells rich in blood vessels. This new structure is the **corpus luteum**, which subsequently secretes progesterone and estrogen.

The **posterior pituitary** is a direct extension of nervous tissue from the hypothalamus. Nerve signals cause direct hormone release. The two hormones secreted by the posterior pituitary are ADH and oxytocin.

- **Antidiuretic hormone** (ADH), also known as vasopressin, acts on the kidney to reduce water loss.
- **Oxytocin** acts on the uterus during birth to cause uterine contraction.

KAPLAN

Thyroid

The thyroid hormone, **thyroxine**, is a modified amino acid that contains four atoms of iodine. It accelerates oxidative metabolism throughout the body. An abnormal deficiency of thyroxine causes goiter, decreased heart rate, lethargy, obesity, and decreased mental alertness. In contrast, hyperthyroidism (too much thyroxine) is characterized by profuse perspiration, high body temperature, increased basal metabolic rate, high blood pressure, loss of weight, and irritability.

Parathyroid Glands

The parathyroid glands are small pea-like organs located on the posterior surface of the thyroid. They secrete parathyroid hormone, which regulates calcium and phosphate balance in blood, bones, and other tissues. Increased parathyroid hormone increases bone formation. Plasma calcium must be maintained at a constant level for the function of muscles and neurons.

Pancreas

The pancreas is a multifunctional organ. It has both an **exocrine** and an **endocrine function**. The exocrine function of the pancreas secretes enzymes through ducts into the small intestine. The endocrine function, on the other hand, secretes hormones directly into the bloodstream. The endocrine function of the pancreas is centered in the **islets of Langerhans**, localized collections of endocrine alpha and beta cells that secrete glucagon and insulin, respectively. **Insulin** stimulates the muscles to remove glucose from the blood when glucose concentrations are high, such as after a meal. Insulin is also responsible for spurring muscles and the liver to convert glucose to glycogen, the stored form of glucose. The islets of Langerhans also secrete **glucagon**, which responds to low concentrations of blood glucose by stimulating the breakdown of glycogen into glucose, keeping the level of glucose in blood high enough to supply tissues. Individuals with diabetes are not able to effectively regulate glucose in the bloodstream.

Adrenal Glands

The adrenal glands are situated on top of the kidneys and consist of the **adrenal cortex** and the **adrenal medulla**.

In response to stress, ACTH stimulates the adrenal cortex to synthesize and secrete the steroid hormones collectively known as **corticosteroids**. Corticosteroids are effective anti-inflammatory medicines, but their use is limited by their alterations of fat metabolism and their suppression of the immune system. The adrenal cortex also secretes small quantities of androgens (male sex hormones) in both males and females. Since testes produce most of the androgens in males, the physiologic effect of the adrenal androgens is quite small. In females, however, overproduction of the adrenal androgens may have masculinizing effects, such as excessive facial hair.

The secretory cells of the adrenal medulla can be viewed as specialized sympathetic nerve cells that secrete hormones into the circulatory system. This organ produces **epinephrine** (adrenaline) and **norepinephrine** (noradrenaline).

Epinephrine increases the conversion of glycogen to glucose in liver and muscle tissue, causing a rise in blood glucose levels and an increase in the basal metabolic rate. Both epinephrine and norepinephrine increase the rate and strength of the heartbeat, as well as dilate and constrict blood vessels. These in turn increase the blood supply to skeletal muscles, the heart, and the brain, while decreasing the blood supply to the kidneys, skin, and digestive tract. These effects prepare the body for stress and are known as the "**fight-or-flight response**." They are elicited by sympathetic nervous stimulation in response to stress. Both of these hormones are also neurotransmitters.

Reproductive Glands

The gonads are important endocrine glands, with testes producing testosterone in males and ovaries producing estrogen in females. See the section on reproduction later in this lesson for more details.

Nervous System

The nervous system enables organisms to receive and respond to stimuli from their external and internal environments. The brain and spinal column regulate breathing, movement, and perception of sight, sound, touch, smell, and taste. They allow organisms not only to perceive their environment but to respond to their experience, and alter their behavior over time through learning.

Functional Units of the Nervous System

To understand the nervous system, it is best to start with the basic functional unit of the nervous system—the **neuron**. Neurons are specialized cells designed to transmit information in the form of electrochemical signals called **action potentials**. These signals are generated when neurons alter the voltage found across their plasma membrane. The excitable membrane is the property that allows neurons to carry an action potential.

Synapses

The nervous system is not simply a network of electrical wires with the brain as the switch-board. There is a strong chemical component to the signals that neurons convey. Neurons do not usually carry the action potential all the way to the membrane of the target cell. When a neuron reaches a target cell, the **axon** ends in a synaptic terminal, with a gap called the **synapse** between the neuron and the target cell. The membrane potential is then converted to a chemical signal, or **neurotransmitter**, that is released across a small gap between the neuron and the target cell. This gap between the neuron and the target cell is called the **synaptic cleft**. The target cell in communication with the neuron then receives the chemical signal by binding the neurotransmitter and starting a signal of its own. There are many types of synapses of neurons with other neurons. For motor neurons in the somatic nervous system, a specialized synapse of motor neurons with skeletal muscle cells is called the **neuromuscular junction**.

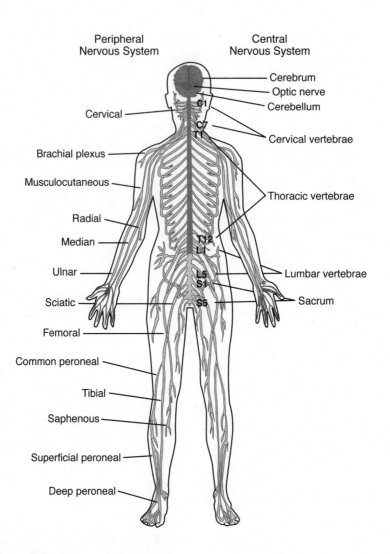

Peripheral Nervous System

Central Nervous System

- Cerebrum
- Optic nerve
- Cerebellum
- Cervical vertebrae
- Cervical
- C1
- C7
- T1
- Brachial plexus
- Musculocutaneous
- Thoracic vertebrae
- Radial
- Median
- T12
- L1
- Ulnar
- L5
- S1
- Lumbar vertebrae
- Sciatic
- S5
- Sacrum
- Femoral
- Common peroneal
- Tibial
- Saphenous
- Superficial peroneal
- Deep peroneal

Organization of the Nervous System

As organisms evolve and become more complex, their nervous systems undergo corresponding increases in complexity. Simple organisms can only respond to simple stimuli, while complex organisms like humans can discern subtle variations of a stimulus, such as a particular shade of color.

Vertebrate Nervous System

Vertebrates have a **brain** enclosed within the **cranium** and a **spinal cord;** together these form the **central nervous system** (CNS) that processes and stores information. The optic nerve, which emerges directly from the brain, is also considered part of the central nervous system. Throughout the rest of the body is the **peripheral nervous system**, containing motor or efferent neurons that carry signals to effector organs, such as muscles and glands, to take actions in response to nervous impulses. Sensory neurons in the peripheral nervous system convey information back to the CNS for processing and storage. Another division of the nervous system is between the autonomic and voluntary components of efferent pathways.

Peripheral Nervous System

The peripheral nervous system carries nerves from the CNS to target tissues of the body and includes all neurons that are not part of the CNS. The peripheral nervous system consists of the cranial nerves (excluding the optic nerve), which primarily innervate the head and shoulders, and 31 pairs of spinal nerves, which innervate the rest of the body. Cranial nerves exit from the brainstem and spinal nerves exit from the spinal cord. The peripheral nervous system has two primary divisions, the somatic and the autonomic nervous systems.

Somatic Motor Nervous System

This system innervates skeletal muscle and is responsible for voluntary movement, generally subject to conscious control. Motor neurons release the neurotransmitter acetylcholine (ACh) onto ACh receptors located on skeletal muscle. This causes depolarization of the skeletal muscle, leading to muscle contraction. In addition to voluntary movement, the somatic nervous system is also important for reflex action via the reflex arc.

Autonomic Nervous System

The autonomic nervous system is neither structurally nor functionally isolated from the CNS or the peripheral system. Its function is to regulate the involuntary functions of the body, including the heart and blood vessels, the gastrointestinal tract, urogenital organs, structures involved in respiration, and the intrinsic muscles of the eye. In general, the autonomic system innervates glands and smooth muscle, but not skeletal muscles. It is made up of the sympathetic nervous system and the parasympathetic nervous system.

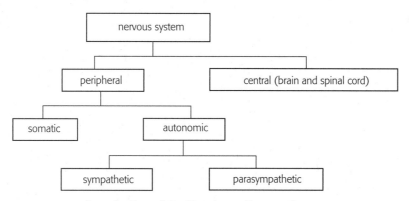

Organization of the Vertebrate Nervous System

Sympathetic Nervous System

This system utilizes norepinephrine as its primary neurotransmitter. It is responsible for activating the body during emergency situations and actions (the fight-or-flight response), including strengthening of heart contractions, increases in heart rate, dilation of the pupils, bronchodilation, and vasoconstriction of vessels feeding the digestive tract.

Tissue regulated by the sympathetic system includes the adrenal glands, which produce adrenaline in response to stimulation. Adrenaline produces many of the same fight-or-flight responses as the sympathetic system alone.

Parasympathetic Nervous System

Acetylcholine serves as the primary neurotransmitter for the parasympathetic nervous system. One of this system's main functions is to deactivate or slow down the activities of muscles and glands (the rest-and-digest response). These activities include pupillary constriction, slowing down of the heart rate, bronchoconstriction, and vasodilation of vessels feeding the digestive tract. The principal nerve of the parasympathetic system is the vagus nerve. Most of the organs innervated by the autonomic system receive both sympathetic and parasympathetic fibers, the two systems being antagonistic to one another.

Homeostasis

Homeostasis is the body's ability to maintain stable internal conditions in terms of temperature, pH, and water concentrations in spite of continually changing external conditions. Although every organ system plays a role, the nervous and endocrine systems are the body's chief communicators of external change. Living cells can function only within a narrow range of such conditions as temperature, pH, and nutrient availability, yet must survive in an environment where these and other conditions can vary from hour to hour, day to day, and season to season. Most bodily functions are aimed at maintaining homeostasis, and failure to maintain it leads to disease and often death.

The usual means of maintaining homeostasis is called a negative feedback mechanism. In this process, the body senses an internal change and activates mechanisms that reverse that change. An example of negative feedback is body temperature regulation. If blood temperature rises too high, specialized neurons in the hypothalamus (part of the brain) sense the temperature abnormality. The neurons signal other nerve centers, which send signals to the blood vessels of the skin to dilate. As these blood vessels dilate, more blood flows close to the body surface, radiating excess heat from the body. If blood vessel dilation is not enough to cool the body to a normal level, the brain activates sweating. Evaporation of moisture from the skin has a strong cooling effect. (You can feel the effect of evaporation by standing in front of a fan when sweaty or damp from a shower.)

If the blood temperature falls too low, on the other hand, the hypothalamus senses this as well and sends signals to the blood vessels supplying the skin to constrict. The effect is that the body keeps its warm blood deeper in the body and loses less surface heat. If blood vessel constriction is not enough to warm the body, the brain activates shivering. Shivering releases heat energy and helps warm the body back toward its optimal temperature of 98.6° F.

Other examples of homeostasis are the body's ability to adjust blood glucose levels and regulate blood carbon dioxide levels. Homeostasis is so important to maintaining health that most disease is regarded as homeostatic imbalance.

The Human Brain

The human brain is divided into several anatomical regions with different functions.

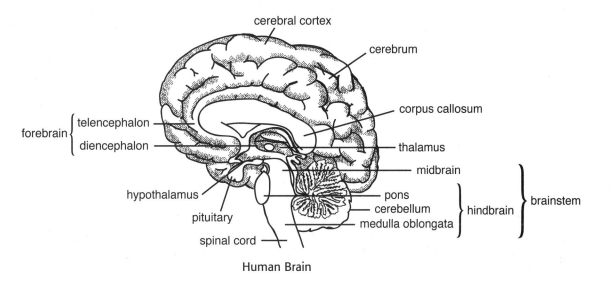

Human Brain

- **Cerebral cortex.** The cerebral cortex controls all voluntary motor activity by initiating the responses of motor neurons present within the spinal cord. It also controls higher functions, such as memory and creative thought. The cortex is divided into hemispheres, left and right, with some specialization of function between them ("left-brain, right-brain"). The cortex consists of an outer portion containing neuronal cell bodies (gray matter) and an inner portion containing axons (white matter).

- **Frontal lobe.** This lobe is considered the cognitive center, processing emotion, expression, memory, language, judgment, and sexual behaviors.

- **Olfactory lobe.** This serves as the center for reception and integration of olfactory input.

- **Thalamus.** Nervous impulses and sensory information are relayed and integrated en route to and from the cerebral cortex by this region.

- **Hypothalamus.** Hunger, thirst, pain, temperature regulation, and water balance are visceral and homeostatic functions controlled by this center.

- **Cerebellum.** Muscle activity is coordinated and modulated here.

- **Pons.** This serves as the relay center for cerebral cortical fibers en route to the cerebellum.

- **Medulla oblongata.** This influential region controls vital functions like breathing, heart rate, and gastrointestinal activity. It has receptors to detect carbon dioxide. When carbon dioxide levels become too high, the medulla oblongata forces you to breathe. When you hold your breath for too long and carbon dioxide levels rise in your body, you pass out. The medulla oblongata makes you breathe involuntarily to bring an influx of oxygen into your body.

- **Reticular activating system.** This network of neurons in the brainstem is involved in processing signals from sensory inputs and transmitting them to the cortex and other regions. This system is also involved in regulating the activity of other brain regions, such as the cortex, in order to alter levels of alertness and attention.

- **Basal ganglia.** Found in various parts of the brain, basal ganglia are associated with many different functions, including voluntary fine motor movement, procedural and habit learning, eye movement, cognition, and emotions.

The **spinal cord** is also part of the CNS. The spinal cord acts as a route for axons to travel out of the brain. It also serves as a center for many reflex actions that do not involve the brain, such as the **knee-jerk reflex**.

Sensory Systems of the Nervous System

All complicated nervous systems are made more useful through input mechanisms that we know as our senses. Sight, hearing, balance, taste, smell, and touch provide an influx of data for the nervous system to assimilate. Other sensory information that we are not consciously aware of is also provided to the CNS, including internal conditions such as the management of temperature and carbon dioxide levels. All of these sensory detection systems use cells that are usually specialized, modified neurons to receive information and alter their membrane potential in response to information. This altered membrane potential can then trigger an action potential to carry information back to the CNS. Some sensory cells detect chemical information (taste and smell), some detect electromagnetic energy (vision), and others detect mechanical information (sound, pressure). All sensation is caused by action potentials that are sent to the CNS by sensory cells. An action potential from the eye is the same as an action potential from the ear. The difference in perception, how we experience the information, is determined by how the information is received and processed by the CNS. An action potential from the eye is perceived as sight because it passes to the visual center of the brain for processing.

Sight

The eye detects light energy and transmits information about intensity, color, and shape to the brain. The transparent **cornea** at the front of the eye bends and focuses light rays. These rays then travel through an opening called the **pupil**, whose diameter is controlled by the pigmented, muscular **iris**. The iris responds to the intensity of light in the surroundings (light makes the pupil constrict). Light continues through the **lens**, which is suspended behind the pupil. This lens focuses the image onto the **retina**, which contains photoreceptors that transduce light into action potentials. The image on the retina is actually upside down but revision and interpretation in the cerebral cortex result in the perception of the image right-side up. The image from each eye is also integrated in the cortex to produce the binocular vision with depth perception that allows us to throw, catch, and drive with improved ability. The shape of the lens is changed to focus images from nearby or far objects. To see nearby objects, the muscles attached to the lens are relaxed and the lens rounds up, focusing light more sharply. If the shape of the eye is either too short or too long, or if the lens becomes stiff with age, then the eye is unable to focus the image and corrective lenses may be required to bring images into focus.

There are two types of specialized **photoreceptor cells** in the eye that respond to light: cones and rods. **Cones** respond to high-intensity illumination and are sensitive to color, while **rods** detect low-intensity illumination and are important in night vision. The optic nerve conducts visual information to the brain.

Hearing and Balance

The ear transduces sound energy into impulses that are perceived by the brain as sound. Sound waves pass through three regions as they enter the ear. First, they enter the outer ear, which consists of the **auricle** (pinna) and the **auditory canal**. Located at the end of the auditory canal is the **tympanic membrane** (eardrum) of the middle ear, which vibrates at the same frequency as the incoming sound. Next, three bones, or **ossicles** (malleus, incus, and stapes), amplify the stimulus, and transmit it through an oval window leading to the fluid-filled inner ear. The amplification of sound in the inner ear induces electrical impulses that travel through auditory nerves to the CNS for interpretation.

Taste and Smell

Taste buds are chemical sensory cells located on the tongue, the soft palate, and the epiglottis. The outer surface of a taste bud contains a taste pore, from which microvilli, or taste hairs, protrude. Interwoven around taste buds is a network of nerve fibers that are stimulated by the taste buds, and these neurons transmit impulses to the brainstem. There are four main kinds of taste sensations: sour, salty, sweet, and bitter.

Olfactory receptors are chemical sensors found in the olfactory membrane, which lies in the upper part of the nostrils over a total area of about 5 cm2. The receptors are specialized neurons from which olfactory hairs called cilia project. When odorous substances enter the nasal cavity, they bind to receptors in the cilia, depolarizing the olfactory receptors. Axons from the olfactory receptors join to form the olfactory nerves, which project to the olfactory bulbs in the base of the brain.

Motor Systems

One of the key systems of the body is the system of muscles that are effectors for the CNS. To exert an effect, muscles also require something to act against, which is the skeletal system.

Vertebrates have an **endoskeleton** as a framework for the attachment of skeletal muscles, permitting movement when a muscle contracts by bringing two bones together—which is the basis for all voluntary movement. The endoskeleton also provides protection, since bones surround delicate, vital organs. For example, the rib cage protects the thoracic organs (heart and lungs), while the skull and vertebral column protect the brain and spinal cord. The vertebrate skeleton contains **cartilage** and **bone**, both formed from connective tissue.

Cartilage, although firm, is also flexible and is not as hard or as brittle as bone. It makes up the skeletons of lower vertebrates, such as sharks and rays. In higher animals, cartilage is the principal component of embryonic skeletons, and is replaced during development by the aptly termed replacement bone. Because cartilage has no vessels or nerves, it takes longer to heal than bone.

Bone makes up most of the skeleton of mature higher vertebrates, including humans; it is made of calcium, phosphate salts, and strands of the protein collagen. A hollow cavity within each long bone is filled with **bone marrow**, the site where the formation of blood cells takes place.

Bones are connected at joints, either immovable, as in the skull, or movable like the hip. In the latter type, ligaments serve as bone-to-bone connectors, while tendons attach skeletal muscle to bones and bend the skeleton at the site of movable joints. Rotation of a movable joint means moving a part around an axis. In the vertebrate skeleton, the **axial skeleton** is the midline basic framework of the body, consisting of the skull, vertebral column, and the rib cage. The **appendicular skeleton**, on the other hand, includes the bones of the appendages, as well as the pectoral and pelvic girdles.

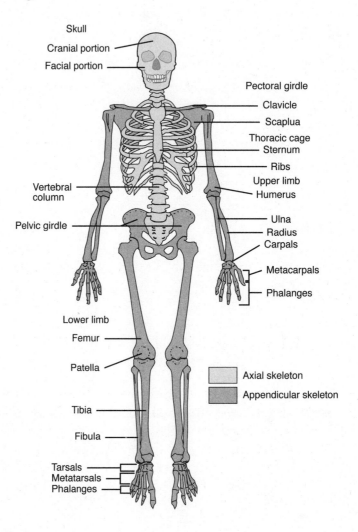

Muscle System

The muscle system serves as an effector of the nervous system. Muscles contract to implement actions after they receive nervous stimuli. For example, your arm muscles will automatically contract if you touch a hot stove. A skeletal muscle originates at a point of attachment to a stationary bone. It is this point that moves during contraction. An **extensor** extends or straightens the bones at a joint—for example, straightening out a limb. A **flexor** is a muscle that serves to bend a joint to an acute angle, as in bending the elbow to bring the forearm and upper arm together. Bones and muscles work together like a lever system.

Types of Muscles

Vertebrates possess three different types of muscle tissues: **smooth**, **skeletal**, and **cardiac**. In all three types, muscles cause movement by contraction, and the sliding of actin and myosin filaments past each other within cells causes the contraction. The differences between the types of muscle include where they are located, what they do, and what the cells look like.

Also known as involuntary muscle, **smooth muscle** is generally found in visceral systems and is innervated by the autonomic nervous system. Each muscle fiber consists of a single cell with one centrally located nucleus. Smooth muscle is nonstriated, meaning it does not have clearly organized arrays of actin and myosin filaments. Smooth muscle is present in the walls of arteries and veins, the walls of the digestive tract, bladder, and uterus. Smooth muscle contracts in response to action potentials, and the contraction is mediated by actin-myosin fibers like in other muscle, although the fibers do not have the clear organization displayed in other muscle types. Smooth-muscle cells in tissue are connected to each other through junctions that allow electrical impulses to pass directly from one cell to the next without passing through chemical synapses.

Skeletal muscles are also known as voluntary muscles; they produce intentional physical movement. A skeletal muscle cell is a single, large multinucleated fiber containing alternating light and dark bands called **striations**. Overlapping strands of thick myosin protein filaments that slide past thin actin protein filaments during muscle contraction cause these bands. The actin and myosin filaments in skeletal muscle are organized into sections called **sarcomeres** that form contractile units within each muscle cell. The somatic nervous system innervates skeletal muscle. Each skeletal muscle fiber is stimulated by nerves through neuromuscular synapses. When a nerve stimulates a muscle cell, an action potential moves over the whole muscle fiber, releasing calcium in the cytoplasm of the cell. This calcium causes the actin and myosin to slide over each other, shortening the fibers and the cell. Many muscle cells are bundled together to create muscle fibers and muscles.

The tissue that makes up the heart is known as cardiac muscle. It has characteristics of both skeletal and smooth muscle. **Cardiac muscle** cells have a single nucleus, like smooth muscle, and are striated, like skeletal muscle. Cardiac muscle cells are connected by gap junctions just like smooth muscles are, so cells can pass action potentials directly throughout the heart and do not require chemical synapses. Cardiac muscle contraction is regulated by the autonomic nervous system, which increases the rate and strength of contractions through sympathetic stimulation and decreases their rate through the parasympathetic system. Cardiac muscle has an internal pacemaker responsible for the heartbeat that is modified by the nervous system but does not require the nervous system to maintain a regular heartbeat.

🅚 🅗 HUMAN REPRODUCTION AND EMBRYONIC DEVELOPMENT

Human Male Reproductive System

The human male produces sperm in the **testes**, gonads located in an outpocketing of the abdominal wall called the **scrotum**. The sperm develop in a series of small, coiled tubes within the testes called the **seminiferous tubules**. **Sertoli cells** in the seminiferous tubules support the sperm and **Leydig cells** make the **testosterone** that supports male secondary sex characteristics.

The **vas deferens** carries sperm to the urethra, which passes through the penis. During ejaculation, the **prostate gland** and **seminal vesicles** along the path add secretions to the sperm that carry and provide nutrients for the sperm as part of **semen**.

As gonads, the testes have a dual function; they produce both sperm and male hormones (such as testosterone). Leydig cells in the testis secrete testosterone beginning in puberty. **Testosterone** and other steroid hormones collectively called **androgens** induce secondary sexual characteristics of the male, such as facial and pubic hair, changes in body shape, and deepening voice changes.

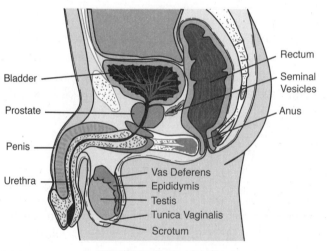

Male Reproductive System

Spermatogenesis is the meiotic development of sperm in males. Sperm production occurs throughout adult life in males, and meiosis in sperm production is continuous, proceeding forward without a significant pause. In the testes, diploid germ cells divide mitotically to create primary **spermatocytes**, which continuously undergo meiosis to form four haploid **spermatids** from each primary spermatocyte. The four spermatids are equivalent in size and function, and all four result in viable gametes. Spermatids must mature further to develop the characteristics held by mature sperm: a head containing DNA and a tail that provides motility. A specialized sac at the tip of the sperm called the **acrosome** is full of enzymes that allow the sperm to break through the protective layers around the egg. One birth control strategy has been to inhibit these enzymes so that sperm cannot reach the egg. The testes are located outside the abdominal cavity because they must remain 2–4° cooler than the rest of the body to ensure proper development of sperm.

Human Female Reproductive System

The **ovum** develops in a discontinuous process called **oogenesis** that is not completed in a single continuous process, unlike spermatogenesis. During development of female children, ova progress to **meiotic prophase I** in the first round of meiotic cell division and then become arrested, stuck at this stage. These ova remain arrested in meiosis throughout the life of a woman, except for the ova that mature during each menstrual cycle and progress through this meiotic block. Women are born with all the **eggs** they will ever have, while males produce fresh sperm daily. This is the reason that genetic anomalies are more common in the eggs of older women; these anomalies have had years to accumulate in ova while sperm have a short life span.

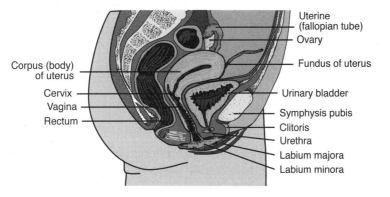

Corpus (body) of uterus
Cervix
Vagina
Rectum

Uterine (fallopian tube)
Ovary
Fundus of uterus
Urinary bladder
Symphysis pubis
Clitoris
Urethra
Labium majora
Labium minora

Female Reproductive System

The completion of the first meiotic cell division by maturing ova preparing for ovulation creates one cell with most of the cytoplasm and another smaller cell that has little cytoplasm. This smaller cell may itself divide later to create two smaller cells, but does not create viable ova and is called a **polar body**. The developing ovum becomes a secondary oocyte that pauses again during the second meiotic cell division, even as it is released during ovulation. The ova in humans do not actually complete oogenesis until after fertilization, at which time the ovum releases the last polar body and joins the nuclei of the male and female cells to create the diploid zygote. The unequal distribution of cytoplasm during oogenesis is another feature that is distinct from spermatogenesis.

Ovaries are paired structures in the lower portion of the abdominal cavity. As part of the menstrual cycle, one ovum develops each month within a follicle in an ovary. The follicle is a collection of cells around the ova that support its development and secrete hormones. Each ovary is accompanied by a **fallopian tube**, also called an **oviduct**. During ovulation, an ovum leaves the ovary through the follicle and is ejected into the upper end of the oviduct. At birth, all the eggs that a female will ovulate during her lifetime are already present in the ovaries, but these eggs develop and ovulate at a rate of one every 28 days (approximately), starting in puberty.

The ovaries also produce female sex hormones such as **estrogen**. Like male sex hormones, the female sex hormones regulate the secondary sexual characteristics of the female, including the development of the **mammary** (milk) **glands** and wider hip bones (pelvis). They also play an important role in the menstrual cycle, which involves the interaction of the pituitary gland, ovaries, and uterus.

Embryonic Development

The first step in development is **fertilization**. If sperm are present in the oviduct during ovulation, and a sperm succeeds in encountering the ovum, then fertilization can occur, forming a **zygote**, a single **diploid** cell. During fertilization, the egg nucleus (containing the **haploid number**, or **n chromosomes**) unites with the sperm nucleus (containing n **chromosomes**). This union produces a zygote of the original diploid or **2n** chromosome number. In this way, the normal somatic number (2n) of chromosomes in a diploid cell is restored, and the cell has two homologous copies of each chromosome.

Everything else in development up to adulthood consists of mitotic divisions. If there are two or more eggs released by the ovaries, more than one can be fertilized. The result of several eggs being fertilized is multiple gestation, producing fraternal twins, triplets, quadruplets, etc., which are produced when two or more separate sperm fertilize two or more eggs.

Fraternal twins are related genetically in the same way that any two siblings are. Drugs to treat infertility often induce multiple ovulation and can lead to multiple-birth pregnancies. If there is only one fertilized egg, twins may still result through separation of identical cells during the early stages of cleavage (for example, the two-, four-, or eight-cell stage) into two or more independent embryos. These develop into identical (**monozygotic**) twins, triplets, and so forth, since they all came from the same fertilized egg and have identical genomes. Identical twins are often used in human genetic studies to determine what traits are genetically inherited, since their environment must cause differences between the twins.

When the egg and the sperm join, they trigger a cascade of events that occur as the zygote begins to divide rapidly. These events, which are part of the process of fertilization, may occur either externally or internally.

🅚 🅗 COMMONLY CONFUSED TERMS IN ANATOMY AND PHYSIOLOGY

Like biology, the study of anatomy and physiology involves a number of terms that are easy to confuse. Following are some of the most commonly confused terms, with explanations to distinguish them from one another.

Don't Confuse These on Test Day

- **mRNA**, or messenger RNA, carries messages that encode proteins.
- **tRNA**, or transfer RNA, carries amino acids to make proteins.
- **rRNA**, or ribosomal RNA, is a structural component of ribosomes.

- **Transcription** involves DNA being read and that information being transcribed or transferred to RNA.
- **Translation** is when RNA is read, leading to the process of protein synthesis.

- **Prokaryotes** have no nucleus and no membrane-bound organelles but do have ribosomes and cell walls made up of peptidoglycans.
- **Eukaryotes** have a nucleus, membrane-bound organelles, and ribosomes. Examples include protists, fungi, plants, and animals. Fungi and plant eukaryotic cells have cell walls made of cellulose.

- **Spermatogenesis** is characterized by several things, including:
  - *The production of four mature sperm; each sperm has an X or Y chromosome and does not donate mitochondria to the embryo.*
  - *The process is continuous.*
  - *Fresh sperm are created daily.*

- **Oogenesis** is characterized by the following:
  - *The process produces one egg and two to three polar bodies.*
  - *Only ova with X chromosomes are produced.*
  - *The process is discontinuous.*
  - *The process produces ova that donate mitochondria to embryos.*
  - *A limited supply of ova is produced early in life and the development of ova is arrested later in life.*

- The **right ventricle** pumps blood to the lungs in the pulmonary artery.
- The **left ventricle** pumps blood through the aorta to the rest of the body.

- **Atria** receive blood from veins.
- **Ventricles** pump blood out of arteries.

KAPLAN

- **Arteries** have the following characteristics and functions:
  - *Thick-walled.*
  - *Oxygenated.*
  - *Conduct blood at high pressures.*
  - *Have a pulse.*
  - *Have no valves to prevent backflow.*

- **Veins** have the following characteristics and functions:
  - *Thin-walled.*
  - *Deoxygenated.*
  - *Conduct blood at low pressures.*
  - *Have no pulse.*
  - *Have valves to prevent backflow.*

- The **sympathetic nervous system** has the following characteristics and functions:
  - *Associated with the fight-or-flight response.*
  - *Increases the heart rate.*
  - *Increases the breathing rate.*
  - *Lowers the digestive rate.*
  - *Causes pupil dilation.*

- The **parasympathetic nervous system** has the following characteristics and functions:
  - *Is associated with the rest-and-digest response.*
  - *Lowers the heart rate.*
  - *Does not affect the breathing rate.*
  - *Increases the digestive rate.*
  - *Does not cause pupil dilation.*

- **Cones** are photoreceptors that respond to high-intensity illumination and color.
- **Rods** respond to low-intensity illumination (they are important in night vision) but do not detect color well.

- **Smooth muscle** is involuntary muscle present in the arteries, gastrointestinal tract, and elsewhere.
- **Skeletal muscles** are voluntary muscles that cause body movement.
- **Cardiac muscle** is the tissue that makes up the heart.

REVIEW QUESTIONS

The following questions are not meant to mimic actual test questions. Instead, these questions will help you review the concepts and terms covered in this chapter.

1. List the five key electrolytes in the body:

    _____

    _____

    _____

    _____

    _____

2. List the four main tissue types in the body:

    _____

    _____

    _____

    _____

3. What directional term means "at or toward the top of the body or head"?

    _____

4. Where does chemical digestion begin?

    _____

5. What is the difference between passive immunity and active immunity in the body?

    _____

    _____

    _____

    _____

6. True or False? Vertebrates have closed circulatory systems.

7. Name at least three of the air passages involved in respiration.

    _____

    _____

    _____

8. What system enables organisms to receive and respond to stimuli from their external and internal environments?

    _____

9. Name the three different muscle types vertebrates possess.

    _____

    _____

    _____

10. Which is a characteristic or function of the parasympathetic nervous system?

    (A) Increases the heart rate.
    (B) Increases the digestive rate.
    (C) Increases the breathing rate.
    (D) Increases the size of the pupils.

REVIEW ANSWERS

1. The five key electrolytes in the body are sodium, potassium, chloride, bicarbonate, and magnesium.

2. The four main tissue types in the body are connective tissue, epithelial tissue, muscle tissue, and nerve tissue.

3. The directional term *superior* means "at or toward the top of the body or head."

4. Chemical digestion begins in the mouth, where enzymes in saliva begin to break down complex starches into simple sugars.

5. *Passive immunity* involves barriers that block potential pathogens from entering the body. The skin is a key element in the body's passive immune defenses. *Active immunity* is the process by which the body identifies and eliminates pathogens from the body; this is done mainly by white blood cells.

6. True.

7. Answers may vary. The air passages involved in respiration consist of the nose, pharynx, larynx, trachea, bronchi, bronchioles, and alveoli.

8. The nervous system enables organisms to receive and respond to stimuli from their external and internal environments.

9. Vertebrates possess three different types of muscle tissues: smooth, skeletal, and cardiac.

10. **B** One characteristic of the parasympathetic nervous system is that it increases the digestive rate. Increases in heart rate, (A), and breathing rate, (C), along with pupil dilation, (D), occur as a result of the sympathetic, not parasympathetic, nervous system.

Chapter Nine: **Physical Science Review**

In the last two chapters, you reviewed all the basics about life sciences: biology and anatomy and physiology. Life science topics appear on both the Kaplan exam and the HESI A2 exam. This chapter reviews the two major subjects of physical science: chemistry and physics.

Physical science topics appear on the HESI exam, but not the Kaplan. If you are taking the Kaplan exam, you may opt to omit this chapter from your review. If you are taking the HESI exam, this chapter is a must. It has a separate lesson for both of those divisions, followed by strategies to help you on the test, as well as a review of topics covered in this chapter. Before you get started, here's some information you may find helpful for tackling chemistry and physics.

Ⓗ MATH FOR SCIENCE

Before starting the following lessons, let's review some of the basic mathematical concepts often used in both chemistry and physics: exponents, the metric system and SI units, scientific notation, and powers of ten.

If you believe your math skills in these areas are strong, and you are confident you do not need to review any further, jump ahead to the chemistry lesson.

Exponents

For any nonzero number a and any integer n:

Exponent of zero: $a^0 = 1$

Exponent of one: $a^1 = a$

Negative exponent: $a^{-n} = \frac{1}{a^n}$

If a, b, x, y, and z are all integers:

Product of powers: $(a^x)(a^y) = a^{x+y}$

Power of powers: $(a^x)^y = a^{xy}$

Quotient of powers: $\frac{a^x}{a^y} = a^{x-y}$

Power of a product: $(ab)^x = a^x b^x$

Power of a monomial: $(a^x b^y)^z = a^{xz} b^{yz}$

The nth root of powers: $\sqrt[y]{a^x} = a^{x/y}$

KAPLAN

Powers of Ten

When $a = 10$, the rules listed on the previous page can also be used. For example:

$$10^0 = 1$$
$$10^1 = 10$$
$$10^2 = 100$$
$$10^3 = 1,000, \text{ and so on. Also:}$$
$$10^{-1} = \frac{1}{10}$$
$$10^{-2} = \frac{1}{100}$$
$$10^{-3} = \frac{1}{1,000}, \text{ and so on.}$$

Scientific Notation

Very large and very small numbers are often used in both chemistry and physics. Scientific notation is a convention for expressing numbers that simplifies the calculation of equations and standardizes their results. To express a number in scientific notation, convert it into a number between 1 and 10 (the **mantissa** or **coefficient**) multiplied by the number 10; raised to the appropriate **exponent** (the power a number is raised to).

For example, with scientific notation, the number 7,000,000,000 would be expressed as: 7×10^9. In this example, the number 7 is the mantissa, and the number 10 is raised to an exponent of 9. Scientific notation can also be used for numbers smaller than one; for example, the number 0.042 would be expressed as 4.2×10^{-2}.

The Metric System and Systeme Internationale (SI) Units

The metric system involves measurement organized in multiples and submultiples related by powers of 10. The system is structured to measure six base units: length, mass, temperature, time, electric current, and substance. The metric system includes other units, but they are all tied to the core six units.

SI Base Units of the Metric System

Base Quantity	Base Unit	Symbol
Length	meter	m
Mass	kilogram	kg
Time	second	s
Temperature	Kelvin	K
Amount of Substance	mole	mol
Electric Current	ampere	A

The metric system employs a system whereby powers of 10 are assigned specific names or prefixes. These prefixes are placed before a unit to indicate the power of 10 that is the fraction or multiplier of that unit.

Common Metric Prefixes

Prefix	Symbol	Power of 10	Example
nano	n	10^{-9}	nanosecond (ns)
micro	μ	10^{-6}	microfarad (mF)
milli	m	10^{-3}	milligram (mg)
centi	c	10^{-2}	centimeter (cm)
kilo	k	10^{3}	kilogram (kg)
mega	M	10^{6}	megawatt (MW)

Now that you have the basics down, let's get started.

H CHEMISTRY LESSON

Atomic Structure

The **atom** is the basic building block of matter, representing the smallest unit of a chemical element. In 1911, Ernest Rutherford provided experimental evidence that an atom has a dense, positively charged **nucleus** that accounts for only a small portion of the volume of the atom. The nucleus, which is the core of the atom, is formed by two subatomic particles, called **protons** and **neutrons**. A third form of subatomic particle known as **electrons** exist outside the nucleus in characteristic regions of space called orbitals. All atoms of an element show similar chemical properties and cannot be further broken down by chemical means.

Subatomic Particles

Protons

Protons carry a single positive charge and have a mass of approximately one atomic mass unit (abbreviated as amu.). The atomic number Z of an element is equal to the number of protons found in an atom of that element. All atoms of a given element have the same atomic number; in other words, the number of protons an atom has defines the element. The atomic number of an element can be found in the periodic table (see the section about the periodic table that is found later in the lesson) as an integer above the symbol for the element.

Neutrons

Neutrons carry no charge and have a mass only slightly heavier than that of protons. The total number of neutrons and protons in an atom, known as the mass number, determines its mass.

KAPLAN

Electrons

Electrons carry a charge equal in magnitude but opposite in charge to that of protons. An electron has a very small mass, approximately $\frac{1}{1,836}$ the mass of a proton or neutron, which is negligible for most purposes. The electrons farthest from the nucleus are known as valence electrons. The further the valence electrons are from the nucleus, the weaker the attractive force of the positively charged nucleus and the more likely the valence electrons are to be influenced by other atoms. Generally, valence electrons and their activity determine the reactivity of an atom. In a neutral atom, the number of electrons is equal to the number of protons. A positive or negative charge on an atom is due to a loss or gain of electrons; the result is called an **ion**. A positively charged ion (one that has lost electrons) is known as a **cation**; a negatively charged ion (one that has gained electrons) is known as an **anion**.

Subatomic Particle	Relative Mass	Charge	Location
Proton	1	1	Nucleus
Neutron	1	0	Nucleus
Electron	0	−1	Electron orbitals

Nuclear Chemistry

Now that you understand atomic structure, it's time to review nuclear chemistry.

The Nucleus

At the center of an atom lies its nucleus, consisting of one or more nucleons (protons or neutrons) held together with considerably more energy than what is needed to hold electrons in orbit around the nucleus. The radius of a nucleus is about 100,000 times smaller than the radius of an atom. Before we go on, let's review some concepts we've just read about.

Atomic Number Z

An element's atomic number is defined by the number of protons in its nucleus; the name *atomic number Z* is used to represent this number. The letter Z represents an integer that is equal to the number of protons in a nucleus. The number of protons is what defines an element: An atom, ion, or nucleus is identified as carbon, for example, only if it has six protons. Each element has a unique number of protons. The letter Z is used as a presubscript to the chemical symbol in isotopic notation; that is, it appears as a subscript before the chemical symbol. The chemical symbols and the atomic numbers of all the elements are given in the periodic table. You will find more information about the periodic table later in the lesson.

Mass Number A

When calculating mass number, **A** is an integer equal to the total number of nucleons (neutrons and protons) in a nucleus. Let **N** represent the number of neutrons in a nucleus. The equation relating **A**, **N**, and **Z** is simply:

$$A = N + Z$$

Isotopes

Different nuclei of the same element will by definition all have the same number of protons. The number of neutrons, however, can be different. Nuclei of the same element can therefore have different mass numbers. For a nucleus of a given element with a particular number of protons (atomic number Z), the various nuclei with different numbers of neutrons are called **isotopes** of that element.

For example, the three isotopes of hydrogen are:

$^1_1$H: A single proton; the nucleus of ordinary hydrogen.

$^2_1$H: A proton and a neutron together; the nucleus of one type of heavy hydrogen called deuterium.

$^3_1$H: A proton and two neutrons together; the nucleus of a heavier type of heavy hydrogen called tritium.

Note that despite the existence of names like deuterium and tritium, they are all considered hydrogen because they have the same number of protons (one). The example shown here is a little bit of an anomaly because in general isotopes do not have specific names of their own.

Atomic Mass and Atomic Mass Unit

Atomic mass is most commonly measured in atomic mass units (abbreviated amu). By definition, 1 amu is exactly one-twelfth the mass of the neutral carbon-12 atom. In terms of more familiar mass units:

$$1 \text{ amu} = 1.66 \times 10^{-27} \text{ kg} = 1.66 \times 10^{-24} \text{ g}$$

Atomic Weight

Elements have different masses because of isotopes. Atomic weight refers to a weighted average of the masses of an element. The average is weighted according to the natural abundances of the various isotopic species of an element. The atomic weight can be measured in amu.

Nuclear Reactions

Nuclear reactions such as fusion, fission, and radioactive decay involve either combining or splitting the nuclei of atoms. Since the binding energy per nucleon is greatest for intermediate-sized atoms, when small atoms combine or large atoms split a great amount of energy is released.

Fusion

Fusion occurs when small nuclei combine into a larger nucleus. As an example, many stars—including the sun—power themselves by fusing four hydrogen nuclei to make one helium nucleus. Through this method, the sun produces 4×10^{26} joules (J) every second. Here on Earth, researchers are trying to find ways to use fusion as an alternative energy source.

KAPLAN)

Fission

Fission is a process in which a large nucleus splits into smaller nuclei. Spontaneous fission rarely occurs. However, by the absorption of a low-energy neutron, fission can be induced in certain nuclei. Of special interest are those fission reactions that release more neutrons, since these other neutrons will cause other atoms to undergo fission. This, in turn, releases more neutrons, creating a chain reaction. Such induced fission reactions power commercial electricity-generating nuclear plants.

Radioactive Decay

Radioactive decay is naturally occurring and spontaneous. It is characterized by the decay of certain nuclei and the emission of specific particles. It could be classified as a certain type of fission. The **reactant** in radioactive decay is known as the **parent isotope** while the product is the daughter isotope.

Alpha Decay

Alpha decay is the emission of an alpha (α) particle, which is a ^{4}He nucleus that consists of two protons and two neutrons. The alpha particle is very massive (compared to a beta particle, see below) and doubly charged. Alpha particles interact with matter very easily; hence they do not penetrate shielding (such as lead sheets) very far.

Beta Decay

Beta decay is the emission of a beta particle (β). Despite the similarity between electrons and beta particles, it is important to realize that these particles are not electrons that would normally be found around the nucleus in a neutral atom. Rather, they are products of decay emitted by the nucleus. This is particularly true when a neutron in the nucleus decays into a proton and an electron. Since an electron is singly charged, and about 1,836 times lighter than a proton, the beta radiation from radioactive decay is more penetrating than alpha radiation.

Gamma Decay

Gamma decay is the emission of gamma rays (γ), which are high-energy photons. They carry no charge and simply lower the energy of the emitting (parent) nucleus without changing the mass number or the atomic number. In other words, the daughter's **A** is the same as the parent's, and the daughter's **Z** is the same as the parent's.

Radioactive Decay Half-Life (t1/2)

In a collection of a great many identical radioactive isotopes, the half-life of a sample is the time it takes for half of the sample to decay. For example: If the half-life of a certain isotope is four years, what fraction of a sample of that isotope will remain after 12 years?

Solution: If four years is one half-life, then 12 years is three half-lives. During the first half-life—the first four years—half of the sample will have decayed. During the second half-life (years five to eight), another half will decay, leaving one-fourth of the original. During the third and final period (years nine to 12), half of the remaining fourth will decay, leaving one-eighth of the original sample.

The fact that different radioactive species have different characteristic half-lives is what enables scientists to determine the age of organic materials. The long-lived radioactive carbon isotope ^{14}C, for example, is generated from nuclear reactions induced by high-energy cosmic rays from outer space. There is always a certain fraction of this isotope in the carbon found on Earth. Living things, like trees and animals, are constantly exchanging carbon with the environment, and thus will have the same ratio of carbon-14 to carbon-12 within them as is present in the atmosphere. Once they die, however, they stop incorporating carbon from the environment, and start to lose carbon-14 because of its radioactivity. The longer the species has been dead, the less carbon-14 it will still have. For example, if a sample is taken from an item or a body and the ratio of ^{14}C to ^{12}C is half of that present in the atmosphere, we would conclude that the species existed about one half-life of ^{14}C ago.

Periodic Table of the Elements

The periodic table has been mentioned earlier in this lesson. Now it's time to find out more about it. The periodic table arranges elements in increasing atomic numbers. Its spatial layout is such that a lot of information about an element's properties can be deduced simply by examining its position. The vertical columns are called **groups**, while the horizontal rows are called **periods**. There are seven periods, representing the principal quantum numbers $n = 1$ to $n = 7$, and each period is filled more or less sequentially. The period an element is in tells us the highest shell that is occupied, or the highest principal quantum number. Elements in the same group (same column) have the same electronic configuration in their valence, or outermost shell. For example, both magnesium (Mg) and calcium (Ca) are in the second column; they both have two electrons in the outermost s subshell, the only difference being that the principal quantum number is different for Ca ($n = 4$) than for Mg ($n = 3$). Because these outermost electrons, or valence electrons, are involved in chemical bonding, they determine the chemical reactivity and properties of the element. In short, elements in the same group will tend to have similar levels of chemical reactiveness.

Valence Electrons and the Periodic Table

The valence electrons of an atom are those electrons in its outer energy shell. The visual layout of the periodic table is convenient for determining the electron configuration of an atom (especially the valence electron configuration).

Periodic Trends of the Elements

The properties of elements exhibit certain trends, which can be explained in terms of the element's position in the periodic table or its electron configuration. In general, elements seek to gain or lose valence electrons so as to achieve the stable octet formation possessed by the inert or noble gases of Group VIII (last column of the periodic table). Two other important general trends exist. First, as one goes from left to right across a period, it becomes clear that the number of electrons for each element increases one at a time; the electrons of the outermost shell experience an increasing amount of nuclear attraction, becoming closer and more tightly bound to the nucleus. Second, scanning a given column for a group element from top to bottom shows that with each element the outermost electrons become less tightly bound to the nucleus. This is because the number of filled principal energy levels (which shield the outermost electrons from attraction by the nucleus) increases downward within each group. These trends help explain elemental properties such as atomic radius, ionization potential, electron affinity, and electronegativity.

Periodic Table of the Elements

Group

Period	1 IA 1A	2 IIA 2A	3 IIIB 3B	4 IVB 4B	5 VB 5B	6 VIB 6B	7 VIIB 7B	8 ------	9 VIII --	10 -----	11 IB 1B	12 IIB 2B	13 IIIA 3A	14 IVA 4A	15 VA 5A	16 VIA 6A	17 VIIA 7A	18 VIIIA 8A
1	1 H 1.008																	2 He 4.003
2	3 Li 6.941	4 Be 9.012											5 B 10.81	6 C 12.01	7 N 14.01	8 O 16.00	9 F 19.00	10 Ne 20.18
3	11 Na 22.99	12 Mg 24.31						------ 8 ------					13 Al 26.98	14 Si 28.09	15 P 30.97	16 S 32.07	17 Cl 35.45	18 Ar 39.95
4	19 K 39.10	20 Ca 40.08	21 Sc 44.96	22 Ti 47.88	23 V 50.94	24 Cr 52.00	25 Mn 54.94	26 Fe 55.85	27 Co 58.47	28 Ni 58.69	29 Cu 63.55	30 Zn 65.39	31 Ga 69.72	32 Ge 72.59	33 As 74.92	34 Se 78.96	35 Br 79.90	36 Kr 83.80
5	37 Rb 85.47	38 Sr 87.62	39 Y 88.91	40 Zr 91.22	41 Nb 92.91	42 Mo 95.94	43 Tc (98)	44 Ru 101.1	45 Rh 102.9	46 Pd 106.4	47 Ag 107.9	48 Cd 112.4	49 In 114.8	50 Sn 118.7	51 Sb 121.8	52 Te 127.6	53 I 126.9	54 Xe 131.3
6	55 Cs 132.9	56 Ba 137.3	57 La* 138.9	72 Hf 178.5	73 Ta 180.9	74 W 183.9	75 Re 186.2	76 Os 190.2	77 Ir 190.2	78 Pt 195.1	79 Au 197.0	80 Hg 200.5	81 Tl 204.4	82 Pb 207.2	83 Bi 209.0	84 Po (210)	85 At (210)	86 Rn (222)
7	87 Fr (223)	88 Ra (226)	89 Ac~ (227)	104 Rf (257)	105 Db (260)	106 Sg (263)	107 Bh (262)	108 Hs (265)	109 Mt (266)	110 --- ()	111 --- ()	112 --- ()		114 --- ()		116 --- ()		118 --- ()

Lanthanide Series*	58 Ce 140.1	59 Pr 140.9	60 Nd 144.2	61 Pm (147)	62 Sm 150.4	63 Eu 152.0	64 Gd 157.3	65 Tb 158.9	66 Dy 162.5	67 Ho 164.9	68 Er 167.3	69 Tm 168.9	70 Yb 173.0	71 Lu 175.0
Actinide Series~	90 Th 232.0	91 Pa (231)	92 U (238)	93 Np (237)	94 Pu (242)	95 Am (243)	96 Cm (247)	97 Bk (247)	98 Cf (249)	99 Es (254)	100 Fm (253)	101 Md (256)	102 No (254)	103 Lr (257)

Atomic Radius

The atomic radius is an indication of the size of an atom. In general, with each element in a period the atomic radius decreases across a period (from left to right on the table). Within each group, the atomic radius increases (from top to bottom on the table). The atoms with the largest atomic radii are found in the last period (bottom line) of Group I (furthest to the left).

As one moves from left to right across a period, the number of electrons in the outer shell increases one at a time. Electrons in the same shell cannot shield one another from the attractive pull of protons very efficiently. As the number of protons increases, a greater positive charge is produced and the effective nuclear charge increases steadily across a period. This means the valence electrons feel an increasingly strong attraction towards the nucleus, which causes the atomic radius to decrease.

As one moves down a group of the periodic table, the number of electrons and filled electron shells will increase, but the number of valence electrons will remain the same. Thus, the outermost electrons in a given group will feel the same amount of effective nuclear charge, but electrons will be found further from the nucleus as the number of filled energy shells increases. Thus, the atomic radius increases.

Ionization Energy

The **ionization energy** (IE), or **ionization potential**, is the energy required to completely remove an electron from an atom or ion. Removing an electron from an atom always requires an input of energy, since it is attracted to the positively charged nucleus. The closer and more tightly bound an electron is to the nucleus, the more difficult it is to remove, and the higher its level of ionization energy. Ionization energies grow successively. The **first ionization energy** is the energy required to remove one valence electron from a parent atom; the **second ionization energy** is the energy needed to remove a second valence electron from an ion with a $+1$ charge to form an ion with a $+2$ charge, and so on.

Ionization energy increases from left to right across a period as the atomic radius decreases. Moving down a group, ionization energy decreases as the atomic radius increases. Group I elements have low ionization energies because the loss of an electron results in the formation of a stable octet.

Electron Affinity

Electron affinity is the energy released when an electron is added to a gaseous atom. It represents the ease with which an atom can accept an electron. The stronger the attractive pull of the nucleus for electrons, the greater the electron affinity will be. A positive electron affinity value represents energy release when an electron is added to an atom.

A casual way of describing the difference between ionization energy and electron affinity is that the former tells us how attached the atom is to the electrons it already has, while the latter tells us how the atom feels about gaining another electron.

Electronegativity

Electronegativity is a measure of the attraction an atom has for electrons in a chemical bond. The greater the electronegativity of an atom, the greater its attraction for bonding electrons. This concept is related to ionization energy and electron affinity: Elements with low ionization energies and low electron affinities will have low levels of electronegativity because their nuclei do not attract electrons strongly, while elements with high ionization energies and high electron affinities will have higher levels of electronegativity because of the strong pull the nucleus has on electrons. Therefore, electronegativity increases from left to right across periods. In any group, electronegativity decreases as the atomic number increases, as a result of the increased distance between the valence electrons and the nucleus—that is, greater atomic radius.

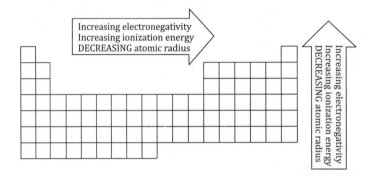

Categories of Elements

The elements of the periodic table may be classified into three categories: metals, located on the left side and the middle of the periodic table; nonmetals, located on the right side of the table; and metalloids (semimetals), found along a diagonal line between the other two.

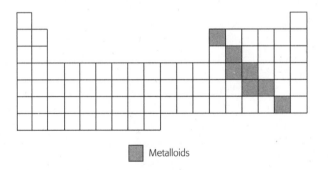

Metals

Metals are shiny solids at room temperature (except for mercury, which is a liquid) and generally have high melting points and densities. Metals have the characteristic ability to be deformed without breaking. Metal's ability to be hammered into shapes is called **malleability;** its ability to be drawn into wires is called **ductility**. Many of the characteristic properties of metals, such as large atomic radius, low ionization energy, and low electronegativity, are due to the fact that the few electrons in the valence shell of a metal atom can easily be removed.

Because valence electrons can move freely, metals are good conductors of heat and electricity. Group IA and IIA represent the most reactive metals. The transition elements are metals that have partially filled **d orbitals**.

Nonmetals

Nonmetals are generally brittle in a solid state and show little or no metallic luster. They have high ionization energies and electronegativities, and are usually poor conductors of both heat and electricity. Most nonmetals share the ability to gain electrons easily (i.e., they tend to form negative ions), but otherwise they display a wide range of chemical behaviors and reactiveness. Nonmetals are located on the upper right side of the periodic table; they are separated from the metals by a line cutting diagonally through the region of the periodic table containing elements with partially filled **p orbitals**.

Metalloids

In the periodic table, the metalloids, or semimetals, are found along the line between the metals and nonmetals. The properties of metalloids vary considerably; their densities, boiling points, and melting points fluctuate widely. Their ionization energies and electronegativities lie between those of metals and nonmetals; therefore, these elements possess characteristics of both those classes. For example, silicon has a metallic luster, yet it is brittle and not an efficient conductor. The reactivity of metalloids is dependent upon the element with which they are reacting. For example, boron (B) behaves as a nonmetal when reacting with sodium (Na) and as a metal when reacting with fluorine (F). The elements classified as metalloids are boron, silicon (Si), germanium (Ge), arsenic (As), antimony (Sb), polonium (Po), and tellurium (Te).

The Chemistry of Groups

Elements in the same group, or column of the periodic table, have the same number of valence electrons, and hence tend to have very similar chemical properties.

Alkali Metals

The alkali metals are the elements of Group IA. They possess most of the physical properties common to metals, yet their densities are lower than those of other metals. The alkali metals have only one loosely bound electron in their outermost shell, giving them the largest atomic radii of all the elements in their respective periods. Their metallic properties and high levels of reactivity are determined by the fact that they have low ionization energies; thus, they easily lose their valence electron to form univalent **cations** (cations with a +1 charge). Alkali metals have low levels of electronegativity and react very readily with nonmetals, especially halogens.

Alkaline Earth Metals

The alkaline earth metals are the elements of Group IIA. They also possess many characteristically metallic properties. Like the alkali metals, these properties are dependent upon the ease with which they lose electrons. The alkaline earth metals have two electrons in their outer shell and thus have smaller atomic radii than the alkali metals. Alkaline earths have low electronegativities and low electron affinities.

KAPLAN

Halogens

The halogens, Group VIIA (second to last column of the periodic table), are highly reactive nonmetals. They have seven valence electrons, one short of the favored octet configuration. Halogens are highly variable in their physical properties. For instance, at room temperature, the halogens range from gaseous (F_2 and Cl_2) to liquid (Br_2) to solid (I_2). Their chemical properties are more uniform: The electronegativities of halogens are very high, and they are particularly reactive with alkali metals and alkaline earth metals that *want* to donate electrons to the halogens to form stable ionic crystals.

Noble Gases

The noble gases, also called inert gases, are found in Group VIII. They are fairly nonreactive because they have a complete valence shell, which is an energetically favored arrangement. As a result, they have high ionization energies. They possess low boiling points and are all gases at room temperature.

Transition Elements

The transition elements are those that are found between the alkaline earth metals (the last six columns of the periodic table). The numbering of the groups can get rather confusing because of the existence of two conventions, but you needn't be too concerned with this. These elements are metals known as transition metals. They are very hard and have both high melting and boiling points. As one moves across a period, the five **d orbitals** become progressively more filled. The **d electrons** are held only loosely by the nucleus and are relatively mobile, contributing to the malleability and high electrical conductivity of these elements. Chemically, transition elements have low ionization energies and may exist in a variety of positively charged forms or oxidation states.

Chemical Bonding

The atoms of many elements can combine to form **molecules**. The atoms in most molecules are held together by strong attractive forces called chemical bonds. These bonds are formed via the interaction of the valence electrons of combining atoms. The chemical and physical properties of the resulting molecules are often very different from those of their constituent elements. In addition to the very strong forces within a molecule, there are weaker intermolecular forces between molecules. These intermolecular forces, although weaker than the intramolecular chemical bonds, are of considerable importance for understanding the physical properties of many substances.

Processes that involve the breaking and forming of chemical bonds are generally considered chemical processes, while those that only involve interactions between molecules are generally considered physical processes.

In the formation of chemical bonds, many molecules contain atoms bonded according to the octet rule, which states that an atom tends to bond with other atoms until it has eight electrons in its outermost shell. These chemical bonds form a stable electron configuration similar to that of noble gas elements. Exceptions to this rule are as follows: hydrogen, which can have only two valence electrons (the configuration of He); lithium and beryllium, which bond to attain two and four valence electrons, respectively; boron, which bonds to attain six; and elements beyond the second row, such as phosphorus and sulfur, which can expand their octets to include more than eight electrons by incorporating **d orbitals**.

When classifying chemical bonds, it is helpful to introduce two distinct types: **ionic bonds** and **covalent bonds**. During ionic bonding, one or more electrons from an atom with a lower level of ionization energy are transferred to an atom with great electron affinity; the resulting ions are held together by electrostatic forces. During covalent bonding, an electron pair is shared between two atoms. In many cases, the bond is partially covalent and partially ionic; such bonds are called polar covalent bonds.

Ionic Bonds and Compounds

When two atoms with large differences in electronegativity react, the atom that is less electronegative completely transfers its electrons to the atom that is more electronegative. The elements with higher degrees of electronegativity remove electrons from less electronegative elements. The atom that loses electrons becomes a positively charged ion, or cation, and the atom that gains electrons becomes a negatively charged ion, or anion. In general, the elements of Groups I and II (low electronegativities) bond ionically to elements of Group VII (high electronegativities).

Ionic compounds have characteristic physical properties. They have high melting and boiling points due to the strong electrostatic forces between ions. They can conduct electricity in liquid and aqueous states, though not in solid states. Ionic solids form crystal lattices consisting of infinite arrays of positive and negative ions. In this arrangement, the attractive forces between ions of opposite charge are maximized, while the repulsive forces between ions of like charge are minimized.

Covalent Bonds

When two or more atoms with similar electronegativities interact, they often achieve a noble gas electron configuration by sharing electrons in what is known as a covalent bond. However, noble gas configuration is not always attained; there are exceptions to this rule. The binding force between two atoms results from the attraction that each electron of the shared pair has for the two positive nuclei. A covalent bond can be characterized by two features: bond length and bond energy. Bond length is the average distance between the two nuclei of atoms involved in forming the bond; bond energy is the energy required to separate two bonded atoms. As bond length decreases, bond strength increases.

Types of Covalent Bonding

The nature of a covalent bond depends on the relative electronegativities of the atoms sharing the electron pairs. Whether or not covalent bonds are considered polar or nonpolar depends on the difference in electronegativities between the atoms. Polar covalent bonding occurs between atoms with small differences in electronegativity. Nonpolar covalent bonding occurs between atoms that have the same electronegativities. This occurs between all of the diatomic elements, such as oxygen, nitrogen, etc.

Chemical Reactions

In the last section, we discussed how atoms combine and are held together by bonds that can be either ionic or covalent. When atoms combine, that process may result in the loss of some individual properties, while new characteristics may be gained. Water, for example, is formed from two hydrogen atoms and an oxygen atom, but it does not really behave like the elements hydrogen or oxygen.

A **compound** is a pure substance that is composed of two or more elements in fixed proportion. Compounds can be broken down chemically to produce their constituent elements or other compounds. All elements, except for some of the noble gases, can form new compounds by reacting with other elements or compounds. These new compounds can also react with elements or compounds to form yet more compounds.

Molecules

A molecule is a combination of two or more atoms held together by covalent bonds. It is the smallest unit of a compound that displays the properties of that compound. Molecules may contain two atoms of the same element, as in N_2 and O_2, or may be comprised of two or more different atoms, as in CO_2 and SOC_{12}.

Earlier, we discussed the concept of atomic weight. Like atoms, molecules can also be characterized by their weight. Molecular weight is simply the sum of the weights of the atoms that make up a molecule.

Types of Chemical Reactions

There are many ways in which elements and compounds can react to form other compounds; memorizing every reaction would be impossible, as well as unnecessary. However, nearly every inorganic reaction can be classified into at least one of four general categories.

Synthesis Reactions

Synthesis reactions are those in which two or more reactants form one product. The formation of sulfur dioxide by burning sulfur in air is an example of a synthesis reaction.

$$S\ (s) + O_2(g) \xrightarrow{\Delta} SO_2\ (g)$$

The letters in parentheses designate the phase of the species: **s** for solid, **g** for gas, **l** for liquid, and **aq** for aqueous solution. The sign Δ represents the addition of heat.

Decomposition Reactions

A decomposition reaction is defined as one in which a compound breaks down into two or more substances, usually as a result of heating. An example of a decomposition reaction is the breakdown of mercury (II) oxide. Typically, energy is released in these types of reactions, known as exothermic reactions.

$$2\ HgO(s) \longrightarrow 2\ Hg(l) + O_2(g) + \Delta$$

Single Displacement Reactions

Single displacement reactions occur when an atom (or ion) of one compound is replaced by an atom of another element. For example, zinc metal will displace copper ions in a copper sulfate solution to form zinc sulfate.

$$Zn\ (s) + CuSO_4(aq) \xrightarrow{\Delta} Cu\ (s) + ZnSO_4\ (aq)$$

Double Displacement Reactions

In double displacement reactions, also called metathesis reactions, elements from two different compounds displace each other to form two new compounds. For example, when solutions of calcium chloride and silver nitrate are combined, insoluble silver chloride forms in a solution of calcium nitrate.

$$CaCl_2\ (aq) + 2\ AgNO_3\ (aq) \xrightarrow{\Delta} Ca(NO_3)_2\ (aq) + 2\ AgCl\ (s)$$

Neutralization reactions are a specific type of double displacement that occurs when an acid reacts with a base to produce a solution of a salt and water. For example, hydrochloric acid and sodium hydroxide react to form sodium chloride and water.

$$HCl\ (aq) + NaOH\ (aq) \xrightarrow{\Delta} NaCl\ (aq) + H_2O\ (l)$$

Combustion Reactions

Combustion reactions occur when a compound reacts with oxygen to form water and carbon dioxide. For example, propane will combust in the presence of oxygen according to the following chemical equation:

$$C_3H_8\ (g) + 5O_2\ (g) - \xrightarrow{\Delta} 3CO_2\ (g) + 4H_2O\ (l)$$

Balanced Equations

Chemical equations express how much and what type of reactants must be used to obtain a given quantity of product. According to the law of conservation of mass, the mass of the reactants must be equal to the mass of the products. More specifically, chemical equations must be balanced with the correct coefficients so that the product contains the same number of atoms as the reactants.

A general method to learn how to balance a chemical equation is the following four-step method:

1. Determine whether the chemical equation is already balanced.
2. If the equation is not balanced, start by balancing the element that occurs in the fewest number of reactant and product molecules. Start with carbon or any atom with a high molar mass.
3. Balance the remaining elements.
4. Make sure that the number of atoms of each element is balanced.

Let's take a look at how to balance the following reaction of iron with water.

$$Fe + H_2O \longrightarrow Fe_3O_4 + H_2$$

When you look at the unbalanced reaction, it is clear that the equation is not already balanced because there are more iron atoms on the right side than on the left side. We can start by balancing Fe, since it is a high molar mass atom and only appears once on the reactant and product sides. There are three Fe atoms on the product side, so we can balance Fe by adding a coefficient of 3 to Fe on the reactant side:

$$3\ Fe + H_2O \longrightarrow 1\ Fe_3O_4 + H_2$$

Having balanced Fe, we can then turn to oxygen, since it occurs with Fe in Fe_3O_4 (and we have already balanced Fe). There are four atoms of oxygen on the product side, so we can balance oxygen by placing a coefficient of 4 in front of H_2O on the reactant side:

$$3\ Fe + 4\ H_2O \longrightarrow 1\ Fe_3O_4 + H_2$$

The last thing left to do is to balance hydrogen. There are now eight H atoms on the left side, so we place a coefficient of 4 in front of H_2 to balance the equation:

$$3\ Fe + 4\ H_2O \longrightarrow 1\ Fe_3O_4 + 4\ H_2$$

Phases of Matter

Matter exists in several phases—gas, liquid, solid and plasma—each with its own characteristics.

The Gaseous Phase

Among the different phases of matter, the gaseous phase is the simplest to understand and model, since all gases, to a first approximation, display similar behavior and follow similar laws, regardless of their identity. The atoms or molecules in a gaseous sample move rapidly and are far apart. In addition, intermolecular forces between gas particles tend to be weak; this results in certain characteristic physical properties, such as the ability to expand in order to fill any volume and to take on the shape of a container. Furthermore, gases are easily, though not infinitely, compressible.

Descriptive Chemistry of Some Common Gases

There are certain miscellaneous facts about the properties of some common gases you should be aware of. These properties are exploited in qualitative tests designed to detect their presence.

- **Oxygen:** Molecular oxygen, O_2, is a reactant in combustion reactions. If a glowing splint is lowered into a test tube containing oxygen, it will reignite.
- **Hydrogen:** When ignited in air, H_2, burns with a blue flame.
- **Nitrogen:** N_2, the largest component of air (a little less than 80% by volume) is relatively inert.
- **Carbon dioxide:** CO_2 produces a moderately acidic solution when dissolved in water because of the reaction:

$$CO_2\ (g)\ 1\ H_2O\ (l)\ \xrightarrow{\Delta}\ H_2CO_3\ (aq)$$

When carbon dioxide is passed through limewater, $Ca(OH)_2$, the solution turns cloudy from the formation of insoluble calcium carbonate:

$$CO_2 + Ca(OH)_2 \xrightarrow{\Delta} CaCO_3 + H_2O$$

The precipitation of calcium carbonate, however, does not go on indefinitely. As just mentioned, water containing CO_2 is slightly acidic, and this causes calcium carbonate to dissolve:

$$CaCO_3\ (s) + H_2O(l) + CO_2\ (g) \xrightarrow{\Delta} Ca_2 + (aq) + 2HCO_3 \xrightarrow{\Delta} (aq)$$

Kinetic Molecular Theory of Gases

All gases show similar physical characteristics and behavior. A theoretical model to explain why gases behave the way they do was developed during the second half of the nineteenth century. The combined efforts of Ludwig Boltzmann, James Clerk Maxwell, and others led to the **kinetic molecular theory of gases**, which gives us an understanding of the behavior of gases on a microscopic, molecular level. Like the gas laws, this theory was developed in reference to ideal gases, although it can be applied with reasonable accuracy to real gases as well. The assumptions of the kinetic molecular theory of gases are as follows:

1. Gases are made up of particles whose volumes are negligible compared to the container volume.
2. Gas atoms or molecules exhibit no intermolecular attractions or repulsions.
3. Gas particles are in continuous, random motion, undergoing collisions with other particles and with the container walls.
4. Collisions between any two gas particles are elastic, meaning that no energy is dissipated or, equivalently, no kinetic energy is conserved.
5. The average kinetic energy of gas particles is proportional to the absolute temperature of the gas and is the same for all gases at a given temperature.

Condensed Phase and Phase Changes

When the attractive forces between molecules overcome the random thermal kinetic energy that keeps molecules apart during the gas phase, molecules cluster together, unable to move about freely and then enter the liquid or solid phase. Because of their smaller volume relative to gases, liquids and solids are often referred to as the condensed phases.

General Properties of Liquids

In a liquid, atoms or molecules are held close together with little space between them. As a result, liquids, unlike gases, have definite volumes and cannot be expanded or compressed easily. However, molecules can still move around and are in a state of relative disorder. Consequently, a liquid can change shape to fit its container, and its molecules are able to diffuse and evaporate.

One of the most important properties of liquids is their ability to mix, both with each other and other phases, forming **solutions**. The degree to which two liquids can mix is called their **miscibility**. Oil and water are almost completely immiscible because of their difference in polarity. When oil and water are mixed, they normally form separate layers, with oil on top because it is less dense. Under extreme conditions, such as violent shaking, two immiscible liquids can form a fairly homogeneous mixture called an emulsion. Although they look like solutions, emulsions are actually mixtures of discrete particles too small to be seen distinctly.

General Properties of Solids

In a solid, the attractive forces between atoms, ions, or molecules are strong enough to hold them together rigidly; thus, the particles' only motion is vibration about fixed positions, and the kinetic energy of solids is predominantly vibrational energy. As a result, solids have definite shapes and volumes.

Phase Equilibria and Phase Changes

The different phases of matter interchange upon the absorption or release of energy, and more than one of them may exist in equilibrium under certain conditions. **Dynamic equilibrium** is a condition that permits two opposing processes to occur in a manner that the outcome's net change is zero. In the next sections, we will discuss some other types of equilibrium.

Gas-Liquid Equilibrium

The temperature of a liquid is related to the average kinetic energy of the liquid molecules; however, the kinetic energy of the individual molecules will vary (just as there is a distribution of molecular speeds in a gas). A few molecules near the surface of the liquid may have enough energy to leave the liquid phase and escape into the gaseous phase. This process is known as **evaporation** (or **vaporization**). Each time liquid loses a high-energy particle, the average kinetic energy of the remaining molecules decreases, which means that the temperature of the liquid decreases. Evaporation is thus a cooling process. Given enough kinetic energy, the liquid will completely evaporate.

If a cover is placed on a beaker of liquid, the escaping molecules are trapped above the solution. These molecules exert a countering pressure, which forces some of the gas back into the liquid phase; this process is called **condensation**.

Atmospheric pressure acts on a liquid in a similar fashion as a solid lid. As evaporation and condensation proceed, a state of equilibrium is reached in which the rates of the two processes become equal; that is, the liquid and vapor are in dynamic equilibrium. The pressure the gas exerts when the two phases are at equilibrium is called the **vapor pressure**. Vapor pressure increases as temperature increases because more molecules will have sufficient kinetic energy to escape into the gas phase. The temperature at which the vapor pressure of the liquid equals the external (most often atmospheric) pressure is called the boiling point. In general, then, the temperature at which a liquid boils is dependent on the pressure surrounding it. We know water boils at 100°C because at this temperature its vapor pressure (or the pressure exerted by the gas phase H_2O molecules) is equal to one atmosphere. At places of high elevation, the surrounding pressure is lower than 1 standard atmospheric pressure (atm), so water boils at a lower temperature. By controlling the ambient pressure, we can change the temperature at which water boils. This is the principle behind pressure cookers. By maintaining high pressure, water can reach a temperature higher than 100°C before it vaporizes, thus making it more effective at heating things.

Liquid-Solid Equilibrium

The liquid and solid phases can also coexist in equilibrium. Even though the atoms or molecules of a solid are confined to definite locations, each atom or molecule can undergo motions about some equilibrium position. These motions (vibrations) increase when energy (most commonly in the form of heat) is supplied. If atoms or molecules in the solid phase absorb enough energy in this fashion, the solid's three-dimensional structure breaks down and the liquid phase begins. The transition from solid to liquid is called **fusion** or **melting**. The reverse process, from liquid to solid, is called **solidification**, **crystallization**, or **freezing**. The temperature at which these processes occur is called the **melting point** or **freezing point**, depending on the direction of the transition.

Whereas pure crystals have very distinct, sharp melting points, amorphous solids such as glass tend to melt over a larger range of temperatures, due to their less-ordered molecular distribution.

Gas-Solid Equilibrium

A third type of phase equilibrium exists between gasses and solids. When a solid goes directly into the gas phase, the process is called **sublimation**. Dry ice (solid CO_2) sublimes under atmospheric pressure; the absence of a liquid phase makes it a convenient refrigerant. The reverse transition, from a gaseous to solid phase, is called **deposition**.

Solution Chemistry

Solutions are homogeneous mixtures of substances that combine to form a single phase, generally the liquid phase. Many important chemical reactions, both in the laboratory and in nature, take place in solution (including almost all reactions in living organisms). A solution consists of a **solute** dissolved in a **solvent**. The solvent is the component of the solution whose phase remains the same after mixing. For example, a solid cube of sugar dissolved in water yields a liquid mixture of water and sugar. In this example, water is the solvent and sugar the solute.

If the two substances are already in the same phase, the solvent is generally taken to be the component present in greater quantity. Solute molecules move about freely in solvent and can interact with other molecules or ions; consequently, chemical reactions occur easily in solution.

Solution Terminology

There are several key ideas and terms relating to solutions you should be familiar with.

Solvation: The interaction between solute and solvent molecules is known as solvation or **dissolution**; when water is the solvent, it is also known as **hydration** and the resulting solution is known as an **aqueous solution**.

Solubility: The solubility of a substance is the maximum amount of that substance that can be dissolved in a particular solvent at a particular temperature.

Percent Composition by Mass: The percent composition by mass of a solution is the mass of the solute divided by the mass of the solution (solute plus solvent), multiplied by 100.

Dilution: A solution is diluted when solvent is added to a solution of high concentration to produce a solution of lower concentration.

Molarity: The number of moles of solute dissolved in 1 liter of solution. Molarity is abbreviated as M.

Acids and Bases

Many important reactions in chemical and biological systems involve two classes of compounds—acids and bases. The presence of acids and bases can often be easily detected because they lead to color changes in certain compounds called indicators, which may be in solution or on paper. A particular common indicator is litmus paper, which turns red in acidic solution and blue in basic solution. A more extensive discussion of the chemical properties of acids and bases is outlined below.

Definitions of Acids and Bases

The first definitions of acids and bases were formulated by Svante Arrhenius toward the end of the nineteenth century. Arrhenius defined an acid as a species that produces H^+ (protons) in an aqueous solution, and a base as a species that produces OH^- (hydroxide ions) in an aqueous solution.

A more general definition of acids and bases was proposed independently by Johannes Brønsted and Thomas Lowry in 1923. A Brønsted-Lowry acid is a species that donates protons, while a Brønsted-Lowry base is a species that accepts protons. At approximately the same time as Brønsted and Lowry, Gilbert Lewis also proposed definitions for acids and bases. Lewis defined an acid as an electron-pair acceptor, and a base as an electron-pair donor. Lewis's are the most inclusive definitions, however; we will focus our attention on Brønsted-Lowry acids and bases.

Properties of Acids and Bases

The behavior of acids and bases in solution is governed by equilibrium considerations. It's important to know that pH (proton concentration) and pOH (hydroxide ion concentration) are not totally independent of each other: Knowing the value of one allows us to calculate the other.

For example, in pure water (H_2O), pH and pOH would be equal, both having a value of 7. A solution with equal concentrations of H^+ and OH^- is neutral. A pH below 7 indicates a relative excess of H^+ ions, and therefore an acidic solution; a pH above 7 indicates a relative excess of OH^- ions, and therefore a basic solution.

Organic Chemistry

Organic chemistry is the study of compounds containing the element carbon. This covers a wide range of compounds, including proteins, alcohols, steroids, sugars, and compounds found in petroleum, just to name a few. The reason we can study them as facets of one subject is because of the unifying bonding properties of carbon.

Hydrocarbons

Hydrocarbons are compounds that contain only carbon and hydrogen atoms. Depending on the kinds of bonds found between carbon atoms (only single bonds can exist between carbon and hydrogen), hydrocarbons can be classified into one of four classes: alkanes, alkenes, alkynes, and aromatics.

Alkanes, Alkenes, and Alkynes

Alkanes are hydrocarbons that contain only single bonds. They are all named by attaching the suffix *-ane* to a prefix that indicates the number of carbon atoms. These prefixes will be used again in the naming of other hydrocarbons and it is therefore worth knowing at least a few.

# of C Atoms	Prefix	Name of Alkane	Molecular Formula
1	*meth-*	methane	CH_4
2	*eth-*	ethane	C_2H_6
3	*prop-*	propane	C_3H_8
4	*but-*	butane	C_4H_{10}
5	*pent-*	pentane	C_5H_{12}
6	*hex-*	hexane	C_6H_{14}

Alkenes are hydrocarbons involving carbon-carbon double bonds. They are named using the same scheme as alkanes, except that their suffix is *-ene*.

Alkynes are hydrocarbons involving carbon-carbon triple bonds. They follow the same naming scheme as alkanes and alkenes, but use the suffix *-yne*.

Aromatics

Certain unsaturated cyclic hydrocarbons are known as aromatics. We need not concern ourselves with exactly what makes a compound aromatic, but all such compounds have a cyclic, planar structure in common and possess a higher degree of stability than expected.

Oxygen-Containing Compounds

Organic compounds that include oxygen in addition to carbon and hydrogen include alcohols, ethers, carbohydrates, and carbonyl compounds such as aldehydes, ketones, esters, and carboxylic acids.

Nitrogen-Containing Compounds

Nitrogen-containing compounds are another large class of organic compounds. The most important nitrogen-containing functional group is the amine group, $-NH_2$, which is found in amino acids, the basic building blocks of proteins.

Ⓗ PHYSICS LESSON

Kinematics

Kinematics is the branch of mechanics dealing with motion. It is the study of how things move: how far things move, how fast they move, and how long it takes them to move.

Distance and Displacement

While **distance** is the total amount of space moved, without a particular direction, displacement is very different. **Displacement** is a vector quantity that describes a change in position, and it has both direction and magnitude.

Speed and Velocity

Average speed is scalar. To calculate the average speed of an object, take the total distance covered, and divide it by the total time it took to cover the distance:

$$\text{Average Speed} = \frac{\text{Total Distance}}{\text{Total Time}}$$

$$V = \frac{D}{T}$$

In the equation above, V stands for speed, D is distance, and T is time. Remember to keep your units consistent: If your data is written in terms of meters and seconds, then your speed should be written in "meters per second," or "m/s." This is the most common way to express speed when calculating. If you need an answer written in "kilometers per hour," you will have to remember to convert your units appropriately.

Average velocity is the ratio of the displacement vector over the change in time and is a vector quantity. **Acceleration** (A) is the rate of change of an object's velocity. To calculate acceleration, divide an object's **change in velocity** (V) by the change in **time** (T):

$$\text{Acceleration} = \frac{\text{Change in Velocity}}{\text{Change in Time}}$$

Note that velocity is generally written in "meters per second," and time is generally recorded in seconds. Since you divide the change in velocity by the change in time, acceleration is generally written in "meters per second squared," or "m/s^2." Remember to make sure your units are consistent; if you are given time data expressed in minutes, you will need to multiply by 60 to convert the data to seconds before calculating.

Newtonian Mechanics

Dynamics is the study of what causes motion; that is, the **forces** that lead to motion, such as pulling or pushing. Dynamics is often referred to as Newtonian mechanics or Newton's laws of motion, after Isaac Newton, who published his groundbreaking three laws of motion in 1687.

Force is a vector quantity. Forces are observed as the push or pull on an object. Forces can either be exerted between bodies in contact (such as the force a person exerts to push a box across the floor), or between bodies not in contact (such as the force of gravity holding the Earth in its orbit). The unit for force, in SI, is the newton (N).

Newton's First Law of Motion

A body either at rest or in motion with constant velocity will remain that way unless a **net force** acts upon it. This law is often known as the law of inertia.

Newton's Second Law of Motion

A net force applied to a body of a mass will result in that body undergoing acceleration in the same direction as the net force. The magnitude of the body's acceleration is directly proportional to the magnitude of the net force and inversely proportional to the body's mass. This can be expressed as:

$$F_{net} = \Sigma F = ma$$

In other words, to calculate net force, multiply an object's mass (in kilograms) by its acceleration (in meters per second squared). The resulting answer will be expressed in terms of "kilogram-meters per second squared," also written "$kg\text{-}m/s^2$." However, usually the term *newton* is sufficient to express force. Important: Ensure that mass is expressed in kilograms before calculating. If you calculate with mass expressed in terms of grams or some other unit instead, your answer could be off by a magnitude of 1,000!

You might be asked to calculate the acceleration of an object subject to two different forces acting upon it in opposing directions. To find the answer, subtract the smaller of the two forces from the greater; the remaining amount is the net force actually being applied in the direction of the greater force. Divide that force by the object's mass to determine the object's acceleration.

Newton's Third Law of Motion

If body A exerts a force (F) on body B, then body B exerts a force (–F), that is equal in magnitude and opposite in direction, back on A. In Newton's own words, "To every action there is always opposed an equal reaction." The concept can be expressed as:

$$F_B = -F_A$$

Gravity

Gravity is an attractive force felt by all forms of matter. The magnitude of the **gravitational force** (F) is given as:

$$F = \frac{Gm^1m^2}{r^2}$$

In this approach, G is the gravitational constant (6.67×10^{-11} N • m^2/kg^2), m^1 and m^2 are the masses of the two objects, and r is the distance between their centers.

Friction

Whenever two objects are in contact, their surfaces rub together creating a friction force. **Static friction** (f_s) is the force that must be overcome to set an object in motion. For example, to make a book that is at rest start to slide across a table, a force greater than the maximum static force is required. However, once the book starts to slide, the friction force is not as strong. This new friction force is called **kinetic friction**.

Work and Energy

There are many words in physics that may be used quite differently outside the context of a physics course—work and energy are two such words.

Work

Essentially, you can think of work as responsible for changing the energy of an object. Work is defined as the scalar product of force (F) and displacement (s):

$$W = Fs$$

Work is expressed in **joules** (J) as it is the product of force and displacement; it has units of newton-meters, or **joules** (J). A joule is a unit of work or energy equal to the work done by a force of one newton acting through a distance of one meter. Work can be written out in the following equation:

$$W = Fd \cos\theta$$

In this approach, θ is the angle between the applied force and the displacement.

Energy

A body in motion possesses energy. This energy of motion is called **kinetic energy**. A body can also possess **potential energy**, which depends on a body's position rather than motion. An example of potential energy is the gravitational potential energy an object has when it is raised to a particular height. Objects on Earth have greater potential energy the further they are from the surface. Kinetic energy (KE) is calculated by the following equation: $KE = \frac{1}{2}mv^2$ where m is the mass of the object and v is the velocity of the object. Potential energy (PE) is calculated as a function of an object's mass (m) and height (h): $PE = mgh$ where g is the acceleration due to gravity.

Conservation of Energy

When the work done by nonconservative forces is equal to zero or there are no nonconservative forces (such as an object falling without air resistance), the total amount of energy, also known as the total mechanical energy, remains constant. In such a situation, there is a conservation of energy.

Power

Equally important as the amount of work required to perform an operation is the amount of time required to do the work. Power is the rate at which work is done. The standard unit of power is the watt; one watt is equivalent to one joule per second. The rate to calculate power is:

$$P = \frac{Work}{Time}$$

Waves

Waves contain individual particles that move back and forth with simple harmonic motion. In **transverse waves**, the particles oscillate perpendicular to the direction of the wave motion. String elements move at right angles to the direction of travel of a wave. In the case of **longitudinal waves**, particles oscillate along the direction of the wave motion.

The high point of a wave is its crest, and the low point is called its trough. The maximum displacement of a wave, measured from the point of equilibrium (conceptualized as a flat line running through the center of the wave), is known as its amplitude. The distance between two crests of a wave is the wavelength. The number of waves that pass a specific point over a specific period of time (generally 1 second) is known as the frequency of the wave; frequency is expressed in hertz.

Traveling waves are best described by an example: If a string that is fixed at one end is moved from side to side, a wave travels down the string. When the wave reaches a fixed boundary, it is reflected and inverted. If the free end of the string is continuously moved from side to side, two waves are created—the original wave moving down the string, and a reflected wave moving the other way. These waves interfere with each other.

If a string is fixed on both ends, and waves are created, certain wave frequencies can result in a waveform remaining in a stationary position—known as **standing waves**.

Sound Waves

Sound is transmitted by the movement of particles along the direction of motion of a sound wave. As such, sound is a longitudinal wave. More generally, sound is a mechanical disturbance that is dependent upon a medium for travel. It can be transmitted through solids, liquids, and gases; it cannot be transmitted through vacuum. The speed of sound in a medium is determined by the spacing of particles. The smaller the spacing between particles, the faster sound will travel in that medium. For this reason, sound travels faster in a solid than in a liquid, and faster in a liquid than in a gas.

KAPLAN

For sound to be produced, there must be a longitudinal movement of air molecules—produced by the vibration of a solid object that sets adjacent molecules into motion, or by means of an acoustic vibration in an enclosed space. Sound produced by string and percussion instruments, such as the guitar, violin, and piano, comes from solid objects. Using these instruments as an example, a string or several strings are set into motion and vibrate at their normal mode frequencies. Since the strings are very thin, they are ineffective in transmitting their vibration to the surrounding air. A solid body is employed to provide a better coupling to the air. In the case of a guitar, the vibration is transmitted through the bridge to the body of the instrument, which vibrates at the same frequency as the string.

Sound created by acoustic vibration includes sound from instruments such as organ pipes, the flute, and the recorder. There are no moving parts—sound is produced by a vibrating motion of air within the instrument. In the case of an organ pipe, pitch is determined by the length of the pipe. However, instruments such as the recorder and the flute are able to generate more than one pitch by the opening and closing of holes. The sound of the human voice is created by air passing between vocal cords. Pitch is controlled by varying tension of the cords.

Electric Charge

Charge may be either positive or negative. A positive charge and a negative charge attract one another; positive repels positive; and negative repels negative. These fundamental concepts are the foundation of Coulomb's law, which is essential to understanding all electrical phenomena. The SI unit of charge is the **coulomb** (C).

Current, Voltage, and Resistance

The flow of a charge is called an **electric current**. There are two types of basic currents: **direct** and **alternating**. The charge of a direct current flows in one direction only; the flow of an alternating current changes periodically. When two points at different electric potentials are connected by a conductor (such as a metal wire), charge flows between the two points. In a conductor, only negatively charged electrons are free to move. These act as charge carriers and move from low to high potentials. The direction of the current is taken as the direction in which positive charge would flow, from high to low. Thus the direction of current is opposite to the direction of electron flow.

Resistance is the opposition within a conductor to the flow of an electric current. The opposition takes the form of an energy loss or drop in potential. **Ohm's law** states the voltage drop across a resistor is proportional to the current it carries.

$$I = \frac{V}{R}$$

I is current, V is voltage, and R is resistance.

Current is unchanged as it passes through a resistor. This is because no charge is lost inside a resistor. The SI derived unit of electrical resistance is the **ohm** (Ω).

Although the topic of electricity may not seem directly related to nursing, you should have a general understanding of it.

Now that you have completed your review of basic chemistry and physics, you're ready to learn some strategies for Test Day.

ⓗ PHYSICAL SCIENCE STRATEGIES

If you read the strategies we present in Chapter Seven, Biology, you know the science portions of the nursing school entrance exams contain knowledge-based questions. You also know that doesn't mean that there are no strategies to use on Test Day. It just means they have a slightly different approach because they have to deal with a test of knowledge. Here are our favorite strategies for knowledge-based test questions.

- Intense review of terms or concepts commonly confused for each other.
- Strategic review of physical science concepts.

Here is how each of these works for Physical Science.

Terms Commonly Confused with Each Other

After long hours of study, you might not even care what the difference between an ionic bond and a covalent bond is. However, you would care if that were something you were facing on Test Day. Here are a few of the terms and concepts in chemistry and physics that are commonly confused or mistaken for each other. Familiarize yourself with them in preparation for the test.

Don't Mix These Up on Test Day

- **Atomic number**: number of protons
- **Mass number**: number of protons and neutrons

- **Ionic bond:** transfer of electron(s)
- **Covalent bond:** sharing of electron(s)

- **Solute**: substance being dissolved (often solid)
- **Solvent**: substance doing the dissolving (often liquid)
- **Solution**: solvent and a dissolved solute

- **Arrhenius** defined an acid as a species that produces H+ in an aqueous solution, and a base as a species that produces OH– in aqueous solution.
- A **Brønsted-Lowry** acid is a species that donates protons, while a **Brønsted-Lowry base** is a species that accepts protons.
- A **Lewis acid** is an electron-pair acceptor, and a **Lewis base** is an electron-pair donor.

- **Mass** is the measure of the amount of substance in an object and is measured in kilograms.
- **Weight** is the gravitational force pulling down on an object and is measured in newtons (N).

KAPLAN

- **Heat** is the kinetic energy of molecules transferred from a warmer substance to a cooler one.
- **Temperature** is a measure of the average kinetic energy of the molecules in a substance.
- The **atomic number Z** is the number of protons.
- The **mass number A** is the number of protons and neutrons.
- **Fusion** is the combining of small nuclei into larger ones, releasing energy.
- **Fission** is the splitting of a large nucleus into smaller ones, with the release of neutrons and energy.

Tips for Answering Physical Science Questions

As with Biology, all of the questions you will be asked are multiple-choice and content-based. Use the following tips to guide your studying of this material:

Use the 4-Step Method for Problem Solving. Physics and chemistry are math-based subjects. You will often be asked to complete calculations or solve a problem. The same principles that you have used in math will also apply in science. The 4-Step Method will help you solve any problem in which you have to use a formula to find the answer. These questions may ask you to calculate speed, acceleration, kinetic energy, potential energy, resistance, current, frequency, wavelength, half-life, force, work, etc. In some cases these formulas will be provided for you, but in others you will need to know them in advance. Spend some time learning and memorizing the formulas, but worry more about how to manipulate them to solve a problem.

Ask if your answer is reasonable. Since this science section of the exam contains only multiple-choice questions, often you will be able to eliminate answers based purely on magnitude or units. Follow these four steps to answer your questions.

1. Read the question stem without looking at the answers first.
2. Predict what the answer should be.
3. Examine each of the answer choices and compare these to your predicted answer. Eliminate unreasonable answer choices.
4. Narrow the answer to one choice based on your deeper knowledge of the concept.

Focus on the trends in the periodic table. In some chemistry classes, your teacher might have required you to memorize the data included on the periodic table. While it is helpful to know some information for the first 20 elements such as the atomic number and atomic mass because they are the most likely to appear on the exam, your time will be better spent focusing on the trends in the periodic table. Atomic radius, electronegativity, ionization energy, and electron affinity are the important trends to understand. These trends will tell you about the structure and reactivity of most elements and compounds.

Outline the main ideas. No comprehensive exam can possibly test you on all of the science content you have learned prior to entering nursing school. As you review the major science concepts in this text, use outlining to identify and review the main ideas (i.e., atomic structure, balancing equations, Newton's laws of motion). It is more important to understand the major concepts of the course than it is to memorize every supporting detail. Focus your studies on these main ideas; they will help you to deduce the answers on many multiple-choice questions.

Actively engage with the material. Make flashcards, create lists, or write notes on what you have studied. You can ask friends or family to quiz you to make sure that you have mastered the concepts and really know the material. At this stage, you may also want to review Chapter Two for a refresher on general test-taking strategies. These include answering easier questions first, making an educated guess, and using the process of elimination to find the right answer.

If you're ready to start reviewing, try to answer as many of the review questions from this chapter as you can.

REVIEW QUESTIONS

The following questions are not meant to mimic actual test questions. Instead, these questions will help you review the concepts and terms covered in this chapter.

1. List the three types of subatomic particles.

_____

_____

_____

2. True or False? The periodic table arranges elements in decreasing atomic numbers.

3. The elements of the periodic table may be classified into three categories; list them below.

_____

_____

_____

4. Define the chemical term **compound**.

_____

_____

5. Which of the following is NOT a gas law?

   The assumptions of the kinetic molecular theory of gases are as follows:

   (A) Gases are made up of particles whose volumes are negligible compared to the container volume.

   (B) Gas atoms or molecules exhibit no intermolecular attractions or repulsions.

   (C) Gas particles are in continuous, random motion, undergoing collisions with other particles and with the container walls.

   (D) Because gases can take on the shape of a container, they are infinitely compressible.

   (E) Collisions between any two gas particles are elastic, meaning that no energy is dissipated or, equivalently, that kinetic energy is conserved.

   (F) The average kinetic energy of gas particles is proportional to the absolute temperature of the gas, and is the same for all gases at a given temperature.

6. Fill in the blank. The transition from liquid to solid is called _____.

7. Define half-life.

   _____

   _____

8. True or False? Kinematics is the study of why things move.

9. Give the equation for acceleration.

   _____

   _____

10. Put Newton's Three Laws of Motion in order.

    _____ Law of action and reaction

    _____ Law of inertia

    _____ Force equals mass times acceleration

11. True or False? The law of conservation of energy states that when work is done on a system, the energy of that system changes from one form to another, but the total amount of energy remains the same.

12. Match the type of wave with its description.

    _____ Transverse wave

    _____ Longitudinal wave

    (A) A wave that vibrates in a direction that is perpendicular to the direction of motion of the wave.

    (B) A wave that vibrates in a direction that is parallel to the direction of motion of the wave.

13. Check all that apply to a sound wave.

    _____ It is a longitudinal wave.

    _____ It is a mechanical wave.

    _____ It is a transverse wave.

    _____ It does not need a medium to travel through.

14. True or False? Heat is the kinetic energy of molecules transferred from a cooler substance to a warmer one.

REVIEW ANSWERS

1. A.   Protons
   B.   Neutrons
   C.   Electrons

2. False. The periodic table arranges the elements in **increasing** atomic numbers.

3. A.   Metals
   B.   Nonmetals
   C.   Metalloids

4. A compound is a pure substance that is composed of two or more elements in a fixed proportion.

5. Option (D) is not a gas law.

6. Possible answers include: solidification, crystallization, or freezing.

7. The half-life of a sample is the time it takes for half of the sample to decay.

8. False. Kinematics is the study of **how** things move. The study of why things move is called dynamism.

9. $\text{Acceleration} = \dfrac{\text{Change in Velocity}}{\text{Change in Time}}$.

10. **1**   Law of inertia.
    2   Force equals mass times acceleration.
    3   Law of action and reaction.

11. True.

12. **A**   Transverse wave
    B   Longitudinal wave

13. The following are true statements about a sound wave:
    It is a longitudinal wave.
    It is a mechanical wave.

14. False. Heat is the kinetic energy of molecules transferred from a warmer substance to a cooler one.

PART SIX

Practice Tests and Explanations

Taking the Practice Tests

You've completed your reviews, and now it's time to take the practice tests. Here are a few tips to help you do your best:

1. Allow 2 hours to take each practice test. Note the number of questions in each section and budget your time accordingly.

2. Remember to follow the test-taking strategies covered in Section One. The more you practice using these strategies, the more comfortable you'll be using them on Test Day.

3. Make sure your practice test environment is quiet and free from distractions. Pretend you're taking an actual test.

4. To make it easier to fill out, tear out or photocopy the answer sheet so you can place it next to the test rather than having to flip back to it.

This is the first full-length practice test in this book. There is an answer sheet on the following page. At the end of the test, you will find an answer key as well as detailed answer explanations. Use these explanations to understand what questions you missed and why. By scoring your test and reading through the answer explanations, you should be able to further diagnose your strengths and weaknesses as you prepare for Test Day.

Nursing School Entrance Exams
Practice Test One, Kaplan
Answer Sheet

Reading Comprehension

1. Ⓐ Ⓑ Ⓒ Ⓓ   4. Ⓐ Ⓑ Ⓒ Ⓓ   7. Ⓐ Ⓑ Ⓒ Ⓓ   10. Ⓐ Ⓑ Ⓒ Ⓓ   13. Ⓐ Ⓑ Ⓒ Ⓓ

2. Ⓐ Ⓑ Ⓒ Ⓓ   5. Ⓐ Ⓑ Ⓒ Ⓓ   8. Ⓐ Ⓑ Ⓒ Ⓓ   11. Ⓐ Ⓑ Ⓒ Ⓓ   14. Ⓐ Ⓑ Ⓒ Ⓓ

3. Ⓐ Ⓑ Ⓒ Ⓓ   6. Ⓐ Ⓑ Ⓒ Ⓓ   9. Ⓐ Ⓑ Ⓒ Ⓓ   12. Ⓐ Ⓑ Ⓒ Ⓓ   15. Ⓐ Ⓑ Ⓒ Ⓓ

Writing

1. Ⓐ Ⓑ Ⓒ Ⓓ   4. Ⓐ Ⓑ Ⓒ Ⓓ   7. Ⓐ Ⓑ Ⓒ Ⓓ   10. Ⓐ Ⓑ Ⓒ Ⓓ   13. Ⓐ Ⓑ Ⓒ Ⓓ

2. Ⓐ Ⓑ Ⓒ Ⓓ   5. Ⓐ Ⓑ Ⓒ Ⓓ   8. Ⓐ Ⓑ Ⓒ Ⓓ   11. Ⓐ Ⓑ Ⓒ Ⓓ   14. Ⓐ Ⓑ Ⓒ Ⓓ

3. Ⓐ Ⓑ Ⓒ Ⓓ   6. Ⓐ Ⓑ Ⓒ Ⓓ   9. Ⓐ Ⓑ Ⓒ Ⓓ   12. Ⓐ Ⓑ Ⓒ Ⓓ

Mathematics

1. Ⓐ Ⓑ Ⓒ Ⓓ   5. Ⓐ Ⓑ Ⓒ Ⓓ   9. Ⓐ Ⓑ Ⓒ Ⓓ   13. Ⓐ Ⓑ Ⓒ Ⓓ   17. Ⓐ Ⓑ Ⓒ Ⓓ

2. Ⓐ Ⓑ Ⓒ Ⓓ   6. Ⓐ Ⓑ Ⓒ Ⓓ   10. Ⓐ Ⓑ Ⓒ Ⓓ   14. Ⓐ Ⓑ Ⓒ Ⓓ

3. Ⓐ Ⓑ Ⓒ Ⓓ   7. Ⓐ Ⓑ Ⓒ Ⓓ   11. Ⓐ Ⓑ Ⓒ Ⓓ   15. Ⓐ Ⓑ Ⓒ Ⓓ

4. Ⓐ Ⓑ Ⓒ Ⓓ   8. Ⓐ Ⓑ Ⓒ Ⓓ   12. Ⓐ Ⓑ Ⓒ Ⓓ   16. Ⓐ Ⓑ Ⓒ Ⓓ

Science

1. Ⓐ Ⓑ Ⓒ Ⓓ   4. Ⓐ Ⓑ Ⓒ Ⓓ   7. Ⓐ Ⓑ Ⓒ Ⓓ   10. Ⓐ Ⓑ Ⓒ Ⓓ   13. Ⓐ Ⓑ Ⓒ Ⓓ

2. Ⓐ Ⓑ Ⓒ Ⓓ   5. Ⓐ Ⓑ Ⓒ Ⓓ   8. Ⓐ Ⓑ Ⓒ Ⓓ   11. Ⓐ Ⓑ Ⓒ Ⓓ   14. Ⓐ Ⓑ Ⓒ Ⓓ

3. Ⓐ Ⓑ Ⓒ Ⓓ   6. Ⓐ Ⓑ Ⓒ Ⓓ   9. Ⓐ Ⓑ Ⓒ Ⓓ   12. Ⓐ Ⓑ Ⓒ Ⓓ

KAPLAN

Practice Test One, Kaplan

READING COMPREHENSION

Questions 1–2 are based on the following passage.

Many mammals instinctively raise their fur when they are cold—a reaction produced by tiny muscles just under the skin that surround hair follicles. When the muscles contract, the hairs stand up, creating an increase in air space under the fur. The air space provides more effective insulation for the mammal's body, thus allowing it to retain more heat for longer periods of time. Some animals also raise their fur when they are challenged by predators or even other members of their own species. The raised fur makes the animal appear slightly bigger, and, ideally, more powerful. Interestingly, though devoid of fur, humans still retain this instinct. So, the next time a horror movie gives you "goosebumps," remember that your skin is following a deep-seated mammalian impulse now rendered obsolete.

1. The increased air space under the fur mentioned in the passage primarily serves which purpose?

   (A) To combat cold.

   (B) To intimidate other animals.

   (C) To render goosebumps obsolete.

   (D) To cool overheated predators.

2. Based on the passage, the author would MOST likely agree with which statement?

   (A) Goosebumps in humans are an unnecessary and unexplained phenomenon.

   (B) Goosebumps in humans are a harmful but necessary measure.

   (C) Goosebumps in humans are an amusing but dangerous feature.

   (D) Goosebumps in humans are a useless but interesting remnant.

Questions 3–4 are based on the following passage.

While it is often helpful to think of humans as simply another successful type of mammal, a vital distinction remains. When a pride of lions enjoys a surfeit of food, they are likely to hunt quickly, eat all they can, and then spend the remainder of the day sleeping. When people enjoy such easy living, we see a markedly different pattern—our big brains cause us to be restless, and we engage in play. This takes the form of art, philosophy, science, even government. So, the intelligence and curiosity that allowed early humans to develop agriculture, and thus a caloric surplus, also led to the use of that surplus as a foundation for culture.

3. Which is the author's purpose in citing the behavior of lions in the passage?

   (A) To provide an example of an even more successful mammalian species.

   (B) To question the efficiency of the lion's feeding behavior.

   (C) To provide a contrast to the image of humans as industrious and resourceful.

   (D) To help illustrate the distinguishing characteristic of humans that led to the development of culture.

4. Which is the main purpose of the final sentence of the passage ("So, the intelligence . . . for culture")?

   (A) Illustrate the significance of a distinction.

   (B) Counter a likely objection.

   (C) Provide an alternative explanation.

   (D) Suggest future implications of a phenomenon.

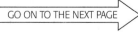
GO ON TO THE NEXT PAGE

KAPLAN

Questions 5–8 are based on the following passage.

City parks were originally created to provide the local populace with a convenient refuge from the crowding and chaos of their surroundings. Until quite recently, these parks served their purpose admirably. Whether city dwellers wanted to sit under a shady tree to think or take a vigorous stroll to get some exercise, they looked forward to visiting these nearby oases. Filled with trees, shrubs, flowers, meadows, and ponds, city parks were a tranquil spot in which to unwind from the daily pressures of urban life. They were places where people met their friends for picnics or sporting events. And they were also places to get some sun and fresh air in the midst of an often dark and dreary environment, with its seemingly endless rows of steel, glass, and concrete buildings.

For more than a century, the importance of these parks to the quality of life in cities has been recognized by urban planners. Yet city parks around the world have been allowed to deteriorate to an alarming extent in recent decades. In many cases, they have become centers of crime; some city parks are now so dangerous that local residents are afraid even to enter them. And the great natural beauty that was once their hallmark has been severely damaged. Trees, shrubs, flowers, and meadows have withered under the impact of intense air pollution and littering, and ponds have been fouled by untreated sewage.

This process of progressive decline, however, is not inevitable. A few changes can turn the situation around. First, special police units, whose only responsibility would be to patrol city parks, should be created to ensure parks remain safe for those who wish to enjoy them. Second, more caretakers should be hired to care for the grounds and, in particular, to collect trash. Beyond the increased staffing requirements, it will also be necessary to insulate city parks from their surroundings. Total isolation is, of course, impossible; but many beneficial measures in that direction could be implemented without too much trouble. Vehicles, for instance, should be banned from city parks to cut down on air pollution. And sewage pipes should be rerouted away from park areas to prevent the contamination of land and water. If urban planners are willing to make these changes, city parks can be restored to their former glory for the benefit of all.

5. The author uses the phrase "convenient refuge" to suggest which aspect about parks?

   (A) They were built in order to preserve plant life in cities.
   (B) They were designed with the needs of city residents in mind.
   (C) They were meant to end the unpleasantness of city life.
   (D) They were supposed to help people make new friends.

6. Which is the reason why the author mentions crime and pollution in the passage?

   (A) To describe how rapidly the city parks have deteriorated.
   (B) To describe how city parks can once again be made safe and clean.
   (C) To explain why people can no longer rest and relax in city parks.
   (D) To explain why urban planners should not be in charge of city parks.

7. In the last paragraph, the author acknowledges which problem in restoring city parks?

   (A) The constant need to collect trash.
   (B) The difficulty in rerouting sewage pipes.
   (C) The congestion caused by banning vehicular traffic.
   (D) The lack of total separation from the surrounding city.

8. Based on the passage, which statement is MOST likely true?

   (A) Modern city parks usually have their own dedicated security forces.
   (B) Most cities were originally designed with future park needs in mind.
   (C) Modern city parks face greater challenges than parks faced in the past.
   (D) Most cities have reduced the number of parks to make room for housing.

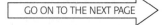
GO ON TO THE NEXT PAGE

Questions 9–12 are based on the following passage.

The relationship between humans and animals dates back to the misty morning of history. The caves of southern France and northern Spain are full of wonderful depictions of animals. Early African petroglyphs depict recognizable mammals, as does much American Indian art. Even without art, we have evidence of the closeness of humans and animals. The bones of dogs lie next to those of humans in the excavated villages of northern Israel and elsewhere. This unity of death is terribly appropriate. It marks a relationship that is the most ancient of all, one that dates back at least to the Mesolithic Era.* With the dog, the hunter acquired a companion and ally very early on, before agriculture, long before the horse and the cat. The companion animals were followed by food animals, and then by those that provided enhanced speed and range, and finally, by those that worked for us.

How did it all come about? A dog of some kind was almost inevitable. Consider its essence: a social carnivore, hunting larger animals across the broad plains it shared with our ancestors. Because of its pack structure, it is susceptible to domination by, and attachment to, a pack leader: the top dog. Its young are born into the world dependent, rearable, without too much skill, and, best of all, they form bonds with the rearers. Dogs have a set of appeasement behaviors that elicit affective reactions from even the most hardened and unsophisticated humans. Puppies share with human babies the power to transform cynics into cooing softies. Furthermore, the animal has a sense of smell and hearing several times more acute than our own, great advantages to a hunting companion and intrusion detector. The dog's defensive behavior makes it an instinctive guard animal.

Mesolithic Era: the Middle Stone Age, between 8,000 and 3,000 years B.C.E.

9. Which statement BEST explains why the author describes the archeological discoveries in paragraph 1 as "terribly appropriate"?

   (A) Dogs were always buried next to their owners in the Mesolithic Era.

   (B) Few animals were of religious significance in prehistoric cultures.

   (C) They illustrate the role of dogs on a typical hunting expedition.

   (D) Our relationship with dogs is older than that with any other animal.

10. According to paragraph 1, which kinds of animals were the first to forge a close relationship with humans?

   (A) Those that acted as companions.

   (B) Those that provided a source of food.

   (C) Those that helped develop agriculture.

   (D) Those that enabled humans to travel farther.

11. According to the author, which is the reason why some kind of dog was "inevitable" as a companion animal for humans?

   (A) It survived by maintaining its independence.

   (B) It was stronger than other large animals.

   (C) It shared its prey with our ancestors.

   (D) It was suited for human domination.

12. Which term BEST defines the word <u>essence</u> as it is used in paragraph 2 of the passage?

   (A) History.

   (B) Nature.

   (C) Scent.

   (D) Success.

GO ON TO THE NEXT PAGE

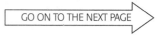

Questions 13–15 are based on the following passage.

The learning behavior of many mammals is dictated by instinct but tempered and refined by experience. Very complex behaviors can be learned through individual trial-and-error or practice, as long as that practice is motivated by instinctive drives. For example, predatory cats aren't born knowing how to hunt, but instinct drives them to stalk, pounce on, and bite things they perceive as prey, and they gradually become more skilled and effective hunters. Wolves aren't born knowing how to get along with other wolves, but the experience of living in the pack, the correction and support they receive from elders, and the survival instinct that drives them to stay in the pack result in their eventually learning to find their place in the hierarchy and to cooperate in group activities, such as hunting and rearing young.

Some kinds of animal learning, however, are not so directly dependent on the need to survive. In the case of primates in particular, evolution seems to have fostered a behavior pattern that encourages restless experimentation and exploration of the environment apart from the search to fulfill basic needs. Among humans, for example, the discovery of the laws of gravity didn't directly bear on the survival of Sir Isaac Newton; nor did the description of the properties of triangles help Pythagoras put food on the table. Although these discoveries may later have indirectly improved the quality of life and survival potential of the discoverers' descendants, the lack of an immediate survival imperative suggests that experimentation, discovery, and sharing the benefits of those discoveries have as much to do with enjoyment as with survival.

13. Which term BEST defines the word *tempered* as it is used in paragraph 1 of the passage?

(A) Angered.

(B) Commanded.

(C) Influenced.

(D) Suppressed.

14. Which example is MOST similar to the pattern of learning described in the first paragraph?

(A) A hobbyist learns how to knit by reading a book on arts and crafts.

(B) Math students learn how to use a geometry formula by watching a teacher demonstrate.

(C) A basketball player improves his ability to shoot free throws by practicing every day.

(D) A leafcutter ant hatches knowing how to find leaves and then learns how to harvest them.

15. Why does the author list famous discoverers in paragraph 2?

(A) To illustrate human superiority over other animals.

(B) To prove an argument about the way that discoveries benefit later generations.

(C) To suggest that discoveries are usually accidental.

(D) To demonstrate that discoveries aren't always inspired by a need to survive.

GO ON TO THE NEXT PAGE

WRITING

Questions 1–5 are based on the following passage.

[1]A major story in recent years has been the triumph of electronic mail, commonly known as email. [2]Since the early 1990s, email users have multiplied exponentially. [3]Many major corporations have chosen email as their primary channel for all communications, internal and external. [4]By 2017, an average of 269 billion emails were being sent every single day around the world—equal to more than 35 messages per day for every single person on the planet. [5]Yet, however affective and inexpensive email may be, it is not without flaws. [6]The medium is impersonal, lacking the intimacy of a letter or the immediacy of a phone call. [7]In centuries past, people wrote letters by hand: and some of those have even survived as historical artifacts. [8]As an interactive medium, email is less than ideal, since messages allow correspondents to politely ignore points they do not wish to address, or indeed not to respond at all.

[9]Email have also brought with it a number of ethical issues. [10]For example, if employers provide email services for their employees, should those employers be allowed to access employee emails without permission? [11]If an employee sends harassing or threatening messages through company email services, should the employer be held responsible?

1. Which sentence should be deleted because it is unrelated to the other sentences in the paragraph?

   (A) Sentence 3.
   (B) Sentence 4.
   (C) Sentence 7.
   (D) Sentence 8.

2. Which word in the first paragraph is incorrect?

   (A) Exponentially.
   (B) Affective.
   (C) Immediacy.
   (D) Correspondents.

3. Which sentence has incorrect subject-verb agreement?

   (A) Sentence 4.
   (B) Sentence 7.
   (C) Sentence 9.
   (D) Sentence 11.

4. Where is the BEST place to add this sentence?

   Despite these potential challenges, email has become an integral part of how humans communicate and is likely to remain with us for years to come.

   (A) Following sentence 5.
   (B) Following sentence 7.
   (C) Following sentence 9.
   (D) Following sentence 11.

5. Which choice describes how to correct a punctuation error in the passage?

   (A) Remove the comma after the word *communications* in sentence 3.
   (B) Add a comma after the word *however* in sentence 5.
   (C) Change the comma after the word *impersonal* in sentence 6 to a semicolon.
   (D) Change the colon after the word *hand* in sentence 7 to a comma.

GO ON TO THE NEXT PAGE

KAPLAN)

Questions 6–10 are based on the following passage.

[1]When commercial fish farming—a technique that applies the breeding structures used for raising animals on land to the ocean—was first introduced, it was seen as a creative alternative to the depletion of the world's large finfish and shellfish populations through conventional harvesting methods. [2]Through careful planning, fish farmers could also reliably project how many fish they would be able to harvest in a certain enclosure over a specific amount of time, eliminated the risk of a potential "bad season" of fishing.

[3]New research however, is causing some to reconsider their initial enthusiasm for fish farming. [4]About 29 million tons of large finfish were farmed in 1997, no doubt a significant contribution to the world's fish supplies. [5]Unfortunately, the cost of this production was roughly 10 million tons of smaller wild fish used as feed, an amount that, if perpetuated, could soon virtually obliterate the world's supply of small fish. [6]Another danger posed by fish farms is a result of placing so many fish in such a small area: diseases and parasites can spread rapidly, devestating an entire population of fish before the problem can be addressed. [7]While fish farming might prove to be a smart way to keep from depleting ocean life, it has also created a whole new realm of challenges that the industry must face to achieve success too.

6. Which sentence includes an unnecessary word?

 (A) Sentence 1 includes the unnecessary word *when.*

 (B) Sentence 3 includes the unnecessary word *however.*

 (C) Sentence 6 includes the unnecessary word *another.*

 (D) Sentence 7 includes the unnecessary word *too.*

7. Which word in the second paragraph is incorrect?

 (A) Enthusiasm.

 (B) Perpetuated.

 (C) Devestating.

 (D) Achieve.

8. Which sentence has an incorrect form of a verb?

 (A) Sentence 2.

 (B) Sentence 4.

 (C) Sentence 5.

 (D) Sentence 7.

9. Where is the BEST place to add this sentence?

 In addition, fish farms could eliminate many of the dangers associated with working in the fishing industry, usually considered one of the most dangerous industries in the world.

 (A) Following sentence 2.

 (B) Following sentence 3.

 (C) Following sentence 5.

 (D) Following sentence 6.

10. Which sentence includes an error in punctuation?

 (A) Sentence 2.

 (B) Sentence 3.

 (C) Sentence 4.

 (D) Sentence 6.

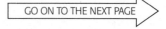
GO ON TO THE NEXT PAGE

KAPLAN

Questions 11–14 are based on the following passage.

[1]With an estimated 200 million cases and nearly a million resulting deaths per year, malaria is the world's number-one public health problem, especially in tropical and subtropical regions. [2]The struggle with this infection is nothing new—malaria is mentioned in some of the earliest medical records of Western civilization. [3]We know for example, that the ancient Greek physician Hippocrates identified three types of malarial fevers in the fifth century B.C.E. [4]By the late fifteenth century, malaria had spread to the Americas, likely as the result of European explorers. [5]In addition to bringing disease, European explorers often devastated indigenous populations through warfare and forced labor.

[6]Two of the most important factors in the proliforation of malaria are climate and poverty. [7]The mosquito that spreads the disease requires a relatively warm and wet environment to flourish. [8]This means that tropical regions are at the greatest risk of the disease. [9]Areas of high poverty are less likely to have proper water drainage or fully enclosed living areas, and may not have access to inexpensive preventatives such as mosquito nets and insect repellents; this puts the poor at greater risk of contracting the disease.

11. Which word in the second paragraph is incorrect?

   (A) Proliforation.
   (B) Environment.
   (C) Flourish.
   (D) Preventatives.

12. Which choice describes how to correct a punctuation error in the passage?

   (A) Change the comma after the word *problem* in sentence 1 to a colon.
   (B) Add a comma after the word *know* in sentence 3.
   (C) Change the comma after the word *Americas* in sentence 4 to a period, and start a new sentence with the word *likely*.
   (D) Change the semicolon after the word *repellents* in sentence 9 to a comma.

13. Where is the BEST place to add this sentence?

   In fact, epidemics in Central America were recorded in 1493, only a year after Columbus's first voyage there.

   (A) Following sentence 2.
   (B) Following sentence 3.
   (C) Following sentence 4.
   (D) Following sentence 7.

14. Which sentence contains unnecessary information and should be removed?

   (A) Sentence 2.
   (B) Sentence 5.
   (C) Sentence 6.
   (D) Sentence 9.

GO ON TO THE NEXT PAGE

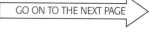

MATHEMATICS

1. $\frac{1}{3} + \frac{1}{6} - \frac{4}{9} =$

   (A) $\frac{1}{18}$

   (B) $\frac{1}{8}$

   (C) $\frac{1}{6}$

   (D) $-\frac{1}{8}$

2. Which is the value of $a(b - 2) + 3c$ if $a = 2$, $b = 6$, and $c = 4$?

   (A) 20

   (B) 12

   (C) 24

   (D) 32

3. Andrew bought a camera on sale at a 20% discount. It was marked down from its regular price of $120. If there is an 8% sales tax on the sale price, how much did Andrew pay for the camera?

   (A) $24.00

   (B) $103.68

   (C) $127.68

   (D) $105.68

4. The integer z is positive. When z is divided by 8, the remainder is 5. Which is the remainder when $4z$ is divided by 8?

   (A) 1

   (B) 3

   (C) 4

   (D) 5

5. Which is the least common multiple of 12 and 8?

   (A) 12

   (B) 24

   (C) 18

   (D) 96

6. Which is the value of x in the equation $6x - 7 = y$, if $y = 11$?

   (A) 12

   (B) 8

   (C) 4

   (D) 3

7. Edward has $400 more than Robert. After Edward spends $60 on groceries, he has 3 times more money than Robert. How much money does Robert have?

   (A) $140

   (B) $120

   (C) $90

   (D) $170

8. John bought a camera on sale that normally costs $160. If the price was reduced 20% during the sale, which was the sale price of the camera?

   (A) $120

   (B) $124

   (C) $128

   (D) $140

9. $\frac{2}{8}$ converted to a percent equals which of the following?

   (A) 0.025%

   (B) 0.25%

   (C) 2.5%

   (D) 25%

GO ON TO THE NEXT PAGE

10. $5\frac{2}{3} \times \frac{1}{2} - \frac{5}{12} =$

    (A) $-\frac{1}{3}$

    (B) $1\frac{7}{8}$

    (C) $2\frac{5}{12}$

    (D) $3\frac{1}{12}$

11. Renée's dress shop is suffering from slow business. Renée decides to mark down all her merchandise. The next day, she sells 33 winter coats. That day Renée sold 30% of the winter coats she had in stock. How many winter coats were in stock before the sale?

    (A) 990

    (B) 99

    (C) 110

    (D) 1,110

12. If $x = \sqrt{3}$, $y = 2$, and $z = \frac{1}{2}$, then $x^2 - 5yz + y^2 = ?$

    (A) 1

    (B) 2

    (C) 4

    (D) 7

13. $120.21 + 8.76 - 72.88 =$

    (A) 38.57

    (B) 56.09

    (C) 62.51

    (D) 121.69

14. What is 25% of 25% of 72?

    (A) 4

    (B) 4.5

    (C) 5

    (D) 12

15. The price of a stock was y dollars, where $y > 0$. The price of the stock then decreased by 20%. By what percent must the price of the stock increase to return to its original value?

    (A) 25%

    (B) 50%

    (C) 20%

    (D) 120%

16. Mrs. Bailer divides the amount of money she has equally between her 4 children. Mr. Bailer then adds $2 to the amount each one receives so that each child now has a total of $5.25. Which equation shows this relationship?

    (A) $4x + 2 = 5.25$

    (B) $\frac{x}{4} + 2 = 5.25$

    (C) $4x = 5.25 + 2$

    (D) $4(x + 2) = 5.25$

17. $\frac{26.88}{19.2} =$

    (A) 0.014

    (B) 0.14

    (C) 1.4

    (D) 14

GO ON TO THE NEXT PAGE

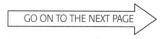

SCIENCE

1. Which answer option facilitates the diffusion of water into and out of cells?

    (A) Carrier proteins.
    (B) Symport systems.
    (C) Ion channels.
    (D) Osmosis.

2. Which association of brain structure and function is false?

    (A) Hypothalamus: Appetite.
    (B) Cerebellum: Motor coordination.
    (C) Cerebral cortex: Higher intellectual function.
    (D) Medulla: Basic emotional drives.

3. The absorption of oxygen from the atmosphere into the blood takes place in which structure?

    (A) Pulmonary artery.
    (B) Pulmonary vein.
    (C) Alveoli.
    (D) Trachea.

4. In which structure does filtration of the blood occur?

    (A) The ureters.
    (B) The nephrons.
    (C) The renal veins.
    (D) The renal arteries.

5. Which blood component transports oxygen?

    (A) Plasma.
    (B) Platelets.
    (C) Leukocytes.
    (D) Erythrocytes.

6. Which structure does NOT transport oxygen-depleted blood to the right atrium of the heart?

    (A) The pulmonary veins.
    (B) The coronary sinus.
    (C) The superior vena cava.
    (D) The inferior vena cava.

7. Hormone regulation in the body is mainly governed by which system?

    (A) Muscular system.
    (B) Endocrine system.
    (C) Nervous system.
    (D) Digestive system.

8. Which term describes a state of low blood pH?

    (A) Acidemia.
    (B) Acidosis.
    (C) Alkalemia.
    (D) Alkalosis.

9. Which answer option is not a function of the large intestine?

    (A) Nutrient absorption.
    (B) Compaction of feces.
    (C) Filtration of damaged or dead blood cells.
    (D) Water reabsorption.

10. Which answer option is the main extracellular electrolyte in the body?

    (A) Potassium.
    (B) Sodium.
    (C) Calcium.
    (D) Chloride.

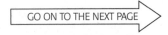

GO ON TO THE NEXT PAGE

11. Which answer option is a function performed by T cells?

    (A) Secreting antibodies to fight pathogens.

    (B) Eliminating old or damaged red blood cells.

    (C) Identifying and destroying infected cells.

    (D) Expressing B-cell receptors.

12. Which part of the respiratory system is the primary means to prevent food from entering the lungs?

    (A) Pharynx.

    (B) Trachea.

    (C) Diaphragm.

    (D) Carina.

13. A patient reports an inability to see at night or in low-light environments. Which is the MOST likely cause for the visual disturbance?

    (A) Abrasion to the cornea.

    (B) Detachment of the retina.

    (C) Degradation of cone cells in the retina.

    (D) Degradation of rod cells in the retina.

14. Where are the ossicles located?

    (A) Larynx.

    (B) Middle ear.

    (C) Kidneys.

    (D) Lungs.

END OF TEST. STOP

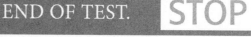

Practice Test One: Answer Key

Reading Comprehension	Writing	Mathematics	Science
1. A	1. C	1. A	1. D
2. D	2. B	2. A	2. D
3. C	3. C	3. B	3. C
4. A	4. D	4. C	4. B
5. B	5. D	5. B	5. D
6. A	6. D	6. D	6. A
7. A	7. C	7. D	7. B
8. C	8. A	8. C	8. A
9. D	9. A	9. D	9. C
10. A	10. B	10. C	10. B
11. D	11. A	11. C	11. C
12. B	12. B	12. B	12. A
13. C	13. C	13. B	13. D
14. C	14. B	14. B	14. B
15. D		15. A	
		16. B	
		17. C	

Answers and Explanations

Reading Comprehension

1. A

The passage states that the air space allows mammals "to retain heat for longer periods of time."

2. D

Because humans are "devoid of fur," the goosebump instinct can be reasonably described as useless. The passage does not suggest that goosebumps are unexplained, harmful, or dangerous, as the other answer choices suggest.

3. C

The description of lion behavior is meant to show the difference between humans and other animals, meaning that the purpose is to provide contrast.

4. A

The final sentence draws a direct connection between curiosity and the development of culture, showing its significance. None of the other answer choices accurately describe this connection.

5. B

The use of the word *convenient* suggests that parks were meant to be easy for residents to access. Although parks may preserve plant life, this would not be considered the primary purpose of parks; although parks might reduce the unpleasantness of city life, nothing in the passage suggests that they were meant to end the unpleasantness of city life.

6. A

The author mentions crime and pollution as supporting details for the assertion that parks "have been allowed to deteriorate to an alarming extent." Although some of the other answer choices sound reasonable, the question asks specifically about the author's purpose in using those examples.

7. A

Although the other problems might exist in park restoration, trash collection is the only one specifically mentioned in the last paragraph.

8. C

The passage mentions that parks "served their purpose admirably" for more than a century but now encounter problems like crime and pollution. This suggests that parks now face greater challenges than they used to.

9. D

The author describes the relationship between humans and dogs as "the most ancient of all."

10. A

The author refers to the dog as a "companion and ally," and notes that companion animals "were followed by food animals" and animals used for other purposes.

11. D

The author describes dogs as being "susceptible to domination by, and attachment to, a pack leader."

12. B

"Nature" is the best definition for the word *essence* as it is used in paragraph 2 of the passage.

13. C

"Influenced" is the best definition for the word *tempered* as it is used in paragraph 1 of the passage.

14. C

There is only one answer choice that illustrates learning through trial-and-error or practice.

15. D

The author notes that the discoveries made by these people occurred without "an immediate survival imperative," and suggests the discoveries may "have as much to do with enjoyment as with survival."

Writing

1. C

Sentence 7 is the only sentence that focuses exclusively on a past form of communication, rather than email.

2. B

The correct spelling of the word is *effective*.

3. C

A singular verb (*has*) is required for the subject *email*.

4. D

The additional sentence begins with the words, "Despite these challenges . . ." which means it should come after the challenges associated with email have already been discussed.

5. D

6. D

The use of the word *also* in sentence 7 makes the inclusion of *too* unnecessary.

7. C

The correct spelling of the word is *devastating*.

8. A

In the sentence's current structure, the verb *eliminated* should be changed to *eliminating*.

9. A

The additional sentence describes one of the potential benefits of fish farming, which are all located in paragraph 1.

10. B

A comma should be added after the word *research* in sentence 3.

11. A

The correct spelling of the word is *proliferation*.

12. B

"For example" should be set off from the rest of the sentence, and therefore requires a comma after the word *know*.

13. C

The additional sentence refers to epidemics in Central America, which are first mentioned in sentence 4.

14. B

Sentence 5 describes how European explorers affected indigenous populations in ways unrelated to malaria.

Mathematics

1. A

Find a common denominator for the fractions $\frac{1}{3}, \frac{1}{6}$, and $\frac{4}{9}$. Notice that 6 is a multiple of 3, since $6 = 2 \times 3$. So you just need to find a number that is a multiple of 9 and 6, since a multiple of 6 is a multiple of 3.

You can find a common multiple of 6 and 9 by starting with the smallest positive multiple of 9, which is $1 \times 9 = 9$, and then looking at the next positive multiples of 9, which are $2 \times 9, 3 \times 9, 4 \times 9, 5 \times 9, \ldots$, until you find a multiple of 6:

- $1 \times 9 = 9$ is not a multiple of 6.
- $2 \times 9 = 18$ is a multiple of 6, since $18 = 3 \times 6$.

So 18 is a multiple of 9, since $18 = 2 \times 9$, and 18 is a multiple of 6, since $18 = 3 \times 6$. You can also see that 18 is a multiple of 3 from $18 = 3 \times 6$.

The positive multiple of 3, 6, and 9 you found, 18, is actually the smallest positive multiple of 3, 6, and 9.

Therefore, $\frac{1}{3} + \frac{1}{6} - \frac{4}{9} = \frac{6}{18} + \frac{3}{18} - \frac{8}{18} = \frac{6 + 3 - 8}{18} = \frac{1}{18}$.

2. A

Substitute the given values for each variable. Since $a = 2$, $b = 6$, and $c = 4$:

$$a(b - 2) + 3c = (2)(6 - 2) + 3(4)$$
$$= 2(4) + 3(4) = 8 + 12 = 20.$$

3. B

Since there is a 20% discount, the marked-down price is $100\% - 20\% = 80\%$ of the original price. Let's convert 80% to a decimal. To convert a percent to a decimal or fraction, divide the percent by 100%: $80\% = \frac{80\%}{100\%} = \frac{80}{100} = \frac{8}{10} = 0.8$. So the marked down price is $0.8 \times \$120 = \$96$. There is an 8% sales tax. Let's convert 8% to a decimal: $8\% = \frac{8\%}{100\%} = \frac{8}{100} = 0.08$. So Andrew paid $1.08 \times \$96$, or \$103.68.

4. C

The easiest way to solve this problem is to substitute an actual number for z. Pick a number that is 5 more than a positive multiple of 8. An easy positive multiple of 8 to work with is 1×8, or 8 itself, so let $z = 8 + 5 = 13$. The number 13 yields a remainder of 5 when divided by 8, since we chose the number 13 because it is 5 more than a multiple of 8. So $(4 \times 13) \div 8 = 52 \div 8 = 6$ with a remainder of 4.

Here is an algebraic solution. Since the remainder when the positive integer z is divided by 8 is 5, $z = 8N + 5$, where N is a nonnegative integer. Since $z = 8N + 5$, $4z = 4(8N + 5) = 32N + 20$. Now 32 is a multiple of 8, since $32 = 4 \times 8$, so when $32N$ is divided by 8, the quotient is $4N$ and the remainder is 0. When 20 is divided by 8, the quotient is 2 and the remainder is 4.

Here is the information we know so far:

- When $32N$ is divided by 8, the remainder is 0.
- When 20 is divided by 8, the remainder is 4.

So when $32N + 20$ is divided by 8, the remainder is $0 + 4 = 4$.

We showed that $4z = 32N + 20$. Therefore, the remainder when $4z$ is divided by 8 is 4.

5. B

Starting with the smallest positive multiple of 12, which is $1 \times 12 = 12$, and then working with the next positive multiples of 12, which are 2×12, 3×12, 4×12, 5×12 ..., work with the positive multiples of 12 until you find a multiple of 8:

- $1 \times 12 = 12$ is not a multiple of 8
- $2 \times 12 = 24$ is a multiple of 8, as $24 = 3 \times 8$.

For the numbers 12 and 8, the least common multiple is 24. That is, the smallest positive integer that can be divided by both 12 and 8 is 24.

6. D

Substitute 11 for y into the equation $6x - 7 = y$. So now you have $6x - 7 = 11$. Add 7 to both sides of the equation: $6x - 7 = 11$, then $6x = 18$. Finally, divide both sides by 6 to find $x = 3$.

7. D

Let x be the number of dollars that Robert has. Then, Edward has $(x + 400)$ dollars. After Edward spends $60, he has $[(x + 400) - 60]$ dollars, which is $(x + 400 - 60)$ dollars, or $(x + 340)$ dollars. You know that after Edward spends $60, he has three times as much as Robert. Therefore, $x + 340 = 3x$. Subtract x from both sides: $340 = 2x$. Divide both sides by 2: $170 = x$. Thus, Robert has $170.

8. C

After the 20% discount, the new price is $100\% - 20\% = 80\%$ of the old price, or 80% of $160. The word "of" means "times," where times means "multiply." To convert a percent to a decimal or fraction, divide the percent by 100%: $80\% = \frac{80\%}{100\%} = \frac{80}{100} = \frac{8}{10} = 0.8$. The discounted price would be 80% of $160, which is $0.8 \times \$160$, or $128.

9. D

$\frac{2}{8}$ is equivalent to $\frac{1}{4}$. To convert a fraction or decimal to a percent, multiply that fraction or decimal by 100%: $\frac{1}{4} = \frac{1}{4} \times 100\% = 25\%$.

10. C

We want the answer choice that equals $5\frac{2}{3} \times \frac{1}{2} - \frac{5}{12}$. Let's begin by converting $5\frac{2}{3}$ to an improper fraction:

$5\frac{2}{3} = \frac{5 \times 3 + 2}{3} = \frac{15 + 2}{3} = \frac{17}{3}$. Thus, $5\frac{2}{3} = \frac{17}{3}$.

Then calculate the first part of the expression:

$5\frac{2}{3} \times \frac{1}{2} - \frac{5}{12} = \frac{17}{3} \times \frac{1}{2} - \frac{5}{12} = \frac{17 \times 1}{3 \times 2} - \frac{5}{12} = \frac{17}{6} - \frac{5}{12}$.

Now let's work with $\frac{17}{6} - \frac{5}{12}$. First you need a common denominator, which here is a multiple of 6 and 12. Since $12 = 2 \times 6$, a common multiple of 6 and 12 is 12, which is actually the smallest positive multiple of 6 and 12.

Calculate the final part of the expression:

$\frac{17}{6} - \frac{5}{12} = \frac{34}{12} - \frac{5}{12} = \frac{34 - 5}{12} = \frac{29}{12} = 2\frac{5}{12}$.

11. C

Let x be the original number of coats. The next day Renée sold 33 coats, which is 30% of the original number of coats. Let's convert 30% to a decimal. To convert a percent to a decimal or fraction, divide the percent by 100%:

$30\% = \frac{30\%}{100\%} = \frac{30}{100} = \frac{3}{10} = 0.3$. So the 33 coats sold the next day are 0.3 of the original number of coats. Thus,

$33 = 0.3x$. Dividing both sides by 0.3, $\frac{33}{0.3} = x$. So $x = \frac{33}{0.3} = \frac{33 \times 10}{0.3 \times 10} = \frac{330}{3} = 110$. Therefore, Renée had 110 coats in stock before the sale.

12. B

Substitute the given values for each variable. Since $x = \sqrt{3}$, $y = 2$, and $z = \frac{1}{2}$, then

$$x^2 - 5yz + y^2 = (\sqrt{3})^2 - 5(2)\left(\frac{1}{2}\right) + 2^2 = 3 - 5 + 4 = 2.$$

13. B

Align the hundredths digits, the tenths digits, and the units digits when adding 120.21 and 8.76. The number 8.76 has no tens digit or hundreds digit:

$$+ \begin{array}{r} 120.21 \\ 8.76 \\ \hline 128.97 \end{array}$$

Align the hundredths digits, the tenths digits, the units digits, and the tens digits when subtracting 72.88 from 128.97. The number 72.88 has no hundreds digit:

$$- \begin{array}{r} 128.97 \\ 72.88 \\ \hline 56.09 \end{array}$$

Thus, $120.21 + 8.76 - 72.88 = 56.09$.

14. B

This question requires you to find a percent of a percent: 25% of 25% of 72. Let's first convert 25% to a decimal. To convert a percent to a decimal or fraction, divide the percent by 100%: $25\% = \frac{25\%}{100\%} = \frac{25}{100} = 0.25$.

Then, multiply by the decimal value:

$$\begin{aligned} 25\% \text{ of } 25\% \text{ of } 72 &= 0.25 \times 0.25 \times 72 \\ &= 0.25 \times (0.25 \times 72) = \\ &= 0.25 \times 18 = 4.5 \end{aligned}$$

Therefore, 25% of 25% of 72 is 4.5.

15. A

If the value of the stock drops by 20%, the new value of the stock is $100\% - 20\% = 80\%$ of the original value. Let's convert 80% to a decimal. To convert a percent to a decimal or fraction, divide the percent by 100%: $80\% = \frac{80\%}{100\%} = \frac{80}{100} = \frac{8}{10} = 0.8$. So the new value of the stock is $0.8y$ dollars.

Let's determine what the percent increase is when the value of the stock goes from $0.8y$ dollars to y dollars. The formula for percent increase is:

$$\text{Percent increase} = \frac{\text{New value} - \text{Original value}}{\text{Original value}} \times 100\%.$$

Be extra careful when using this formula. When the stock dropped 20% from y dollars to $0.8y$ dollars, y dollars was the *original* value of the stock and $0.8y$ dollars was the new value of the stock. However, for the purpose of finding the percent increase in the value of the stock when the value of the stock goes from $0.8y$ dollars to y dollars, $0.8y$ dollars is the original value of the stock and y dollars is the *new* value of the stock. Find the percent increase necessary for the dropped value of $0.8y$ dollars of the stock to go back up to the value of y dollars of the stock:

$$\frac{y \text{ dollars} - 0.8y \text{ dollars}}{0.8y \text{ dollars}} \times 100\% = \frac{y - 0.8y}{0.8y} \times 100\%$$

$$= \frac{0.2y}{0.8y} \times 100\% = \frac{2}{8} \times 100\%$$

$$= \frac{1}{4} \times 100\% = 25\%$$

16. B

Let x dollars be the amount of money Mrs. Bailer has for the 4 children. When Mrs. Bailer divides the amount of money equally among the 4 children, each child has $\frac{x}{4}$ dollars. When Mr. Bailor then adds 2 dollars to the amount each child has, each child now has $\left(\frac{x}{4} + 2\right)$ dollars. Each child now has 5.25 dollars, yielding the equation $\frac{x}{4} + 2 = 5.25$.

17. C

You can find this solution through simple division; however, one quicker way to choose the correct answer here is to come up with a rough estimate of the answer. Because the numerator and denominator are both positive, and the numerator is larger than the denominator, you know the answer will be greater than 1. Therefore, choices (A) and (B) can be eliminated. This leaves only answer choices (C) and (D). Because the numerator and denominator are both positive, the numerator is larger than the denominator, and the numerator is smaller than twice the denominator, you can estimate that the answer is between 1 and 2. Choice (D) can be eliminated, and only choice (C) remains. Choice (C) is correct.

Science

1. D

Osmosis is a process by which molecules—such as water—pass through a cell's membrane.

2. D

The medulla oblongata, located in the brainstem, controls involuntary functions such as breathing and the pumping of the heart.

3. C

The *alveoli* are tiny, capillary-filled chambers in the lungs where carbon dioxide is released from the blood and oxygen enters the blood through the process of diffusion.

4. B

Although all the answer choices are part of the renal system, actual blood filtration takes place in the *nephrons*, which are microscopic structures inside the kidneys.

5. D

Erythrocytes are more commonly known as red blood cells; their primary function is transporting oxygen through the blood by binding hemoglobin to oxygen molecules.

6. A

Veins are usually thought of as vessels that bring oxygen-depleted blood back to the heart, but the *pulmonary veins* bring oxygen-rich blood back to the left atrium of the heart for distribution throughout the body.

7. B

Although hormones play a role in many different systems, the *endocrine system* is a collection of glands that generate and regulate many of the most important hormones in the body.

8. A

Acidemia is the term to describe a state of low blood pH, while *alkalemia* describes a state of high blood pH. *Acidosis* and *alkalosis* are processes or conditions that can result in acidemia and alkalemia, respectively.

9. C

Filtration of damaged or dead blood cells takes place mainly in the liver and spleen, though waste product from dead blood cells is excreted through the large intestine.

10. B

The main extracellular electrolyte is *sodium*. Potassium is the main intracellular electrolyte.

11. C

One of the functions performed by T cells is identifying and destroying infected cells.

12. A

The *pharynx* is where food is diverted to the esophagus during swallowing, thanks to the epiglottis.

13. D

Rod cells in the retina are responsible for low-light vision sensitivity.

14. B

The ossicles are three bones located in the *middle ear* that help transmit sound to the cochlea.

Nursing School Entrance Exams
Practice Test Two, Kaplan
Answer Sheet

Reading Comprehension

1. Ⓐ Ⓑ Ⓒ Ⓓ   4. Ⓐ Ⓑ Ⓒ Ⓓ   7. Ⓐ Ⓑ Ⓒ Ⓓ   10. Ⓐ Ⓑ Ⓒ Ⓓ   13. Ⓐ Ⓑ Ⓒ Ⓓ

2. Ⓐ Ⓑ Ⓒ Ⓓ   5. Ⓐ Ⓑ Ⓒ Ⓓ   8. Ⓐ Ⓑ Ⓒ Ⓓ   11. Ⓐ Ⓑ Ⓒ Ⓓ   14. Ⓐ Ⓑ Ⓒ Ⓓ

3. Ⓐ Ⓑ Ⓒ Ⓓ   6. Ⓐ Ⓑ Ⓒ Ⓓ   9. Ⓐ Ⓑ Ⓒ Ⓓ   12. Ⓐ Ⓑ Ⓒ Ⓓ   15. Ⓐ Ⓑ Ⓒ Ⓓ

Writing

1. Ⓐ Ⓑ Ⓒ Ⓓ   4. Ⓐ Ⓑ Ⓒ Ⓓ   7. Ⓐ Ⓑ Ⓒ Ⓓ   10. Ⓐ Ⓑ Ⓒ Ⓓ   13. Ⓐ Ⓑ Ⓒ Ⓓ

2. Ⓐ Ⓑ Ⓒ Ⓓ   5. Ⓐ Ⓑ Ⓒ Ⓓ   8. Ⓐ Ⓑ Ⓒ Ⓓ   11. Ⓐ Ⓑ Ⓒ Ⓓ   14. Ⓐ Ⓑ Ⓒ Ⓓ

3. Ⓐ Ⓑ Ⓒ Ⓓ   6. Ⓐ Ⓑ Ⓒ Ⓓ   9. Ⓐ Ⓑ Ⓒ Ⓓ   12. Ⓐ Ⓑ Ⓒ Ⓓ

Mathematics

1. Ⓐ Ⓑ Ⓒ Ⓓ   5. Ⓐ Ⓑ Ⓒ Ⓓ   9. Ⓐ Ⓑ Ⓒ Ⓓ   13. Ⓐ Ⓑ Ⓒ Ⓓ   17. Ⓐ Ⓑ Ⓒ Ⓓ

2. Ⓐ Ⓑ Ⓒ Ⓓ   6. Ⓐ Ⓑ Ⓒ Ⓓ   10. Ⓐ Ⓑ Ⓒ Ⓓ   14. Ⓐ Ⓑ Ⓒ Ⓓ

3. Ⓐ Ⓑ Ⓒ Ⓓ   7. Ⓐ Ⓑ Ⓒ Ⓓ   11. Ⓐ Ⓑ Ⓒ Ⓓ   15. Ⓐ Ⓑ Ⓒ Ⓓ

4. Ⓐ Ⓑ Ⓒ Ⓓ   8. Ⓐ Ⓑ Ⓒ Ⓓ   12. Ⓐ Ⓑ Ⓒ Ⓓ   16. Ⓐ Ⓑ Ⓒ Ⓓ

Science

1. Ⓐ Ⓑ Ⓒ Ⓓ   4. Ⓐ Ⓑ Ⓒ Ⓓ   7. Ⓐ Ⓑ Ⓒ Ⓓ   10. Ⓐ Ⓑ Ⓒ Ⓓ   13. Ⓐ Ⓑ Ⓒ Ⓓ

2. Ⓐ Ⓑ Ⓒ Ⓓ   5. Ⓐ Ⓑ Ⓒ Ⓓ   8. Ⓐ Ⓑ Ⓒ Ⓓ   11. Ⓐ Ⓑ Ⓒ Ⓓ   14. Ⓐ Ⓑ Ⓒ Ⓓ

3. Ⓐ Ⓑ Ⓒ Ⓓ   6. Ⓐ Ⓑ Ⓒ Ⓓ   9. Ⓐ Ⓑ Ⓒ Ⓓ   12. Ⓐ Ⓑ Ⓒ Ⓓ

Practice Test Two, Kaplan

READING COMPREHENSION

Questions 1–2 are based on the following passage.

Until quite recently, hypnosis has been a specialized—and often controversial—technique used only in marginal areas of medicine. However, hypnosis is now increasingly finding mainstream use. For example, mental health experts have found that the suggestions of a skilled therapist are often remarkably effective in countering anxiety and depression. The benefits of hypnosis, though, are not limited to the emotional and psychological realm. Hypnosis helps burn center patients manage excruciating pain, and a recent research study found that hypnosis can dramatically shorten the time required for bone fractures to heal, often by several weeks.

1. Which answer option BEST expresses the main idea of the passage?

   (A) Hypnosis has become established as one of the most effective means to manage pain.

   (B) Despite its controversial history, hypnosis has proven useful across many areas of medicine.

   (C) Hypnosis remains controversial, especially when used to treat anxiety and depression.

   (D) The benefits of hypnosis have been shown to be limited to certain areas, but nonetheless effective.

2. Which term or phrase best defines the word <u>manage</u> as it is used in the passage?

   (A) Direct.

   (B) Administer.

   (C) Bring about.

   (D) Cope with.

GO ON TO THE NEXT PAGE

KAPLAN

Questions 3–4 are based on the following passage.

In recent years, shark attacks in U.S. waters have received wide attention. Are such attacks a growing threat to swimmers and surfers? Statistics suggest not. The rate of attacks per number of swimmers has not increased over time. What *has* increased is the popularity of aquatic sports, such as surfing, sail boarding, and kayaking. More people are in the water these days, and therefore the chances of a shark encounter increase. Still, to keep the issue in perspective we should remember there were only six fatal shark attacks in U.S. coastal waters from 1990 to 2000.

3. According to the author, which of the following has NOT increased over time?

   (A) The total number of shark attacks in U.S. waters.

   (B) The popularity of aquatic sports.

   (C) The number of fatal shark attacks in U.S. coastal waters.

   (D) The rate of shark attacks per number of people in the water.

4. Why does the author MOST likely provide the statistic in the final sentence?

   (A) To point out that U.S. coastal waters are safer than those of other countries.

   (B) To illustrate that relatively few fatal shark attacks have occurred in U.S. waters.

   (C) To show that the period 1990–2000 marked a decrease in the number of fatal shark attacks.

   (D) To caution swimmers and surfers against dangers.

GO ON TO THE NEXT PAGE

Questions 5–6 are based on the following passage.

Although much about dolphin communication remains a mystery, scientists have discovered three distinct sounds that dolphins frequently make: chirps, clicks, and whistles. Scientists have learned that dolphins use clicks to create a sonar map, which allows them to navigate and hunt. But, apart from possibly transmitting location, the clicks do not appear to serve any communication purpose. Rather, research indicates that dolphins communicate with each other by whistling. This discovery has necessitated further investigation, as scientists are not yet sure whether the whistles comprise a complex system of linguistic communication or a simple set of sonic cues like the ones used by other animal species.

5. Why does the author mention whistles in the passage?

   (A) To show that dolphins are capable of expressing emotion.
   (B) To prompt questions about the complexity of dolphin communication.
   (C) To illustrate how they aid dolphins in navigating and hunting.
   (D) To continue to spur research into their unknown purpose.

6. Which is implied about dolphins in the passage?

   (A) They are not the only animal species that communicates sonically.
   (B) They never use clicks for communication.
   (C) They are more intelligent than other animal species.
   (D) They use a system of communication similar to that of other animal species.

GO ON TO THE NEXT PAGE

KAPLAN

Questions 7–12 are based on the following passage.

Until recently, patients with progressive diseases that eventually lead to blindness have had little in the way of treatment, let alone a cure. Conditions such as retinitis pigmentosa and macular degeneration still stump doctors, and even the latest treatments, such as prescribing massive doses of vitamin A, only temporarily slow the progress of the disease in some patients. Currently, there is no failsafe way to reverse or even stop the progress of these diseases. Mechanical devices such as retinal implants seem to work with only a limited number of patients—really, only those whose vision loss is caused by a retinal disorder.

However, one new treatment is showing some promise, although it hasn't been thoroughly tested yet. Instead of focusing on dietary solutions, some doctors are attempting to develop an electronic one: a bionic eye that enables the user's brain to translate light impulses and create a virtual black-and-white "picture" of his or her surroundings. The picture, although accurate, only reflects a very limited field of vision, as if the patient had blinders on. Also, the picture moves fairly slowly, as if the patient were watching a film in very slow motion. But, being able to locate and identify objects is a definite first step in achieving everyday functional mobility for the visually impaired.

Rather than the glass eye one might imagine, this artificial vision system consists of an elaborate apparatus that looks like a pair of binoculars, as well as a series of wires that are implanted directly into the patient's brain. The wires electrically stimulate the visual cortex, producing phosphenes, which blind people perceive as small points of light. The device then maps these phosphenes, gradually training the patient's brain to "see." One major advantage of the system, as opposed to other proposed treatments such as retinal implants, is that it is not condition-specific: Patients can use it regardless of the cause of vision loss. For example, patients with genetic conditions such as retinitis pigmentosa, as well as patients with vision loss resulting from illness or accident, can use the device, since it directly stimulates the brain's vision center. In addition, its construction is fairly flexible and portable (the wires, in fact, are said to be hardly noticeable), and its utilities are far-reaching: One could envision a number of useful additional features, including zoom and night vision functions.

7. Why does the author MOST likely refer to retinal implants in paragraph 1?

(A) To provide an example of an electronic artificial vision device.

(B) To describe one way in which mechanical vision devices are limited.

(C) To imply that all degenerative eye diseases are too advanced for most doctors.

(D) To describe one extremely effective artificial vision device.

8. In paragraph 2, why does the author use the phrase definite first step to describe the bionic eye?

(A) It hasn't been thoroughly tested yet, and should not be viewed as a "cure" for blindness.

(B) The device provides only limited vision, but it could be enough to improve mobility for users.

(C) Advances in the bionic eye might lead to the development of more effective retinal implants.

(D) It provides a viable alternative to dietary treatments.

9. In paragraph 3, what does the phrase functional mobility refer to?

(A) The ability to perform daily activities.

(B) The usefulness of electrical devices.

(C) The ability to read road signs.

(D) The theory that electrical vision devices work better than mechanical ones.

GO ON TO THE NEXT PAGE ▷

10. In the final paragraph, why does the author suggest that the uses of the bionic eye are far-reaching?

   (A) The device could be provided with capabilities beyond even those of normal eyesight.

   (B) A wide variety of visually impaired people could be treated with the device.

   (C) The device could be provided at a low cost for people all over the world.

   (D) Technological developments required for the bionic eye could kick-start other industries.

11. Which statement BEST expresses the main idea of the passage?

   (A) An artificial vision system will likely take many years to develop and refine and may prove to be too limited in its capabilities for most visually impaired people.

   (B) A "bionic" artificial vision system relies on electrical impulses to stimulate the user's brain into "seeing."

   (C) The development of a "bionic" artificial vision system could bring functional sight to people who previously had little hope of ever seeing again.

   (D) Some medical conditions that cause visual impairment are much more difficult to treat than visual impairments caused by injury.

12. Based on the passage, which statement is MOST likely true about macular degeneration?

   (A) It is a progressive disease that eventually leads to a complete loss of vision.

   (B) It is the most common cause of vision loss among the elderly.

   (C) It cannot be treated by a "bionic" artificial vision system.

   (D) It is more difficult to treat than retinitis pigmentosa.

GO ON TO THE NEXT PAGE

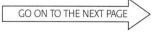

Questions 13–15 are based on the following passage.

On a stormy June day in 1752, Benjamin Franklin carried out the famous experiment in which he channeled lightning down a kite string and stored the electric charge in a Leyden jar, the precursor to the modern capacitor. The consequences could not have been more pronounced. Franklin proved that electricity was a force of nature, like Newton's gravity, and the subsequent invention of the lightning rod (based on Franklin's theories) sharply reduced risk of fire to tall buildings. Franklin's experiment had cultural repercussions as well. It showed that scientific research could have practical benefits, and it impugned the superstitious belief—widespread at the time—that lightning resulted from divine displeasure.

13. For which purpose does the author include the sentence, "The consequences could not have been more pronounced"?

    (A) To show that it was difficult to describe the results of the experiment.

    (B) To suggest that Franklin became famous because of the experiment.

    (C) To illustrate the importance of conducting experiments.

    (D) To stress that Franklin's experiment had far-reaching effects.

14. Based on the passage, in which of these did Franklin's kite experiment play a part?

    (A) Promoting superstitious beliefs.

    (B) Explaining the force of gravity.

    (C) Developing the Leyden jar.

    (D) Illustrating the utility of scientific research.

15. Which answer option best defines the word <u>impugned</u> as it is used in the passage?

    (A) Reinforced.

    (B) Cast doubt upon.

    (C) Popularized.

    (D) Called attention to.

GO ON TO THE NEXT PAGE

WRITING

Questions 1–5 are based on the following passage.

[1]One of the hazards of swimming in the ocean is an unexpected encounter with a jellyfish. [2]Contact with the poison in a jellyfish's tentacles can result in sharp, lingering pain, or even death if the person stung is highly allergic. [3]While everyone, including the jellyfish, would like to avoid these encounters, they are not uncommon. [4]In fact, I was stung twice when I lived in Australia. [5]This is hardly surprising considering that jellyfish lives in every ocean in the world and have done so for more than 650 million years. [6]The animals are likely so widespread because of their extreme adaptability—they are quite hardy and can withstand a wide range of temperatures and conditions in their environment.

[7]Although a jellyfish sting is unpleasant, the mechanics behind the sting are fascinating. [8]The jellyfish is able to administor its sting thanks to tiny organelles known as nematocysts. [9]Each tentacle on a jellyfish can contain thousands of nematocysts. [10]When a nematocyst is triggered generally by potential prey brushing against the surface of the tentacle, it fires out a tiny, sharp barb to pierce the skin of the prey and inject toxin. [11]If hundreds or thousands of nematocysts are all triggered at once by a single victim, they can cause excruciating pain or even death.

1. Which answer option describes how to correct a punctuation error in the passage?

   (A) Change the comma after the word *pain* in sentence 2 to a semicolon.
   (B) Change the dash after the word *adaptability* in sentence 6 to a comma.
   (C) Add a comma after the word *triggered* in sentence 10.
   (D) Change the comma after the word *victim* in sentence 11 to a colon.

2. Which sentence should be deleted because it provides unnecessary information?

   (A) Sentence 2.
   (B) Sentence 4.
   (C) Sentence 7.
   (D) Sentence 9.

3. Which word in paragraph 2 is incorrect?

   (A) Unpleasant.
   (B) Administor.
   (C) Potential.
   (D) Excruciating.

4. Where is the BEST place to add this sentence?

   Nematocysts are only found in sea organisms such as jellyfish, corals, and sea anemones.

   (A) Following sentence 4.
   (B) Following sentence 7.
   (C) Following sentence 8.
   (D) Following sentence 11.

5. Which sentence has incorrect subject-verb agreement?

   (A) Sentence 3.
   (B) Sentence 5.
   (C) Sentence 8.
   (D) Sentence 10.

GO ON TO THE NEXT PAGE

KAPLAN

Questions 6–10 are based on the following passage.

[1]In addition to being the largest planet in the Solar System, Jupiter holds the distinction of having the most moons of any planet in the Solar System. [2]Currently, 69 celestial objects are recognized as moons of Jupiter. [3]The four earliest of these to be discovered were, not surprisingly, the largest: Callisto, Europa, Ganymede, and Io. [4]They are collectively known as the Galilean satellites because they were first identified by astronomer Galileo Galilei in 1610. [5]Galileo is recognized as one of the most important figures in the development of physics and the scientific method, but he spent many years under house arrest because he was accused of heresy by the Roman Catholic Church.

[6]The four Galilean satellites of Jupiter probably experienced early, intense bombardment by other celestial objects. [7]Thus, the very ancient surface of Callisto remains scarred by impact craters. [8]The younger, more varied surface of Ganymede reveals distinct light and dark areas, the light areas featuring networks of intersecting grooves and ridges, probably resulting from later iceflows. [9]The impact sites of Europa have been almost completely erased; apparently by water outflowing from the interior and instantly forming vast, low, frozen seas. [10]Satellite photographs of Io, the closest of the four to Jupiter, were revelatory. [11]They showed a landscape dominated by volcanos, many actively erupting, making Io the most tectonically active object in the solar system. [12]Since a body as small as Io cannot supply the energy for such a notable affect, the accepted explanation has been that, forced into a highly excentric orbit, Io is engulfed by tides stemming from a titanic contest between the other three Galilean moons and Jupiter.

6. Which word in paragraph 2 is incorrect?

   (A) Bombardment.
   (B) Intersecting.
   (C) Apparently.
   (D) Excentric.

7. Which sentence includes an unnecessary word?

   (A) Sentence 2 includes the unnecessary word *currently*.
   (B) Sentence 7 includes the unnecessary word *very*.
   (C) Sentence 8 includes the unnecessary word *probably*.
   (D) Sentence 11 includes the unnecessary word *many*.

8. Which sentence should be deleted because it provides unnecessary information?

   (A) Sentence 2.
   (B) Sentence 4.
   (C) Sentence 5.
   (D) Sentence 8.

9. Which sentence contains an error in punctuation?

   (A) Sentence 3.
   (B) Sentence 5.
   (C) Sentence 9.
   (D) Sentence 12.

10. Which word is incorrect in its sentence?

   (A) The word *distinction* in sentence 1.
   (B) The word *collectively* in sentence 4.
   (C) The word *revelatory* in sentence 10.
   (D) The word *affect* in sentence 12.

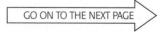
GO ON TO THE NEXT PAGE

Questions 11–14 are based on the following passage.

[1]Coral reefs are created over the course of hundreds or even thousands of years. [2]The main architect in coral reef formation is the stony coral, a relative of sea anemones that lives in tropical climates and secretes a skeleton, of almost pure calcium carbonate. [3]It is partnered by green algae, tiny unicellular plants that live within the tissues of coral. [4]The two organisms form a mutually benificial, symbiotic relationship, with the algae consuming carbon dioxide given off by the coral, and the coral thriving on the abundant oxygen produced photosynthetically by the algae. [5]When the coral dies, its skeleton is left, and other organisms grow on top of it; some estimates suggest that coral reefs provide habitat for around one-fourth of all marine species in the world. [6]Over the years, the mass of the coral skeletons and the associated organisms combine to form the petrified underwater forest that divers find so fascinating. [7]In the United States alone, over three million people go scuba diving every year.

[8]The largest coral reef system in the world, the Great Barrier Reef, is found off the northeastern coast of Australia. [9]It covers an area of more than 100,000 square miles. [10]Although much of the reef is protected as a marine park by the Australian government, some scientists fear that such protection could prove futile in the face of global climate change. [11]According to researchers, between 1985 and 2012, the Great Barrier Reef has lost more than half of it's total coral cover, with warmer ocean temperatures shouldering much of the blame for the dramatic loss.

11. Which sentence should be deleted because it provides unnecessary information?

    (A) Sentence 3.
    (B) Sentence 7.
    (C) Sentence 9.
    (D) Sentence 11.

12. Which word in paragraph 1 is incorrect?

    (A) Secretes.
    (B) Benificial.
    (C) Abundant.
    (D) Petrified.

13. Which choice describes how to correct a punctuation error in the passage?

    (A) Add a comma after the word *hundreds* in sentence 1.
    (B) Remove the comma after the word *skeleton* in sentence 2.
    (C) Replace the semicolon after the word *it* in sentence 5 with a comma.
    (D) Replace the comma after the word *cover* in sentence 11 with a semicolon.

14. Which word is incorrect in its sentence?

    (A) The word *lives* in sentence 2.
    (B) The word *species* in sentence 5.
    (C) The word *futile* in sentence 10.
    (D) The word *it's* in sentence 11.

GO ON TO THE NEXT PAGE

MATHEMATICS

1. If $\frac{x}{5} - 3 = -1\frac{4}{5}$, then which of the following is equal to x?

   (A) $\frac{1}{2}$

   (B) 4

   (C) 6

   (D) 8

2. A worker earns $16 per hour for the first 40 hours she works each week, and one and a half times this much for every hour over 40 hours. If she earned $700 for one week's work, how many hours of overtime did she work?

   (A) 3.3

   (B) 3

   (C) 2.5

   (D) 4

3. How many ounces of a liquid medication should a nurse add to 12 ounces of water so that the solution will contain 20% medication?

   (A) 2.5

   (B) 3

   (C) 3.6

   (D) 4

4. $2^3(3-1)^2 + (-4)^2 =$

   (A) 48

   (B) 32

   (C) 136

   (D) -48

5. A test contains 3 sections. Section A contains $\frac{3}{8}$ of the total number of questions on the test. Section B contains $\frac{1}{10}$ of the total number of questions on the test. What fraction of the total number of questions on the test is the number of questions in both Section A and Section B?

   (A) $\frac{1}{10}$

   (B) $\frac{1}{2}$

   (C) $\frac{19}{40}$

   (D) $\frac{36}{80}$

6. If $\frac{90}{x} = 9n$, then what is the value of nx?

   (A) 10

   (B) $9x$

   (C) 900

   (D) $90xn$

7. $\frac{2}{3} + \frac{3}{8} - \frac{5}{12} =$

   (A) $\frac{5}{12}$

   (B) $\frac{1}{2}$

   (C) $\frac{5}{8}$

   (D) $\frac{2}{3}$

8. A machine labels 150 bottles in 20 minutes. At this rate, how many minutes does it take to label 60 bottles?

   (A) 2

   (B) 4

   (C) 6

   (D) 8

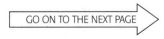

GO ON TO THE NEXT PAGE

KAPLAN

9. If a woman earns $600 for her first 40 hours of work in a week and then is paid one-and-one-half times her regular rate for any additional hours, how many hours must she work to make $690 in a week?

   (A) 43
   (B) 44
   (C) 45
   (D) 46

10. In a group of 25 students, 16 are female. What percent of the group is female?

    (A) 16%
    (B) 40%
    (C) 60%
    (D) 64%

11. If a barrel has the capacity to hold 75 gallons, how many gallons does it contain when it is $\frac{3}{5}$ full?

    (A) 45
    (B) 48
    (C) 54
    (D) 60

12. If $13 + a = 25 + b$, then $b - a =$

    (A) 38
    (B) 12
    (C) 8
    (D) −12

13. If a kilogram is equal to approximately 2.2 pounds, which of the following is the best approximation of the number of kilograms in one pound?

    (A) $\frac{5}{11}$
    (B) $\frac{3}{7}$
    (C) $\frac{3}{8}$
    (D) $\frac{1}{3}$

14. Brad bought a music player on sale at a 20% discount from its regular price of $118. If there is an 8% sales tax that is calculated on the sale price, how much did Brad pay for the music player?

    (A) $86.85
    (B) $94.40
    (C) $101.95
    (D) $127.44

15. If the ratio of males to females in a group of students is 3:5, which of the following could be the total number of students in the group?

    (A) 148
    (B) 150
    (C) 152
    (D) 154

16. If 48 of the 60 seats on a bus were occupied, what percent of the seats were not occupied?

    (A) 12%
    (B) 15%
    (C) 20%
    (D) 25%

17. A delivery service charges $25.00 per pound for making a delivery. If there is an additional 8% sales tax, what is the cost of delivering an item that weighs $\frac{4}{5}$ of a pound?

    (A) $20.00
    (B) $21.60
    (C) $22.60
    (D) $24.00

GO ON TO THE NEXT PAGE

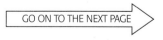

SCIENCE

1. Which is a function of bone?

    I. Formation of blood cells.
    II. Protection of vital organs.
    III. Framework for movement.

    (A) I only.
    (B) II only.
    (C) III only.
    (D) I, II, and III.

2. The rate of breathing is controlled by involuntary centers in which part of the brain?

    (A) Cerebrum.
    (B) Cerebellum.
    (C) Medulla oblongata.
    (D) Spinal cord.

3. Which phrase accurately describes the function of the hormone oxytocin?

    (A) Increases uterine contractions during childbirth.
    (B) Stimulates the release of glucose to the blood.
    (C) Induces water resorption in the kidneys.
    (D) Prepares the uterus for implantation of the fertilized egg.

4. Which blood type can be donated to anyone?

    (A) A
    (B) B
    (C) O
    (D) AB

5. Where in the body is insulin created?

    (A) Adrenal glands.
    (B) Kidneys.
    (C) Pancreas.
    (D) Thymus.

6. Which is the term for the tough elastic tissues found in the joints that connect bones to bones?

    (A) Ligaments.
    (B) Tendons.
    (C) Cartilage.
    (D) Muscles.

7. In which part of the eye are the light-sensitive cells known as rods and cones located?

    (A) Cornea.
    (B) Iris.
    (C) Pupil.
    (D) Retina.

8. Which muscle is controlled by conscious thought?

    (A) Smooth.
    (B) Striated.
    (C) Cardiac.
    (D) All of the above.

9. Where are most of the nutrients in food absorbed?

    (A) Stomach.
    (B) Pylorus.
    (C) Small intestine.
    (D) Large intestine.

10. Which statement about red blood cells in adult humans is true?

    (A) They have no nucleus.
    (B) They are replaced in the liver.
    (C) They are outnumbered by white blood cells in the circulatory system.
    (D) They are generated in the spleen.

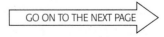
GO ON TO THE NEXT PAGE

11. If a patient diagnosed with diabetes mellitus accidentally overdosed on insulin, which would be likely to occur?

    (A) Increased levels of glucose in the blood.

    (B) Increased glucose concentration in urine.

    (C) Dehydration due to increased urine excretion.

    (D) Increased conversion of glucose to glycogen.

12. Saliva in the mouth begins the process of breaking down which of these?

    (A) Starch.

    (B) Fat.

    (C) Protein.

    (D) All of the above.

13. Which statement accurately describes the function of the hormone progesterone?

    (A) It increases human growth.

    (B) It stimulates the release of glucose to the blood.

    (C) It induces water resorption in the kidneys.

    (D) It prepares the uterus for implantation of the fertilized egg.

14. Which statement is true about dendrites?

    (A) They repair damaged neurons.

    (B) They exist only in the central nervous system.

    (C) They transmit nerve impulses away from the cell body.

    (D) They transmit nerve impulses toward the cell body.

END OF TEST. STOP

Practice Test Two: **Answer Key**

Reading Comprehension	Writing	Mathematics	Science
1. B	1. C	1. C	1. D
2. D	2. B	2. C	2. C
3. D	3. B	3. B	3. A
4. B	4. C	4. A	4. C
5. B	5. B	5. C	5. C
6. A	6. D	6. A	6. A
7. B	7. B	7. C	7. D
8. B	8. C	8. D	8. B
9. A	9. C	9. B	9. C
10. A	10. D	10. D	10. A
11. C	11. B	11. A	11. D
12. A	12. B	12. D	12. A
13. D	13. B	13. A	13. D
14. D	14. D	14. C	14. D
15. B		15. C	
		16. C	
		17. B	

Answers and Explanations

Reading Comprehension

1. B

The passage refers to the controversial history of hypnosis but lists the many areas in which it is being used effectively.

2. D

"Cope with" is the best definition of the word *manage* as it is used in the passage.

3. D

The author states that "the rate of attacks per number of swimmers has not increased over time."

4. B

The author uses the statistic to show that the risk of shark attack is very low.

5. B

The author indicates that whistling may or may not constitute a complex communication system.

6. A

The final sentence refers to other animal species using sonic cues to communicate.

7. B

The author mentions retinal implants to indicate that they can help only a small proportion of patients, which represents a significant limitation of existing mechanical devices.

8. B

While the author describes limited nature of the advantages offered by current bionic eye systems, they can still have significant impact, and they herald greater successes down the road.

9. A

In paragraph 3, the author uses the phrase "functional mobility" to refer to the ability to perform daily activities.

10. A

The author specifically lists possible capabilities beyond normal sight, including zoom and night vision.

11. C

The passage not only focuses on the development of a bionic vision system, but also on how such a system could help people with otherwise incurable vision disabilities. While some answer options include accurate information, they do not cover both of these aspects of the passage.

12. A

While some of the other answer choices could be true, the passage does not provide enough information to infer that they are indeed true. However, the passage clearly suggests that macular degeneration is a progressive disease that leads to vision loss in the first paragraph, when the author states that other treatments "only temporarily slow the progress of the disease."

13. D

The passage goes on to describe the far-reaching effects of Franklin's experiment.

14. D

The author states that the experiment "showed that scientific research could have practical benefits."

15. B

"Cast doubt upon" is the best definition for the word *impugned* as it is used in the passage.

Writing

1. C

The clause "generally by potential prey brushing against the surface of the tentacle" should be set off from the rest of the sentence; it requires a comma after the word *triggered*.

2. B

Sentence 4 includes a personal anecdote only tangentially related to the rest of the passage.

3. B

The correct spelling of the word is *administer*.

4. C

Nematocysts are defined in sentence 8, so the additional sentence should be placed after that.

5. B

As used in the sentence, the word *jellyfish* is plural and requires the singular form of the verb, *live*, rather than the singular form, *lives*.

6. D

The correct spelling of the word is *ec̲centric*.

7. B

The word *ancient* means "extremely old." The word *very*, which modifies it in sentence 7 ("very ancient"), is therefore duplicative and unnecessary.

8. C

The sentence includes information about Galileo's life, but it does not relate directly to the topic of the Galilean satellites.

9. C

Because the semicolon after the word *erased* does not separate two independent clauses, it should be replaced with a comma.

10. D

The correct word is *effect*.

11. B

The sentence provides statistics on scuba diving, but no information directly related to coral reefs.

12. B

The correct spelling of the word is *benef̲icial*.

13. B

The comma in sentence 2 incorrectly divides a clause that should remain undivided.

14. D

As used in the sentence, "its" is a possessive pronoun and does not require an apostrophe.

Mathematics

1. C

Add 3 to both sides of the equation $\frac{x}{5} - 3 = -1\frac{4}{5}$:

$\frac{x}{5} = -1\frac{4}{5} + 3$. Then, convert the $1\frac{4}{5}$ in $-1\frac{4}{5}$ to an improper fraction: $1\frac{4}{5} = \frac{1 \times 5 + 4}{5} = \frac{5+4}{5} = \frac{9}{5}$. Remember the negative sign: $-1\frac{4}{5} = -\frac{9}{5}$. So the equation $\frac{x}{5} = -1\frac{4}{5} + 3$ becomes $\frac{x}{5} = -\frac{9}{5} + 3$. Now let's add $-\frac{9}{5}$ and 3. Write 3 so it has a denominator of 5: $3 = 3 \times \frac{5}{5} = \frac{3 \times 5}{5} = \frac{15}{5}$. Then $-\frac{9}{5} + 3 = -\frac{9}{5} + \frac{15}{5} = \frac{-9+15}{5} = \frac{6}{5}$. Thus, the equation $\frac{x}{5} = -\frac{9}{5} + 3$ becomes $\frac{x}{5} = \frac{6}{5}$, and multiplying both sides by 5 yields $x = 6$.

2. C

For the first 40 hours of work, the worker earns ($16 dollars per hour) × (40 hours) = $640 dollars. Therefore, $700 − $640 = $60 of overtime pay is earned. The overtime rate is $16 \times 1\frac{1}{2}$ dollars per hour. Let's convert $1\frac{1}{2}$ to an improper fraction: $1\frac{1}{2} = \frac{1 \times 2 + 1}{2} = \frac{2+1}{2} = \frac{3}{2}$. Then $16 \times 1\frac{1}{2} = 16 \times \frac{3}{2} = 8 \times 3 = 24$. The overtime rate is 24 dollars per hour.

Here is the information we know so far:

• $60 dollars of overtime was earned.
• The overtime rate was $24 dollars per hour.

So the number of hours of overtime worked was ($60 dollars) ÷ ($24 dollars per hour), which is $\frac{60}{24}$ hours, or 2.5 hours.

3. B

Let's say x ounces of the liquid medication will be added to the 12 ounces of water. Then the total number of ounces of solution, which is made up of liquid medication and water, is $x + 12$. The number of ounces of liquid medication is x, so the fraction of the solution that is liquid medication is $\frac{x}{x + 12}$.

You know that 20% of the solution is medication. Let's convert 20% to a fraction. To convert a percent to a fraction or decimal, divide the percent by 100%: $20\% = \frac{20\%}{100\%} = \frac{20}{100} = \frac{1}{5}$. So the fraction of the solution that is medication is $\frac{1}{5}$. Since you know that the fraction of the solution that is medication is $\frac{x}{x+12}$, you can create the equation $\frac{x}{x+12} = \frac{1}{5}$. Solve this equation for x:

$$\frac{x}{x+12} = \frac{1}{5}$$

Cross-multiply: $\quad (x)(5) = (x+12)(1)$

Simplify each side: $\quad 5x = x+12$

Subtract x from both sides: $\quad 4x = 12$

Divide both sides by 4: $\quad x = 3$

Therefore, 3 ounces of liquid medication should be added to the 12 ounces of water for the solution to contain 20% medication.

4. A

Solve using the order of operations (PEMDAS):
$2^3(3-1)^2 + (-4)^2 = 8\,(2^2) + 16$
$= 8(4) + 16 = 32 + 16 = 48$.

5. C

The fraction of the total number of test questions in both Section A and Section B is $\frac{3}{8} + \frac{1}{10}$. Let's add $\frac{3}{8}$ and $\frac{1}{10}$. To add these fractions, you need a common denominator, which you can find by starting with the smallest positive multiple of 10, which is $1 \times 10 = 10$, and then looking at the next positive multiples of 10, which are 2×10, 3×10, 4×10, 5×10, ..., until you find a multiple of 8:

- $1 \times 10 = 10$ is not a multiple of 8.
- $2 \times 10 = 20$ is not a multiple of 8.
- $3 \times 10 = 30$ is not a multiple of 8.
- $4 \times 10 = 40$ is a multiple of 8, since $40 = 5 \times 8$.

The positive multiple of 8 and 10 you found, 40, is actually the smallest positive multiple of 8 and 10.

Add the fractions with the common denominator:
$\frac{3}{8} + \frac{1}{10} = \frac{15}{40} + \frac{4}{40} = \frac{15+4}{40} = \frac{19}{40}$. The fraction of the total number of questions in the test that are in Section A and Section B is $\frac{19}{40}$.

6. A

Multiplying both sides of the equation $\frac{90}{x} = 9n$ by x yields $x\left(\frac{90}{x}\right) = x(9n)$, or $90 = 9nx$. Dividing both sides of the equation $90 = 9nx$ by 9 yields $10 = nx$. The value of nx is 10.

7. C

Let's find a common denominator for the fractions $\frac{2}{3}$, $\frac{3}{8}$, and $\frac{5}{12}$. Notice that 12 is a multiple of 3, since $12 = 4 \times 3$. Thus, a multiple of 12 is a multiple of 3. So to find a multiple of 3, 8, and 12, determine a number that is a multiple of 8 and 12, because 12 is already a multiple of 3.

You can find a common multiple of 8 and 12 by starting with the smallest positive multiple of 12, which is $1 \times 12 = 12$, and then looking at the next positive multiples of 12, which are 2×12, 3×12, 4×12, 5×12, ..., until you find a multiple of 8:

- $1 \times 12 = 12$ is not a multiple of 8.
- $2 \times 12 = 24$ is a multiple of 8, since $24 = 3 \times 8$.

So 24 is a multiple of 12, since $24 = 2 \times 12$, and 24 is a multiple of 8, since $24 = 3 \times 8$.

Since 12 is a multiple of 3, it is also true that a common multiple of 3, 8, and 12 is 24. In fact, 24 is the smallest positive multiple of these three numbers.

Calculate the expression with the common denominator:

$$\frac{2}{3} + \frac{3}{8} - \frac{5}{12} = \frac{16}{24} + \frac{9}{24} - \frac{10}{24}$$
$$= \frac{16+9-10}{24} = \frac{25-10}{24}$$
$$= \frac{15}{24} = \frac{5}{8}.$$

8. D

The machine labels bottles at a rate of (150 bottles) ÷ (20 minutes), or 7.5 bottles per minute. So the machine will label 60 bottles in (60 bottles) ÷ (7.5 bottles per minute) = 8 minutes.

9. B

The woman's normal hourly salary is (600 dollars) ÷ (40 hours) = 15 dollars per hour. Since her overtime rate is $1\frac{1}{2}$ times her normal rate, her overtime rate is (15 dollars per hour) $\times 1\frac{1}{2} = \left(15 \times 1\frac{1}{2}\right)$ dollars per hour.

Convert $1\frac{1}{2}$ to an improper fraction:
$1\frac{1}{2} = \frac{1 \times 2 + 1}{2} = \frac{2+1}{2} = \frac{3}{2}$. Then multiply:
$15 \times 1\frac{1}{2} = 15 \times \frac{3}{2} = \frac{45}{2} = 22.5$. Therefore, her overtime rate is 22.5 dollars per hour.

KAPLAN

She must earn $690 − $600 = $90 in overtime. To earn $90 in overtime, she must work (90 dollars) ÷ (22.5 dollars per hour) overtime, which is 4 hours overtime.

The total number of hours she must work to make $690 is 40 + 4 = 44.

10. D

Since there are 16 female students in the group of 25 students, the fraction of people in the group who are female is $\frac{16}{25}$. To convert a fraction or decimal to a percent, multiply that fraction or decimal by 100%:

$\frac{16}{25} = \frac{16}{25} \times 100\% = 16 \times 4\% = 64\%$.

Note that multiplying by 100% is the same as multiplying by 1—the symbol % represents $\frac{1}{100}$, so $100\% = 100\left(\frac{1}{100}\right) = 1$. So when multiplying by 100%, the value of what we're multiplying doesn't change. Therefore, when multiplying a fraction or decimal by 100%, we're going to have a percent symbol, but the value of that fraction or decimal will not change.

In this question, you converted $\frac{16}{25}$ to a percent:

$\frac{16}{25} = \frac{16}{25} \times 1 = \frac{16}{25} \times \left[(100)\left(\frac{1}{100}\right)\right] = \frac{16}{25} \times 100\% = 16 \times 4\% = 64\%$.

11. A

The number of gallons the barrel contains when it is $\frac{3}{5}$ full is $\frac{3}{5} \times 75 = 3 \times 15 = 45$.

12. D

Subtracting a from both sides of the original equation $13 + a = 25 + b$ yields $13 = 25 + b - a$. Subtracting 25 from both sides then yields $-12 = b - a$. Thus, $b - a = -12$.

13. A

The number of kilograms in one pound is $\frac{1}{2.2}$, or $\frac{10}{22}$. This can be reduced to $\frac{5}{11}$.

14. C

Since the discount from the regular price is 20%, the sale price is 100% − 20% = 80% of the regular price. Let's convert 80% to a decimal. To convert a percent to a decimal or fraction, divide the percent by 100%:

$80\% = \frac{80\%}{100\%} = \frac{80}{100} = \frac{8}{10} = 0.8$. So the sale price is 0.8 × $118, or $94.40. There is an 8% sales tax on the

discounted price. Let's convert 8% to a decimal:

$8\% = \frac{8\%}{100\%} = \frac{8}{100} = 0.08$. Brad would pay 1.08 × $94.40 = $101.952, which to the nearest hundredth of a dollar is $101.95. (A hundredth of a dollar is a penny.)

15. C

With a ratio of 3:5, the total number of students in the group must be a multiple of 3 + 5, that is, the total number of students in the group must be a multiple of 8. Only choice (C), 152, is a multiple of 8: 152 = 19 × 8.

16. C

Since 48 of the seats were occupied, 60 − 48 = 12 seats were not occupied. The fraction of the seats that were not occupied is $\frac{12}{60}$, which can be reduced to $\frac{1}{5}$. Let's convert $\frac{1}{5}$ to a percent. To convert a fraction or decimal to a percent, multiply that fraction or decimal by 100%:

$\frac{1}{5} = \frac{1}{5} \times 100\% = 20\%$.

17. B

The delivery service charge would be:

$(\$25.00 \text{ per pound}) \times \left(\frac{4}{5} \text{ pound}\right) = (\$5.00)(4) = \$20.00$.

There is an additional 8% sales tax. Let's convert 8% to a decimal. To convert a percent to a decimal or fraction, divide the percent by 100%: $8\% = \frac{8\%}{100\%} = \frac{8}{100} = 0.08$. Therefore, the cost of delivering this item is:

$$(\$20.00) + (0.08 \times \$20.00) = (1 + 0.08) \times \$20.00$$
$$= 1.08 \times \$20.00 = \$21.60.$$

Science

1. D

Bone generates blood cells (in the marrow), protects organs from exterior force, and serves as a foundation for muscles and tendons, allowing for movement.

2. C

The medulla oblongata controls involuntary functions such as breathing.

3. A

The two main functions of oxytocin are increasing uterine contractions during childbirth and regulating lactation.

4. **C**

The blood type "O" is considered the "universal donor."

5. **C**

Insulin is a hormone produced in the pancreas that regulates blood glucose.

6. **A**

Ligaments connect bones to bones (or cartilage), while tendons connect muscles to bones.

7. **D**

Rods and cones are found in the retina of the eye.

8. **B**

Skeletal muscles are under voluntary control, while cardiac and smooth muscles are involuntary.

9. **C**

Most nutrients are absorbed in the small intestine.

10. **A**

Red blood cells in adult humans have no nucleus, allowing space to carry oxygen molecules throughout the body.

11. **D**

Insulin causes the liver to convert glucose into glycogen in a process known as glycogenesis.

12. **A**

Saliva contains an enzyme—amylase—that can break down some starches to sugars.

13. **D**

Progesterone causes the uterine lining to thicken in anticipation of a fertilized egg.

14. **D**

Dendrites transmit impulses toward the cell body, while axons transmit impulses away from the cell body.

Nursing School Entrance Exams
Practice Test Three, HESI
Answer Sheet

Reading Comprehension

1. Ⓐ Ⓑ Ⓒ Ⓓ   4. Ⓐ Ⓑ Ⓒ Ⓓ   7. Ⓐ Ⓑ Ⓒ Ⓓ   10. Ⓐ Ⓑ Ⓒ Ⓓ

2. Ⓐ Ⓑ Ⓒ Ⓓ   5. Ⓐ Ⓑ Ⓒ Ⓓ   8. Ⓐ Ⓑ Ⓒ Ⓓ

3. Ⓐ Ⓑ Ⓒ Ⓓ   6. Ⓐ Ⓑ Ⓒ Ⓓ   9. Ⓐ Ⓑ Ⓒ Ⓓ

Vocabulary

1. Ⓐ Ⓑ Ⓒ Ⓓ   4. Ⓐ Ⓑ Ⓒ Ⓓ   7. Ⓐ Ⓑ Ⓒ Ⓓ   10. Ⓐ Ⓑ Ⓒ Ⓓ

2. Ⓐ Ⓑ Ⓒ Ⓓ   5. Ⓐ Ⓑ Ⓒ Ⓓ   8. Ⓐ Ⓑ Ⓒ Ⓓ

3. Ⓐ Ⓑ Ⓒ Ⓓ   6. Ⓐ Ⓑ Ⓒ Ⓓ   9. Ⓐ Ⓑ Ⓒ Ⓓ

Grammar

1. Ⓐ Ⓑ Ⓒ Ⓓ   4. Ⓐ Ⓑ Ⓒ Ⓓ   7. Ⓐ Ⓑ Ⓒ Ⓓ   10. Ⓐ Ⓑ Ⓒ Ⓓ

2. Ⓐ Ⓑ Ⓒ Ⓓ   5. Ⓐ Ⓑ Ⓒ Ⓓ   8. Ⓐ Ⓑ Ⓒ Ⓓ

3. Ⓐ Ⓑ Ⓒ Ⓓ   6. Ⓐ Ⓑ Ⓒ Ⓓ   9. Ⓐ Ⓑ Ⓒ Ⓓ

Mathematics

1. Ⓐ Ⓑ Ⓒ Ⓓ   4. Ⓐ Ⓑ Ⓒ Ⓓ   7. Ⓐ Ⓑ Ⓒ Ⓓ   10. Ⓐ Ⓑ Ⓒ Ⓓ

2. Ⓐ Ⓑ Ⓒ Ⓓ   5. Ⓐ Ⓑ Ⓒ Ⓓ   8. Ⓐ Ⓑ Ⓒ Ⓓ

3. Ⓐ Ⓑ Ⓒ Ⓓ   6. Ⓐ Ⓑ Ⓒ Ⓓ   9. Ⓐ Ⓑ Ⓒ Ⓓ

Biology

1. Ⓐ Ⓑ Ⓒ Ⓓ   3. Ⓐ Ⓑ Ⓒ Ⓓ   5. Ⓐ Ⓑ Ⓒ Ⓓ

2. Ⓐ Ⓑ Ⓒ Ⓓ   4. Ⓐ Ⓑ Ⓒ Ⓓ

KAPLAN

Chemistry

1. Ⓐ Ⓑ Ⓒ Ⓓ   3. Ⓐ Ⓑ Ⓒ Ⓓ   5. Ⓐ Ⓑ Ⓒ Ⓓ

2. Ⓐ Ⓑ Ⓒ Ⓓ   4. Ⓐ Ⓑ Ⓒ Ⓓ

Anatomy and Physiology

1. Ⓐ Ⓑ Ⓒ Ⓓ   3. Ⓐ Ⓑ Ⓒ Ⓓ   5. Ⓐ Ⓑ Ⓒ Ⓓ

2. Ⓐ Ⓑ Ⓒ Ⓓ   4. Ⓐ Ⓑ Ⓒ Ⓓ

Physics

1. Ⓐ Ⓑ Ⓒ Ⓓ   3. Ⓐ Ⓑ Ⓒ Ⓓ   5. Ⓐ Ⓑ Ⓒ Ⓓ

2. Ⓐ Ⓑ Ⓒ Ⓓ   4. Ⓐ Ⓑ Ⓒ Ⓓ

Practice Test Three, HESI

READING COMPREHENSION

Questions 1−10 are based on the following passage, which was written in 1992 by France Bequette, a writer who specializes in environmental issues.

The ozone layer, the fragile layer of gas surrounding our planet between 7 and 30 miles above the Earth's surface, is being rapidly depleted. Seasonally occurring holes have appeared in it over the Poles and, recently, over densely populated temperate regions of the northern hemisphere. The threat is serious because the ozone layer protects the Earth from the sun's ultraviolet radiation, which is harmful to all living organisms.

Even though the layer is many miles thick, the atmosphere in it is tenuous and the total amount of ozone, compared with other atmospheric gases, is small. Ozone is highly reactive to chlorine, hydrogen, and nitrogen. Of these, chlorine is the most dangerous since it is very stable and long-lived. When chlorine compounds reach the stratosphere, they bond with and destroy ozone molecules, with consequent repercussions for life on Earth.

In 1958, researchers began noticing seasonal variations in the ozone layer above the South Pole. Between June and October the ozone content steadily fell, followed by a sudden increase in November. These fluctuations appeared to result from the natural effects of wind and temperature. But while the low October levels remained constant until 1979, the total ozone content over the Pole was steadily diminishing. In 1985, public opinion was finally roused by reports of a "hole" in the layer.

The culprits responsible for the hole were identified as compounds known as chlorofluorocarbons, or CFCs. CFCs are compounds of chlorine and fluorine. Nonflammable, nontoxic, and noncorrosive, they have been widely used in industry since the 1950s, mostly as refrigerants and propellants and in making plastic foam and insulation.

In 1989 CFCs represented a sizeable market valued at over $1.5 billion and a labor force of 1.6 million. But with CFCs implicated in ozone depletion, the question arose as to whether we were willing to risk an increase in cases of skin cancer, eye ailments, even a lowering of the human immune defense system—all effects of further loss of the ozone layer. And not only humans would suffer. So would plant life. Phytoplankton, the first link in the ocean food chain and vital to the survival of most marine species, would not be able to survive near the ocean surface, which is where these organisms grow.

In 1990, 70 countries agreed to stop producing CFCs by the year 2000. In late 1991, however, scientists noticed a depletion of the ozone layer over the Arctic. In 1992 it was announced that the layer was depleting faster than expected and that it was also declining over the northern hemisphere. Scientists believe that natural events are making the problem worse. The Pinatubo volcano in the Philippines, which erupted in June 1991, released 12 million tons of damaging volcanic gases into the atmosphere.

Even if the whole world agreed today to stop all production and use of CFCs, this would not solve the problem. A single chlorine molecule can destroy 10,000−100,000 molecules of ozone. Furthermore, CFCs have a lifespan of 75−400 years and they take ten years to reach the ozone layer. In other words,

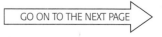

GO ON TO THE NEXT PAGE

KAPLAN

what we are experiencing today results from CFCs emitted ten years ago. Researchers are working hard to find substitute products. Some are too dangerous because they are highly flammable; others may prove to be toxic and to contribute to the greenhouse effect—to the process of global warming. Nevertheless, even if here is no denying that the atmosphere is in a state of disturbance, nobody can say that the situation will not improve, either in the short or the long term, especially if we ourselves lend a hand.

1. Which is the main idea of the second paragraph?

   (A) The ozone layer is fragile and needs protection.
   (B) Ozone is highly reactive to chlorine, hydrogen, and nitrogen.
   (C) Chlorine compounds pose a significant risk to the ozone layer.
   (D) Chlorine is stable and long-lived.

2. Which is the meaning of the word *repercussions* as used in the second paragraph?

   (A) Conclusions.
   (B) Effects.
   (C) Injuries.
   (D) Questions.

3. Which information is not given as a detail in the passage?

   (A) CFCs take ten years to reach the ozone layer.
   (B) Phytoplankton live near the surface of the ocean.
   (C) Loss of the ozone layer could lead to an increase in skin cancer rates.
   (D) CFCs were phased out as a result of the Montreal Protocol.

4. Which answer option is the best summary of the passage?

   (A) The ozone layer is located between 7 and 30 miles above the surface of the Earth, and it is in danger as a consequence of global warming.
   (B) Depletion of the ozone layer can lead to higher rates of skin cancer and widespread loss of ocean life, and banning CFCs will help solve this problem.
   (C) The ozone layer is at risk of significant depletion due to the presence of CFCs in the atmosphere, even if further CFC use were to stop completely. However, humans can improve the situation if they rise to the challenge.
   (D) CFCs are chemical compounds widely used in refrigerants and propellants. The compounds are dangerous to the ozone layer but represent more than $1.5 billion in revenue to plastics and chemical companies.

5. Why does the author mention phytoplankton in the fifth paragraph?

   (A) To show that a depleted ozone layer affects more than just humans.
   (B) To show how fragile ocean life can be.
   (C) To compare the value of marine species to the value of CFCs.
   (D) To explain where much of the planet's photosynthesis occurs.

6. Which is the author's primary purpose in writing this piece?

   (A) To convince readers to stop using CFCs.
   (B) To inform readers about the dangers of CFCs.
   (C) To argue that the planet is warming due to a depleted ozone layer.
   (D) To explain the nature of the ozone layer.

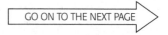
GO ON TO THE NEXT PAGE

7. Which statement is an opinion?

   (A) The ozone layer has shown steady depletion for several decades.

   (B) Chlorine-based compounds can be especially dangerous to the ozone layer because of chlorine's stability and longevity.

   (C) CFCs represented more than $1.5 billion in market value in 1989.

   (D) CFCs pose a greater long-term threat to human well-being than any other risk factor.

8. Which detail supports the idea that CFCs pose a long-term threat to the ozone layer?

   (A) A single chlorine molecule can destroy 10,000–100,000 ozone molecules.

   (B) CFCs have been in wide use since the 1950s.

   (C) CFCs have a lifespan of 75–400 years and take ten years to reach the ozone layer.

   (D) The ozone layer protects the Earth from the sun's ultraviolet radiation.

9. Why does the author mention the Arctic in the sixth paragraph?

   (A) To illustrate how ozone depletion has worsened and spread.

   (B) To provide a counterargument to the idea that ozone depletion is a global problem.

   (C) To show that natural phenomena can also play a role in ozone depletion.

   (D) To explain how weather patterns affect the ozone layer.

10. Which is the meaning of the word *fluctuations* as used in the second paragraph?

    (A) Damages.

    (B) Depletions.

    (C) Variations.

    (D) Uncertainties.

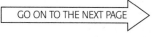

GO ON TO THE NEXT PAGE

KAPLAN

VOCABULARY

1. Select the meaning of the underlined word in the following sentence.

   Through simple diffusion, oxygen can <u>permeate</u> the cell membrane.

   (A) Pass through.
   (B) Dissolve.
   (C) Damage.
   (D) Reinforce.

2. Select the meaning of the underlined word in the following sentence.

   After tests were completed, he was told that the growth on his leg was <u>benign</u>.

   (A) Spreading.
   (B) Cancerous.
   (C) Harmless.
   (D) Common.

3. Which is the best definition of the word *vascular*?

   (A) Pertaining to breathing.
   (B) Pertaining to blood vessels.
   (C) Pertaining to dementia.
   (D) Pertaining to the heart.

4. Select the meaning of the underlined word in the following sentence.

   After noting that the patient's mood was <u>labile</u>, the nurse discovered that he had stopped taking his prescribed antipsychotic medication.

   (A) Elevated.
   (B) Depressed.
   (C) Hostile.
   (D) Unstable.

5. Which word meaning "provided evidence against" best fits in the sentence?

   The patient's continued dizziness and slurred speech _____ his discharge from the hospital.

   (A) Conducted.
   (B) Contraindicated.
   (C) Contracted.
   (D) Constricted.

6. Select the meaning of the underlined word in the following sentence.

   Although the victim was struck by a cyclist at high speed, she was <u>ambulatory</u> when she arrived at the emergency room.

   (A) Able to walk.
   (B) Able to be carried.
   (C) Losing consciousness.
   (D) Transported by a vehicle.

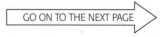
GO ON TO THE NEXT PAGE

7. Which is the best definition of the word *transdermal*?

   (A) Through or by way of the skin.

   (B) Through or by way of the mouth.

   (C) Through or by way of the blood.

   (D) Through or by way of the extremities.

8. Which word meaning "sample" best fits in the sentence?

   The nurse took the patient's tissue _____ to the lab for testing.

   (A) Necropsy.

   (B) Specimen.

   (C) Example.

   (D) Spectrum.

9. Which is the best definition of the word *therapeutic*?

   (A) Toxic.

   (B) Prescribed.

   (C) Additional.

   (D) Curative.

10. Which word meaning "open" best fits in the following sentence?

    The nurse had to ensure that the victim maintained a/an _____ airway during the procedure.

    (A) Occluded.

    (B) Constricted.

    (C) Patent.

    (D) Latent.

GO ON TO THE NEXT PAGE

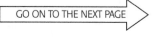

GRAMMAR

1. Which sentence is grammatically correct?

   (A) There are not nearly enough sterile needles to administer the vaccination to everyone.

   (B) Despite the doctor's warning, he was not ready for the strong affects of the medication.

   (C) Her and me both took patients up to Radiology at around the same time.

   (D) The couple claimed that the unattended backpack turned in to the reception desk was their's.

2. Select the best words for the blanks in the following sentence.

   Anyone who _____ drive a manual transmission vehicle _____ also be able to drive an automatic transmission vehicle.

   (A) Shall; shall not.

   (B) Might; must not.

   (C) Should; can.

   (D) Can; should.

3. Which word is used incorrectly in this sentence?

   The difference among ibuprofen and aspirin is significant, particularly with regard to side effects.

   (A) Difference.

   (B) Among.

   (C) Is.

   (D) With.

4. Which sentence is grammatically incorrect?

   (A) The gurney which was in the hallway belonged to the ambulance service, while the gurney in the drop-off bay belonged to the hospital.

   (B) There was a large amount of paperwork still incomplete when he was admitted.

   (C) Hannah thought she did badly on her test, but she ended up scoring near the top of her class.

   (D) The nurse read off the list of potential side effects to the blind patient.

5. Which word from the following sentence is an adverb?

   Gerry often found himself checking in with other night-shift staff during his off-hours.

   (A) Often.

   (B) In.

   (C) Other.

   (D) During.

6. Which word is used incorrectly in this sentence?

   The patients in the urgent care facility had been waiting for hours and was growing impatient.

   (A) Facility.

   (B) Had.

   (C) Waiting.

   (D) Was.

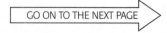
GO ON TO THE NEXT PAGE

7. Which word from the following sentence is a conjunction?

   The nurse could not find an available examination room, so he conducted the screening in an empty office.

   (A) Could.
   (B) Available.
   (C) So.
   (D) In.

8. Which sentence contains sexist language?

   (A) The man helped the elderly woman complete her medical history forms.
   (B) If a fireman wants to stand a good chance of survival, he needs to have properly maintained safety equipment.
   (C) The server presented the lunch bill to Harvey, even though Sandra was the manager of the department.
   (D) If a person is interested in becoming a medical examiner, he or she should research the amount of schooling required for such a job.

9. Select the best word for the blank in the following sentence.

   Ms. Parker was the patient _____ medication was incorrectly dosed.

   (A) Who.
   (B) Whom.
   (C) Who's.
   (D) Whose.

10. Which word from the following sentence is a preposition?

    The third-shift crew all arrived very late, but within ten minutes of each other.

    (A) All.
    (B) Very.
    (C) Within.
    (D) Each.

GO ON TO THE NEXT PAGE

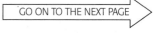

KAPLAN

MATHEMATICS

1. The number 16 is 25% of which number?

    (A) 4

    (B) 48

    (C) 64

    (D) 96

2. Which of the following is $\frac{3}{8}$ written as a percent?

    (A) 32%

    (B) 37.5%

    (C) 42.5%

    (D) 45%

3. Convert the following 12-hour clock time to military time: 7:41:23 PM

    (A) 07:41:23 hours

    (B) 17:41:23 hours

    (C) 19:41:23 hours

    (D) 20:41:23 hours

4. Solve for x: $-2x + 3 = x - 15$

    (A) −6

    (B) −3

    (C) 3

    (D) 6

5. Which of the following ratios accurately expresses $\frac{9}{24}$?

    (A) 3:8

    (B) 5:9

    (C) 6:18

    (D) 9:33

6. Which of the following is 0.75 expressed as a fraction?

    (A) $\frac{4}{5}$

    (B) $\frac{7}{9}$

    (C) $\frac{9}{12}$

    (D) $\frac{8}{11}$

7. What is $\frac{3}{5} \div \frac{1}{8}$?

    (A) $\frac{3}{20}$

    (B) $\frac{3}{40}$

    (C) $\frac{5}{24}$

    (D) $\frac{24}{5}$

8. What is $5\frac{1}{8} - 3\frac{1}{6}$?

    (A) $2\frac{1}{12}$

    (B) $1\frac{23}{24}$

    (C) $8\frac{7}{24}$

    (D) $1\frac{1}{4}$

9. Solve for x: $5x - 7 = x + 5$

    (A) −4

    (B) 2

    (C) 3

    (D) 12

10. If $x = 5$, $y = 8$, and $z = 10$, what is the value of the expression $x^2 + 3(y - z)$?

    (A) 19

    (B) 31

    (C) 39

    (D) 79

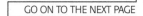
GO ON TO THE NEXT PAGE

BIOLOGY

1. Which of these is a distinguishing characteristic of eukaryotic cells?

    (A) The ability to reproduce.

    (B) A defined, membrane-enclosed nucleus.

    (C) An outer cell membrane.

    (D) The presence of ribosomes for protein production.

2. Which is the best definition of *mitosis*?

    (A) The simplest form of asexual reproduction.

    (B) A five-stage process of cell division.

    (C) A process that mainly occurs in mammals.

    (D) The process used for sex cell production.

3. Which answer option is not one of the four nitrogenous bases of DNA?

    (A) Adenine.

    (B) Cholosyne.

    (C) Guanine.

    (D) Thymine.

4. In the scientific method, which step comes first?

    (A) Conclusion.

    (B) Experiment.

    (C) Hypothesis.

    (D) Observation.

5. Which is the most inclusive level of classification?

    (A) Class.

    (B) Family.

    (C) Phylum.

    (D) Species.

GO ON TO THE NEXT PAGE

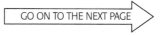

CHEMISTRY

1. Which statement about bases is true?

   (A) They are electron donors.

   (B) They are electron acceptors.

   (C) They are proton donors.

   (D) They are proton acceptors.

2. Which is the process by which the liver can create glucose from proteins and fats?

   (A) Glycolysis.

   (B) Gluconeogenesis.

   (C) Double replacement.

   (D) Oxidative phosphorylation.

3. Which is the simplest form of a carbohydrate?

   (A) Disaccharide.

   (B) Monosaccharide.

   (C) Oligosaccharide.

   (D) Polysaccharide.

4. To which other DNA base is adenine always bound?

   (A) Cytosine.

   (B) Deoxyribose.

   (C) Guanine.

   (D) Thymine.

5. Which statement about redox reactions is true?

   (A) Oxidation involves the loss of electrons, while reduction involves the gain of electrons.

   (B) Oxidation involves the gain of electrons, while reduction involves the loss of electrons.

   (C) A substance that is oxidized gains a positive charge.

   (D) An element in its natural state can have a positive or negative charge.

GO ON TO THE NEXT PAGE

ANATOMY AND PHYSIOLOGY

1. If a patient is described as having a distal leg fracture, where is the injury most likely to be located?

   (A) At the top of the thigh.

   (B) Along the outside of the thigh.

   (C) Near the ankle.

   (D) Near the knee.

2. Which tissue is not one of the four fundamental tissues of the human body?

   (A) Connective tissue.

   (B) Epithelial tissue.

   (C) Cardiac tissue.

   (D) Nerve tissue.

3. Which anatomical system creates blood cells and stores minerals?

   (A) Digestive system.

   (B) Endocrine system.

   (C) Muscular system.

   (D) Skeletal system.

4. Which is the outermost layer of the epidermis called?

   (A) Stratum basale.

   (B) Stratum corneum.

   (C) Stratum granulosum.

   (D) Stratum spinosum.

5. Which structure is part of the peripheral nervous system?

   (A) Cerebellum.

   (B) Optic nerve.

   (C) Spinal cord.

   (D) Vagus nerve.

GO ON TO THE NEXT PAGE

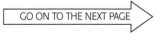

PHYSICS

1. A car travels for 15 minutes and covers a distance of 27 kilometers. Which is the average speed of the car in meters per second?

    (A) 3.0
    (B) 18
    (C) 30
    (D) 40.5

2. A skateboard is rolled down a large hill. Its initial speed is 2 m/s, and it travels down the hill for 30 seconds. The skateboard's final speed is 8 m/s. Which is the magnitude of the skateboard's acceleration in meters per second squared?

    (A) 0.2
    (B) 0.33
    (C) 1.5
    (D) 2

3. A box with a mass of 10 kg rests on a surface. The box is being pushed to the right by a force of 48N against a horizontal frictional force of 36N. Which is the magnitude of acceleration of the box in meters per second squared?

    (A) 0.12
    (B) 0.84
    (C) 1.2
    (D) 8.4

4. In waves, the maximum displacement from equilibrium is known as which of these?

    (A) Amplitude.
    (B) Crest.
    (C) Frequency.
    (D) Wavelength.

5. A circuit contains several resistors placed in series. If the circuit is wired to a 200V power supply and the current is measured at 4 amps, which is the total resistance in the circuit in ohms?

    (A) 20
    (B) 50
    (C) 100
    (D) 800

END OF TEST. STOP

KAPLAN

THE ANSWER KEY APPEARS ON THE FOLLOWING PAGE.

Practice Test Three: **Answer Key**

Reading Comprehension

1. C
2. B
3. D
4. C
5. A
6. B
7. D
8. C
9. A
10. C

Vocabulary

1. A
2. C
3. B
4. D
5. B
6. A
7. A
8. B
9. D
10. C

Grammar

1. A
2. D
3. B
4. A
5. A
6. D
7. C
8. B
9. D
10. C

Mathematics

1. C
2. B
3. C
4. D
5. A
6. C
7. D
8. B
9. C
10. A

Biology

1. B
2. B
3. B
4. D
5. C

Chemistry

1. D
2. B
3. B
4. D
5. A

Anatomy and Physiology

1. C
2. C
3. D
4. B
5. D

Physics

1. C
2. A
3. C
4. A
5. B

Answers and Explanations

Reading Comprehension

1. C

The main idea of the paragraph is to show that chlorine compounds are especially dangerous to the ozone layer. The ozone layer's fragility and need for protection (A), ozone's high reactivity to other atmospheric gases (B), and the stability and longevity of chlorine (D) all support this main idea.

2. B

The word *repercussions* is closest in meaning to "effects."

3. D

The Montreal Protocol is not mentioned in the passage.

4. C

The passage is about CFCs and their harmful effects on the atmosphere, as well as potential human efforts to reverse the damage. The first three paragraphs describe the harmful effects of CFCs, and the final four paragraphs describe the challenges in stopping their use. All the answer choices include details from the passage, but only (C) includes these "big picture" ideas that make up the most important elements of the passage.

5. A

Just before the author mentions phytoplankton, she states that "not only humans would suffer." The paragraph does not discuss the fragility of ocean life (B), the economic value of marine species (C), or the proportion of the planet's photosynthesis undertaken by phytoplankton (D).

6. B

The author does not try to persuade readers not to use CFCs (A), because these compounds are already being phased out. The author also does not present any argument regarding global warming (C). While the author does explain the nature of the ozone layer (D), the primary purpose of this essay is to describe how CFCs threaten the ozone layer.

7. D

The statements about the steady depletion of ozone (A), the particular destructiveness of chlorine-based compounds on ozone (B), and the market value of CFCs (C) can be

measured and verified as fact. By contrast, the assertion that CFCs pose a long-term threat to humans greater than any other (D) is a subjective interpretation.

8. C

Only (C) mentions the long-term nature of CFCs, which last 75–400 years. The other options relate to the destructive power of a chlorine molecule (A), the widespread use of CFCs (B), and the insulating properties of the ozone layer (D).

9. A

The sixth paragraph focuses on how the problem of ozone depletion is getting worse, and the information about the Arctic is a detail that supports the main idea of the paragraph.

10. C

The word *fluctuations* is closest in meaning to "variations."

Vocabulary

1. A

The word *permeate* means "pass through."

2. C

The word *benign* means "harmless."

3. B

The word *vascular* can technically refer to other vessels as well, but is most often used to describe blood vessels.

4. D

The word *labile* means "changing" or "unstable."

5. B

The meaning "provided evidence against" is best represented by the word *contraindicated*.

6. A

The word *ambulatory* means "able to walk."

7. A

The word *transdermal* means "through or by way of the skin."

8. B

The meaning "sample" is best represented by the word *specimen*.

9. D

The word *therapeutic* is best represented by the definition "curative."

10. C

The meaning "open" is best represented by the word *patent*.

Grammar

1. A

Choice (B) uses the incorrect word *affect*; *effect* would be correct in this context. (C) incorrectly uses the objective pronouns *Her and me* as the subject of the sentence; the subjective pronouns *She and I* are needed instead. (D) includes an unnecessary apostrophe in *theirs*.

2. D

The answer choices in this question are all modal auxiliary verbs; they work with the existing verbs in the sentence to express possibility or obligation. Reading the sentence, *can* and *should* are the auxiliary verbs that make the most logical sense; the use of "be able to drive" in the second half of the sentence indicates that *should* makes more sense there as an expression of likelihood, so (D) is correct.

3. B

The preposition *among* should be used in reference to three or more nouns. In this sentence, there are only two nouns (ibuprofen and aspirin), so the correct preposition is *between*.

4. A

The word *which* is used incorrectly; it should be replaced with the word *that*. The clause "that/which was in the hallway" is a nonrestrictive clause; it is essential to describing the gurney, distinguishing it from the other gurney in the drop-off bay. For nonrestrictive clauses, *that* should be used to introduce the clause.

5. A

Often is considered an adverb of frequency, because it describes the rate at which something occurs. The words *in* (B) and *during* (D) are prepositions; *other* (C) is used as an adjective in this sentence.

6. D

The subject of the sentence is "patients," which is a plural noun. For subject-verb agreement, the sentence requires the plural verb form *were*, not *was* (which is the singular form of the verb *to be*).

7. C

Conjunctions are used to connect clauses, as *so* does in this sentence. *Could* (A) is a verb; *available* (B) is an adjective; *in* (D) is a preposition.

8. B

The firefighter in the sentence is a hypothetical person rather than a specific person; using the male pronoun *he* in this situation is sexist, because it assumes that every firefighter who might exist is male. (A) and (C) describe behavior that might be regarded as sexist, but they do not use sexist language. (D) uses neutral language (*he or she*).

9. D

The sentence refers to medication belonging to the patient, so the possessive pronoun *whose* is correct. The word *who* (A) is a subjective pronoun; *whom* (B) is an objective pronoun; and *who's* (C) can be used as a contraction standing for the words *who is*.

10. C

The word *within* is a preposition, which is a part of speech indicating the position or relation between things. Both *all* (A) and *each* (D) are adjectives, which modify nouns; *very* (B) is an adverb, the part of speech that modifies a verb.

Mathematics

1. C

Let's call the unknown number x.

Convert 25% to a fraction by dividing the percent by 100%: $25\% = \frac{25\%}{100\%} = \frac{25}{100} = \frac{1}{4}$. Therefore, you can write the equation $16 = \frac{1}{4}x$, or $16 = \frac{x}{4}$. Multiply both sides by 4: $16 \times 4 = x$, and $64 = x$. Thus, $x = 64$.

When converting a percent to a fraction or decimal, divide the percent by 100%. The symbol % represents $\frac{1}{100}$, so $100\% = 100\left(\frac{1}{100}\right) = 1$. In other words, dividing by 100% is the same as dividing by 1; the value of what you are dividing does not change. Likewise, when dividing a percent by 100%, the % symbols will cancel out.

Here, you converted 25% to a fraction: $25\% = \frac{25\%}{100\%}$.

The symbol % means $\frac{1}{100}$, so $25\% = \frac{25\%}{100\%}$ means

$25\left(\frac{1}{100}\right) \div 100\left(\frac{1}{100}\right)$. You can cancel the factors $\frac{1}{100}$ from

$25\left(\frac{1}{100}\right)$ and $100\left(\frac{1}{100}\right)$. Therefore, $\frac{25\%}{100\%}$ equals $\frac{25}{100}$,

which can be reduced to $\frac{1}{4}$.

The key to understanding why to divide the percent by 100% when converting a percent to a fraction or decimal is to know that % means $\frac{1}{100}$.

2. B

To convert a fraction or decimal to a percent, multiply that fraction by 100%: $\frac{3}{8} = \frac{3}{8} \times 100\% = \frac{3}{2} \times 25\% = \frac{75}{2}\% = 37.5\%$.

3. C

For times between noon and midnight, you must add 12:00:00 to the 12-hour clock time. Therefore, 7:41:23 PM is equivalent to 19:41:23 hours.

4. D

Subtracting x from both sides of the equation $-2x + 3 = x - 15$ yields $-3x + 3 = -15$. Subtracting 3 from each side yields $-3x = -18$. Dividing both sides by -3 yields $x = 6$.

5. A

The ratio 9:24 is not listed as an answer choice, so reduce the fraction $\frac{9}{24}$ to the simpler fraction $\frac{3}{8}$. The fraction $\frac{3}{8}$ is equivalent to the ratio 3:8.

6. C

The decimal 0.75 is equivalent to $\frac{75}{100}$, which you can reduce to $\frac{3}{4}$. Although this is not an answer choice, one of the answer choices, $\frac{9}{12}$, can also be reduced to $\frac{3}{4}$.

7. D

To divide by a fraction, invert the fraction and then multiply: $\frac{3}{5} \div \frac{1}{8} = \frac{3}{5} \times \frac{8}{1} = \frac{3 \times 8}{5 \times 1} = \frac{24}{5}$.

8. B

Let's convert $5\frac{1}{8}$ and $3\frac{1}{6}$ to improper fractions:

$$5\frac{1}{8} = \frac{5 \times 8 + 1}{8} = \frac{40 + 1}{8} = \frac{41}{8}$$

$$3\frac{1}{6} = \frac{3 \times 6 + 1}{6} = \frac{18 + 1}{6} = \frac{19}{6}$$

Therefore, $5\frac{1}{8} - 3\frac{1}{6} = \frac{41}{8} - \frac{19}{6}$. Next, to work with $\frac{41}{8} - \frac{19}{6}$ you need a common denominator, which here is a multiple of 8 and 6.

You can find a positive multiple of 8 and 6 by starting with the smallest positive multiple of 8, which is $1 \times 8 = 8$, and then looking at the next positive multiples of 8, which are $2 \times 8, 3 \times 8, 4 \times 8, 5 \times 8, ...$, until we find a multiple of 6:

- $1 \times 8 = 8$ is not a multiple of 6.
- $2 \times 8 = 16$ is not a multiple of 6.
- $3 \times 8 = 24$ is a multiple of 6, since $24 = 4 \times 6$.

The positive multiple of 8 and 6 you found, 24, is actually the smallest positive multiple of 8 and 6.

Finally, subtract using the new common denominator: $\frac{41}{8} - \frac{19}{6} = \frac{123}{24} - \frac{76}{24} = \frac{123 - 76}{24} = \frac{47}{24} = 1\frac{23}{24}$.

9. C

Subtracting x from both sides of the equation $5x - 7 = x + 5$ yields $4x - 7 = 5$. Adding 7 to each side yields $4x = 12$. Dividing both sides by 4 yields $x = 3$.

10. A

Let's substitute the given values. If $x = 5$, $y = 8$, and $z = 10$, then $x^2 + 3(y - z) = 5^2 + 3(8 - 10)$
$$= 25 + 3(-2) = 25 - 6 = 19.$$

Biology

1. B

What distinguishes eukaryotic cells from prokaryotic cells is a defined, membrane-enclosed nucleus. Both prokaryotic and eukaryotic cells have the ability to reproduce (A), an outer membrane (C), and ribosomes (D).

2. B

Mitosis is a five-stage process of cell division that results in two daughter cells identical to the original cell. The simplest form of asexual reproduction (A) is binary fission. Mitosis occurs in mammals, but also occurs in most other plants and animals, making (C) incorrect. The process used for sex cell production (D) is meiosis.

3. B

The four nitrogenous bases of DNA are adenine (A), guanine (C), thymine (D), and cytosine (not cholosyne).

4. D

The first step of the scientific process is observation. It is followed by forming a hypothesis (C), conducting an experiment (B), and reaching a conclusion (A).

5. C

Phylum is the most inclusive level of the available answer choices offered. From most to least inclusive, the eight levels of biological classification are: domain, kingdom, phylum (C), class (A), order, family (B), genus, species (D).

Chemistry

1. D

Bases are proton acceptors, while acids are proton donors.

2. B

Gluconeogenesis is the process by which the liver creates glucose from proteins and fats. Glycolysis (A) is the process of breaking down glucose. Double replacement (C) occurs when two ionic compounds switch the elements they are bound to as part of a chemical reaction, creating two new ionic compounds. Oxidative phosphorylation (D) is a step in glycolysis during which pyruvate is broken down to create ATP, water, and carbon dioxide.

3. B

Although disaccharides (A), oligosaccharides (C), and polysaccharides (D) are also carbohydrates, monosaccharides are the simplest form of carbohydrate.

4. D

In DNA, adenine and thymine (D) are always bound to each other, while cytosine (A) is always bound to guanine (C). Deoxyribose (B) is a monosaccharide that is integral to the structure of DNA molecules.

5. A

A redox reaction is one in which electrons are transferred between elements. Oxidation always involves electron loss, while reduction always involves electron gain. A substance that is oxidized actually becomes more negatively charged. Elements in their natural state are electrically neutral, meaning the number of protons and electrons is equal.

Anatomy and Physiology

1. C

"Distal" means away from the point of attachment of a limb, so a distal leg fracture would be located near the ankle (C), not at the top of the thigh (A), outside the thigh (B), or near the knee (D).

2. C

Cardiac tissue (C) is not one of the four fundamental tissues. The four fundamental tissues are connective tissue (A), epithelial tissue (B), nerve tissue (D), and muscle tissue.

3. D

The skeletal system performs a wide variety of functions, including production of blood cells (in marrow) and the storage of minerals like calcium (in bone).

4. B

The stratum corneum is the outermost layer of the epidermis, followed by the stratum lucidum, stratum granulosum (C), stratum spinosum (D), and stratum basale (A).

5. D

The vagus nerve is part of the peripheral nervous system, while the cerebellum (A), optic nerve (B), and spinal cord (C) are considered part of the central nervous system.

Physics

1. C

Average speed is equal to total distance divided by total time. The average speed, in meters per second, is required, so the given units in the question must be converted:

15 minutes = (15 minutes) × (60 seconds/minute) = 900 seconds

27 kilometers = (27 kilometers) × (1,000 meters/kilometer) = 27,000 meters

Therefore, the average speed is 27,000 meters ÷ 900 seconds = 270 meters ÷ 9 seconds = 30 meters per second.

2. A

Acceleration is calculated as the change in velocity divided by the change in time. The change in velocity is (8 meters per second) − (2 meters per second) = 6 meters per second. The change in time is (30 seconds) − (0 seconds) = 30 seconds. Then the acceleration is the change in speed divided by the change in time, which is (6 meters per second) ÷ (30 seconds) = 0.2 meters per second squared.

3. C

Acceleration is calculated as the net force on an object divided by the object's mass. The net force on the box is 48 N − 36 N = 12 N. The object's mass is 10 kg. So the acceleration is $\frac{12\ N}{10\ kg}$ = (12 kg-m/s²)/(10 kg) = 1.2 m/s².

The acceleration is 1.2 meters per second squared.

4. A

The maximum displacement from equilibrium in a wave is known as its amplitude. The crest (B) is the maximum displacement in one direction; frequency (C) refers to the number of crests passing a given point within a specific time frame; and wavelength (D) refers to the distance between crests.

5. B

Resistance (in ohms) is calculated as the voltage divided by the current (in amperes, or amps). In this problem, 200 volts divided by 4 amps = 50 ohms.

Nursing School Entrance Exams
Practice Test Four, HESI
Answer Sheet

Reading Comprehension

1. (A) (B) (C) (D)   4. (A) (B) (C) (D)   7. (A) (B) (C) (D)   10. (A) (B) (C) (D)

2. (A) (B) (C) (D)   5. (A) (B) (C) (D)   8. (A) (B) (C) (D)

3. (A) (B) (C) (D)   6. (A) (B) (C) (D)   9. (A) (B) (C) (D)

Vocabulary

1. (A) (B) (C) (D)   4. (A) (B) (C) (D)   7. (A) (B) (C) (D)   10. (A) (B) (C) (D)

2. (A) (B) (C) (D)   5. (A) (B) (C) (D)   8. (A) (B) (C) (D)

3. (A) (B) (C) (D)   6. (A) (B) (C) (D)   9. (A) (B) (C) (D)

Grammar

1. (A) (B) (C) (D)   4. (A) (B) (C) (D)   7. (A) (B) (C) (D)   10. (A) (B) (C) (D)

2. (A) (B) (C) (D)   5. (A) (B) (C) (D)   8. (A) (B) (C) (D)

3. (A) (B) (C) (D)   6. (A) (B) (C) (D)   9. (A) (B) (C) (D)

Mathematics

1. (A) (B) (C) (D)   4. (A) (B) (C) (D)   7. (A) (B) (C) (D)   10. (A) (B) (C) (D)

2. (A) (B) (C) (D)   5. (A) (B) (C) (D)   8. (A) (B) (C) (D)

3. (A) (B) (C) (D)   6. (A) (B) (C) (D)   9. (A) (B) (C) (D)

Biology

1. (A) (B) (C) (D)   3. (A) (B) (C) (D)   5. (A) (B) (C) (D)

2. (A) (B) (C) (D)   4. (A) (B) (C) (D)

KAPLAN

Chemistry

1. Ⓐ Ⓑ Ⓒ Ⓓ   3. Ⓐ Ⓑ Ⓒ Ⓓ   5. Ⓐ Ⓑ Ⓒ Ⓓ

2. Ⓐ Ⓑ Ⓒ Ⓓ   4. Ⓐ Ⓑ Ⓒ Ⓓ

Anatomy and Physiology

1. Ⓐ Ⓑ Ⓒ Ⓓ   3. Ⓐ Ⓑ Ⓒ Ⓓ   5. Ⓐ Ⓑ Ⓒ Ⓓ

2. Ⓐ Ⓑ Ⓒ Ⓓ   4. Ⓐ Ⓑ Ⓒ Ⓓ

Physics

1. Ⓐ Ⓑ Ⓒ Ⓓ   3. Ⓐ Ⓑ Ⓒ Ⓓ   5. Ⓐ Ⓑ Ⓒ Ⓓ

2. Ⓐ Ⓑ Ⓒ Ⓓ   4. Ⓐ Ⓑ Ⓒ Ⓓ

Practice Test Four, HESI

READING COMPREHENSION

Questions 1–10 are based on the following passage.

In a world where modern technology can render certain jobs—such as switchboard operator—obsolete, some economic scholars have looked at ways to ensure that such workers are not left behind. One idea that has enjoyed increasing popularity, and has also generated controversy, is the idea of a universal basic income. A universal basic income is a guaranteed base dividend, paid to every eligible citizen, regardless of whether or not they hold a job.

The idea of a universal basic income dates back at least until the eighteenth century. In 1796, British reformist Thomas Spence called for all profits from lands and rent to be redistributed among "all the living souls in the parish," calling such redistribution "the imprescriptible right of every human being in civilized society." At the same time in the United States, activist Thomas Paine called for landowners to be taxed as a way of providing funds for those with no land. Both ideas share some similarity with modern ideas of social welfare programs. In the early twentieth century, British reformers like Clifford Douglas and Dennis Milner renewed calls for a basic income.

Supporters of a universal basic income argue that it could alleviate many of the problems of the poorest citizens, and in so doing, benefit all citizens. For example, studies have shown that low-income citizens are, by necessity, more likely to spend any money they receive on goods and services, such as food, clothing, or rent. This type of spending contributes directly to economic growth. Wealthier citizens, by contrast, spend a comparatively smaller amount of their money on goods and services. Advocates also point to the simplicity of a universal basic income, noting that it is more efficient and transparent than the patchwork of means-tested social welfare programs that currently exist in many countries. In addition, a guaranteed basic income would eliminate the stigmatization of those receiving welfare benefits and services.

Critics of a universal basic income argue against the notion from several different angles. Some argue that such an income would cause citizens to become "lazy," though studies of pilot programs have not supported this idea. Critics also argue that giving out free money to poor people would simply allow them to waste it on things like alcohol or drugs—again, without supporting evidence from pilot program studies. In addition, if a single country were to approve a basic universal income, it might become flooded with immigrants hoping to take advantage of the new system. From an economic perspective, some critics have expressed concern that giving away free money would simply increase inflation, so that the price of goods would rise to absorb the additional money being supplied to citizens. In the United States, the idea of a basic income has been characterized as "anti-capitalist" and an affront to the strong work ethic that defines the nation.

Although the efficacy of a universal basic income remains open to debate, the debate itself is gaining more attention around the world. In the United States, where wealth inequality is at its highest level since the 1920s, some lawmakers have voiced their support for the idea despite its controversial nature. Some high-profile technology executives have predicted that the issue will become more urgent as automation technology takes the place of more and more human workers. In 2017, Finland began a two-year trial program where it gave 2,000 unemployed people a basic income. When the results from Finland are finally published in 2019, perhaps the critics will discover that a universal basic income is not something to fear, but something to embrace.

GO ON TO THE NEXT PAGE

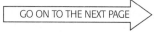

KAPLAN

1. Which is the main idea of the second paragraph?

   (A) The earliest support for a universal basic income came from British reformists.

   (B) The idea of a universal basic income has been around for over 200 years.

   (C) Thomas Paine brought the idea of a universal basic income to the United States.

   (D) Although some fringe intellectuals have supported a universal basic income, the idea has never enjoyed mainstream support.

2. Which is the meaning of the word *obsolete* as used in the second paragraph?

   (A) Ignored.

   (B) Without success.

   (C) No longer needed.

   (D) Unable to prepare.

3. Which answer option is not listed as a detail in the passage?

   (A) Spending on goods and services directly contributes to economic growth.

   (B) Thomas Spence wrote about universal basic income in 1796.

   (C) Clifford Douglas and Dennis Milner were twentieth-century British reformers.

   (D) Finland provided nearly $700 per month to citizens in its basic income trial.

4. Which answer option represents the best summary of the passage?

   (A) A universal basic income is money given to all citizens without any conditions on its use, and the idea has been around for centuries.

   (B) The arguments in favor of a universal basic income include: a more streamlined and efficient way to provide support to citizens; greater economic growth through spending on goods and services; and less stigmatization of the poor.

   (C) The idea of a universal basic income, or a sum of money given without conditions to all citizens, remains controversial but could play an important part in future discussions about employment in an increasingly automated workforce.

   (D) A universal basic income, given out to every citizen even if they do not work, would allow people to become lazy, spend government-provided money on indulgences like alcohol, and erode the longstanding value of a work ethic.

5. Why does the author mention wealthier citizens in the third paragraph?

   (A) To illustrate how lower-income citizens can become wealthy.

   (B) To contrast their spending with the spending of lower-income citizens.

   (C) To explain how wealth transfers between individuals.

   (D) To argue that wealthy people do not deserve to keep their money.

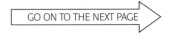

6. Which is the author's primary purpose in writing this piece?

   (A) To examine the pros, cons, and possible future impact of a universal basic income.

   (B) To provide a comprehensive definition of universal basic income for the reader.

   (C) To argue that eighteenth-century activists should be given credit for coming up with the idea of a universal basic income.

   (D) To entertain the reader with anecdotes about how universal basic income has been viewed through the years.

7. Which answer option is an opinion?

   (A) The idea of a universal basic income dates back until at least the eighteenth century.

   (B) Studies have shown that low-income citizens are, by necessity, more likely to spend any money they receive on goods and services, such as food, clothing, or rent.

   (C) In the United States, where wealth inequality is at its highest level since the 1920s, some lawmakers have voiced their support for the idea despite its controversial nature.

   (D) When the results from Finland are finally published in 2019, perhaps the critics will discover that a universal basic income is not something to fear, but something to embrace.

8. Which detail supports the idea that the concept of universal basic income is becoming more widely accepted?

   (A) Finland launched a two-year trial in 2017 to gauge the effects of a universal basic income.

   (B) Inequality in the United States has reached its highest levels since the 1920s.

   (C) British reformers in the early twentieth century pushed for a basic income.

   (D) Automation technology threatens the jobs of an unknown percentage of the workforce.

9. Based on the final sentence of the passage, which statement can be inferred about the author's views on universal basic income?

   (A) The author thinks a universal basic income will not be necessary due to increasing automation technology.

   (B) The author thinks that the results from the Finland trial will not offer conclusive support for either side of the issue.

   (C) The author supports a universal basic income.

   (D) The author does not support a universal basic income.

10. Which is the meaning of the word *efficacy* as used in the fifth paragraph?

   (A) Likelihood.

   (B) Future.

   (C) Concept.

   (D) Effectiveness.

GO ON TO THE NEXT PAGE

VOCABULARY

1. Select the meaning of the underlined word in the sentence.

    Tests revealed that the patient's hearing was severely <u>impaired</u> by the accident.

    (A) Diminished.
    (B) Affected.
    (C) Sensitized.
    (D) Made irregular.

2. Select the meaning of the underlined word in the sentence.

    The nurse discovered an <u>occlusion</u> in the patient's central venous catheter.

    (A) Toxin.
    (B) Blockage.
    (C) Defect.
    (D) Hole.

3. Which is the best definition of the word *abrupt*?

    (A) Sudden.
    (B) Terminal.
    (C) Unpredictable.
    (D) Explosive.

4. Select the meaning of the underlined word in the sentence.

    The quarterly report on communicable diseases was surprisingly <u>succinct</u> and easy to understand.

    (A) Entertaining.
    (B) Cursory.
    (C) Comprehensive.
    (D) Concise.

5. Which word meaning "took into the body" best fits in the sentence?

    The patient with stomach pain reported that he had _____ approximately 50 paper clips.

    (A) Egested.
    (B) Congested.
    (C) Ingested.
    (D) Digested.

6. Select the meaning of the underlined word in the sentence.

    The patient's electrolyte imbalance suggested that he was suffering from <u>acute</u> kidney injury.

    (A) Early.
    (B) Severe.
    (C) Sensitive.
    (D) Likely.

7. Which is the best definition of the word *precipitous*?

    (A) Covered in moisture.
    (B) Without evidence.
    (C) Extremely steep.
    (D) Very high.

8. Which word meaning "cause of a disease" best fits in the sentence?

    By studying the circumstances surrounding each patient's infection, the doctor was able to theorize about the _____ of the outbreak.

    (A) Histology.
    (B) Logy.
    (C) Chronology.
    (D) Etiology.

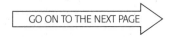
GO ON TO THE NEXT PAGE

9. Which is the best definition of the word *assent*?

    (A) Climb.

    (B) Delivery.

    (C) Agreement.

    (D) Denial.

10. Which word meaning "omnipresent" best fits in the sentence?

    One of the biggest technological advancements in nursing is the rise of _____ computing in the care environment.

    (A) Eponymous.

    (B) Ubiquitous.

    (C) Analogous.

    (D) Synchronous.

GO ON TO THE NEXT PAGE

GRAMMAR

1. Which sentence is grammatically incorrect?

   (A) Whether or not the needle had been used, the fact that it had been opened was enough to warrant its disposal.

   (B) The safety inspector declared that there were to many people gathered in the satellite waiting area.

   (C) She and I were equally alarmed by the presence of the armed officers in the room.

   (D) Please go to the fourth floor and pick up the results of the blood panel.

2. Select the best word for the blank in the following sentence.

   The map that shows the emergency exits on all floors of the hospital _____ incorrect and should be reprinted.

   (A) Are.

   (B) Is.

   (C) Have been.

   (D) Were.

3. Which word is used incorrectly in this sentence?

   Neither the doctor or the nurse was able to determine what happened to the three patients' blood samples.

   (A) Or.

   (B) Was.

   (C) What.

   (D) Patients'.

4. Which sentence is grammatically incorrect?

   (A) Both of the nursing school students were surprised by the number of different medications that they were required to know.

   (B) In the event of a fire, please proceed to the nearest marked exits.

   (C) For Shahir, turning in an incomplete answer sheet was the same as giving up.

   (D) He found that memorizing the names of bones in the human body was far more harder than learning the stages of the cardiac cycle.

5. Which word in the sample sentence is a pronoun?

   The tired trainees all left their notebooks at the front desk during lunch.

   (A) Tired.

   (B) All.

   (C) Their.

   (D) During.

6. Which word is used incorrectly in this sentence?

   The authorities had some difficulty establishing to who the mysterious package was addressed.

   (A) Had.

   (B) Establishing.

   (C) Who.

   (D) Was.

7. Which word from the sample sentence is a participle?

   The three researchers decided to have a working lunch and discuss their findings.

   (A) Three.

   (B) Decided.

   (C) Working.

   (D) Findings.

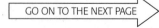
GO ON TO THE NEXT PAGE

8. Which sentence contains a cliché?

   (A) Although Jeff did not want to lose his job, the writing was on the wall after he failed to complete his safety certification.

   (B) After the accident, the passenger in the back seat had to remain hospitalized for much longer than the driver.

   (C) The elderly swimmer was able to complete the race more quickly than some swimmers who were forty years younger.

   (D) Matthijs missed his work shift because his dog swallowed a sock and had to be taken to the veterinary clinic.

9. Select the best word for the blank in the following sentence.

   Ellen _____ playing the trumpet since she was 10 years old.

   (A) Been.

   (B) Has been.

   (C) Have been.

   (D) Is.

10. Which word from the sample sentence is a conjunction?

    She took her break while the wing was relatively quiet, knowing it would be difficult to take one later.

    (A) While.

    (B) Knowing.

    (C) Would.

    (D) Later.

GO ON TO THE NEXT PAGE

KAPLAN

MATHEMATICS

1. If $5(x - 2) = 3x + 6$, what is the value of x?

   (A) -4

   (B) 4

   (C) 8

   (D) 12

2. Convert the following 12-hour clock time to military time: 2:17:08 PM

   (A) 02:17:08 hours

   (B) 12:17:08 hours

   (C) 14:17:08 hours

   (D) 15:17:08 hours

3. Which of the following is $\frac{12}{15}$ written as a percent?

   (A) 76%

   (B) 80%

   (C) 82.5%

   (D) 87.5%

4. Which of the following is 5% of 10% of 200?

   (A) 0.1

   (B) 0.5

   (C) 1

   (D) 2

5. The number 12 is 30% of what number?

   (A) 30

   (B) 32

   (C) 36

   (D) 40

6. Which of the following is 0.6 expressed as a fraction?

   (A) $\frac{3}{5}$

   (B) $\frac{5}{8}$

   (C) $\frac{2}{3}$

   (D) $\frac{3}{4}$

7. What is $\frac{5}{6} \times (-1\frac{1}{4})$?

   (A) $-1\frac{1}{2}$

   (B) $-1\frac{1}{24}$

   (C) $1\frac{1}{24}$

   (D) $1\frac{1}{2}$

8. What is $3\frac{4}{9} - 1\frac{5}{6}$?

   (A) $2\frac{1}{12}$

   (B) $1\frac{11}{18}$

   (C) $2\frac{2}{9}$

   (D) $1\frac{8}{9}$

9. Which of the following is $\frac{15}{18}$ expressed as a ratio?

   (A) 5:6

   (B) 5:9

   (C) 3:4

   (D) 2:3

10. If $x = 8$, $y = 0.3$, and $z = 1.5$, what is the value of the expression $(4 - x)^2 - 8y + 2(z + 3)$?

    (A) 22.6

    (B) 1

    (C) -9.4

    (D) -12

GO ON TO THE NEXT PAGE

BIOLOGY

1. Which is not a characteristic of water?

   (A) High specific heat value.

   (B) Strong polarity that facilitates intermolecular bonds.

   (C) Ability to dissolve many substances.

   (D) Very low adhesion.

2. Which term describes an individual who carries two different alleles for a specific gene?

   (A) Dominant.

   (B) Recessive.

   (C) Heterozygous.

   (D) Homozygous.

3. Which of these is not a lipid?

   (A) Fatty acids.

   (B) Amino acids.

   (C) Steroids.

   (D) Phospholipids.

4. Which organelle is chiefly responsible for respiration and energy production?

   (A) Golgi apparatus.

   (B) Endoplasmic reticulum.

   (C) Mitochondrion.

   (D) Nucleus.

5. Which substance is a product of photosynthesis?

   (A) Glucose.

   (B) Water.

   (C) Carbon dioxide.

   (D) Photons.

GO ON TO THE NEXT PAGE

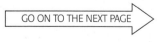

CHEMISTRY

1. Which value does the scientific notation 8.323×10^5 represent?

   (A) 0.00008323
   (B) 83,230
   (C) 832,300
   (D) 8,323,000

2. Which temperature is equivalent to 273K (273 degrees Kelvin)?

   (A) 0 degrees Fahrenheit.
   (B) 0 degrees Celsius.
   (C) 100 degrees Celsius.
   (D) 212 degrees Fahrenheit.

3. Which particles are found in the nucleus of an atom?

   (A) Protons and neutrons.
   (B) Protons and electrons.
   (C) Neutrons and electrons.
   (D) Protons, neutrons, and electrons.

4. Which are the products in the following chemical reaction?

   $$C_3H_8 + 5\,O_2 \rightarrow 3\,CO_2 + 4\,H_2O$$

   (A) Propane and oxygen.
   (B) Carbon and hydrogen.
   (C) Oxygen and hydrogen.
   (D) Water and carbon dioxide.

5. Which type of chemical reaction involves the breaking down of a compound into its component elements?

   (A) Synthesis.
   (B) Decomposition.
   (C) Combustion.
   (D) Single replacement.

GO ON TO THE NEXT PAGE

ANATOMY AND PHYSIOLOGY

1. Which body plane cuts horizontally through the midsection?

   (A) Frontal plane.
   (B) Sagittal plane.
   (C) Transverse plane.
   (D) Median plane.

2. Which term is not a section of the vertebral column?

   (A) Lumbar.
   (B) Sacral.
   (C) Thoracic.
   (D) Cranial.

3. Which of these connects the pituitary gland to the hypothalamus?

   (A) Adrenal cortex.
   (B) Infundibulum.
   (C) Adenohypophysis.
   (D) Neurohypophysis.

4. The male and female sex organs in humans undertake which function?

   (A) Production of gametes.
   (B) Production of hormones.
   (C) Both A and B.
   (D) None of the above.

5. Where does gas exchange take place in the respiratory system?

   (A) Bronchi.
   (B) Trachea.
   (C) Alveoli.
   (D) Larynx.

GO ON TO THE NEXT PAGE

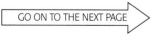

PHYSICS

1. A train travels 9.2 kilometers over a period of 3 minutes and 50 seconds. What is the average speed of the train in meters per second?

   (A) 0.4
   (B) 2.1
   (C) 4
   (D) 40

2. A toy car is rolled down a hill. Its initial speed is 0.4 m/s, and it travels down the hill for 1 minute. At the end of 1 minute, the car's speed is 8.2 m/s. What is the magnitude of the car's acceleration in meters per second squared?

   (A) 0.13
   (B) 0.26
   (C) 2.6
   (D) 7.8

3. Which of these is another way of expressing 14N (14 newtons of force)?

   (A) 14 m/s
   (B) 14 m/s^2
   (C) 14 kg-m/s^2
   (D) 14 net m/s^2

4. A spinning wheel accelerates from 3 revolutions per second to 15 revolutions per second over a period of 1 minute. What is the angular acceleration of the wheel in revolutions per second squared?

   (A) 0.2
   (B) 2
   (C) 4
   (D) 12

5. A storage cart has a mass of 600 kg and is traveling at a speed of 5 m/s. How much kinetic energy, in joules, does the cart have as a result of its motion?

   (A) 1,200
   (B) 7,500
   (C) 12,000
   (D) 15,000

END OF TEST. **STOP**

THE ANSWER KEY APPEARS ON THE FOLLOWING PAGE.

Practice Test Four: **Answer Key**

Reading Comprehension	**Vocabulary**	**Grammar**	**Mathematics**
1. B	1. A	1. B	1. C
2. C	2. B	2. B	2. C
3. D	3. A	3. A	3. B
4. C	4. D	4. D	4. C
5. B	5. C	5. C	5. D
6. A	6. B	6. C	6. A
7. D	7. C	7. C	7. B
8. A	8. D	8. A	8. B
9. C	9. C	9. B	9. A
10. D	10. B	10. A	10. A

Biology	**Chemistry**	**Anatomy and Physiology**	**Physics**
1. D	1. C	1. C	1. D
2. C	2. B	2. D	2. A
3. B	3. A	3. B	3. C
4. C	4. D	4. C	4. A
5. A	5. B	5. C	5. B

Answers and Explanations

Reading Comprehension

1. B

The main idea of the second paragraph is to show the long history of the idea of a universal basic income. Advocacy by Thomas Spence (A) and Thomas Paine (C) in the 18th century are details supporting this main idea. The paragraph does not address whether the idea of universal basic income has had mainstream support (D).

2. C

The word *obsolete* means "no longer needed."

3. D

The passage discusses the impact of consumer spending on economic growth (A), Thomas Spence's ideas on universal basic income (B), and the reformers Clifford Douglas and Dennis Milner (C). The amount of money provided in the Finland trial (D) is not mentioned in the passage.

4. C

The passage lays out arguments for and against a universal income, and speculates on how the topic has become more relevant in recent times. All the answer choices include details from the passage, but (A) offers only a brief definition of universal income, and (B) and (D) each offer only one side of the debate over universal income.

5. B

The author mentions wealthier citizens to contrast their spending with that of lower-income citizens (B), and the sentence on this topic specifically uses the words "by contrast," giving a clue to the purpose. The passage does not explain how to become wealthy (A) or transfer wealth (C) or argue whether wealthy people deserve their money (D).

6. A

Although the author also provides a definition of universal basic income (B), most of the passage discusses the pros, cons, and possible future impact of universal basic income (A), indicating that this is the author's primary purpose in writing this piece. The passage does not demonstrate a controversy concerning who originated the idea (C). The tone of the passage is serious and informative rather than entertaining (D).

7. D

The statements about the origin of the idea (A), spending habits of lower-income citizens (B), and recent support by U.S. lawmakers (C), can be verified. By contrast, the assertion that critics will come to see the desirability of universal basic income (D) is an opinion.

8. A

Finland's trial of universal basic income to evaluate its effects (A) supports the idea that universal basic income is gaining in popularity. While U.S. income inequality (B), British reform (C), and the threat to job security presented by automation are all mentioned in the passage, they do not indicate support for implementing universal basic income.

9. C

The author suggests that critics might rethink the idea of a universal basic income and come to see it as "something to embrace." This suggests that the author supports the idea of a universal basic income.

10. D

The word *efficacy* means "effectiveness."

Vocabulary

1. A

The word *impaired* means "diminished."

2. B

The word *occlusion* means "blockage."

3. A

The word *abrupt* means "sudden."

4. D

The word *succinct* means "concise."

5. C

The meaning "took into the body" is best represented by the word *ingested*.

6. B

The word *acute* means "severe."

7. C

The word *precipitous* means "extremely steep."

8. D

The meaning "cause of a disease" is best represented by the word *etiology*.

9. C

The word *assent* means "agreement."

10. B

The meaning "omnipresent" is best represented by the word *ubiquitous*.

Grammar

1. B

The preposition *to* is used incorrectly in the phrase "there were to many people"; it should be replaced with the adverb *too*.

2. B

Although it may appear that "floors" is the subject of the sentence, it is actually the object of the preposition "on." The true subject of the sentence is "map," which requires a singular verb. Three answer options are plural verbs: *are* (A), *have been* (C), and *were* (D). Only *is* (B) is a singular verb.

3. A

When the correlative conjunction "neither" is used, it is always paired with *nor*. Therefore, the word "or" should be replaced with *nor*.

4. D

The word *more* is unnecessary in combination with the adjective *harder*, which is already in comparative form.

5. C

Their is a possessive pronoun referring to "the tired trainees." *Tired* (A) is an adjective; *all* (B) is an adjective; *during* (D) is a preposition.

6. C

The word *to* is a preposition, and the word that follows is its object. An object needs to be in the objective case, so "who" (a subjective pronoun), is incorrect; it should be replaced with "whom."

7. C

A participle is a word formed from a verb, but used as an adjective. This is how "working" is used in "a working lunch."

8. A

"The writing was on the wall" is a cliché, which should be avoided in written communication.

9. B

By itself, *been* (A) is an incorrect verb form. The subject ("Ellen") is singular; this rules out *have been* (C), a plural verb form. The sentence describes action occurring from the past into the present ("since she was 10 years old"); this rules out *is* (D), because the verb phrase "is playing" describes action occurring from the present into the future.

10. A

In this sentence, "while" serves as a subordinating conjunction that expresses position in time. *Knowing* (B) is a participle, *would* (C) is a verb, and *later* (D) is an adverb.

Mathematics

1. C

Multiplying out the left side of the equation $5(x - 2) = 3x + 6$ yields $5x - 10 = 3x + 6$; subtracting $3x$ from each side yields $2x - 10 = 6$; and adding 10 to each side yields $2x = 16$. Dividing each side by 2 yields $x = 8$.

2. C

In military time, for times after 12 noon, you must add 12:00:00 hours to the PM time. Therefore, 2:17:08 PM is 14:17:08 hours in military time.

3. B

The fraction $\frac{12}{15}$ can be reduced to $\frac{4}{5}$. Now let's convert $\frac{4}{5}$ to a percent. To convert a fraction or a decimal to a percent, multiply that fraction or decimal by 100%:
$\frac{4}{5} = \frac{4}{5} \times 100\% = 4 \times 20\% = 80\%$.

4. C

First convert the percents in this question to fractions. To convert a percent to a fraction or decimal, divide the percent by 100%:

$$5\% = \frac{5\%}{100\%} = \frac{5}{100} = \frac{1}{20}$$

$$10\% = \frac{10\%}{100\%} = \frac{10}{100} = \frac{1}{10}$$

Therefore, 5% of 10% of $200 = \frac{1}{20} \times \frac{1}{10} \times 200 = \left(\frac{1}{20} \times \frac{1}{10}\right) \times 200 = \frac{1 \times 1}{20 \times 10} \times 200 = \frac{1}{200} \times 200 = 1$.

5. D

Let x be the unknown number that 12 is 30% of. Convert 30% to a decimal. To convert a percent to a decimal or fraction, divide the percent by 100%:

$30\% = \frac{30\%}{100\%} = \frac{30}{100} = \frac{3}{10} = 0.3$. So $12 = 0.3x$. Divide both sides by 0.3, and simplify: $\frac{12}{0.3} = x$, $\frac{12 \times 10}{0.3 \times 10} = x$, $\frac{120}{3} = x$, and $40 = x$. Therefore, $x = 40$.

6. A

The number 0.6 is equivalent to $\frac{6}{10}$, which can be reduced to $\frac{3}{5}$.

7. B

Convert $-1\frac{1}{4}$ to an improper fraction. $1\frac{1}{4} = \frac{1 \times 4 + 1}{4} = \frac{4 + 1}{4} = \frac{5}{4}$. So $1\frac{1}{4} = \frac{5}{4}$. Remember the negative sign, so $-1\frac{1}{4} = -\frac{5}{4}$, or $-\frac{5}{4} = \frac{-5}{4}$. So $\frac{5}{6} \times \left(-1\frac{1}{4}\right) = \frac{5}{6} \times \frac{-5}{4}$.

Work with $\frac{5}{6} \times \left(\frac{-5}{4}\right)$. Multiply the numerators, multiply the denominators, simplify if necessary, and then convert back to a mixed fraction: $\frac{5}{6} \times \left(\frac{-5}{4}\right) = \frac{5 \times (-5)}{6 \times 4} = \frac{-25}{24}$. Now $\frac{25}{24} = 1\frac{1}{24}$, so $-\frac{25}{24} = -1\frac{1}{24}$. Therefore, $\frac{5}{6} \times \left(-1\frac{1}{4}\right) = -1\frac{1}{24}$.

8. B

To solve this problem, first convert the mixed numbers to improper fractions: $3\frac{4}{9} = \frac{3 \times 9 + 4}{9} = \frac{27 + 4}{9} = \frac{31}{9}$ and $1\frac{5}{6} = \frac{1 \times 6 + 5}{6} = \frac{6 + 5}{6} = \frac{11}{6}$.

Therefore, $3\frac{4}{9} - 1\frac{5}{6} = \frac{31}{9} - \frac{11}{6}$. Now let's work with $\frac{31}{9} - \frac{11}{6}$. To continue, find a common denominator. You can find a positive common multiple of 9 and 6 by starting with the smallest positive multiple of 9, which is $1 \times 9 = 9$, and then looking at the next positive multiples of 9, which are $2 \times 9, 3 \times 9, 4 \times 9, 5 \times 9, \ldots$, until you find a multiple of 6.

- $1 \times 9 = 9$ is not a multiple of 6.
- $2 \times 9 = 18$ is a multiple of 6, since $18 = 3 \times 6$.

Solve using the common denominator:
$\frac{31}{9} - \frac{11}{6} = \frac{62}{18} - \frac{33}{18} = \frac{62 - 33}{18} = \frac{29}{18} = 1\frac{11}{18}$.

9. A

By dividing both numerator and denominator by 3, you can reduce the fraction $\frac{15}{18}$ to $\frac{5}{6}$, which is equivalent to a ratio of 5:6.

10. A

We want to find the value of the expression $(4 - x)^2 - 8y + 2(z + 3)$ when $x = 8$, $y = 0.3$, and $z = 1.5$. First substitute the given values, $x = 8$, $y = 0.3$, and $z = 1.5$, into the expression; this yields $(4 - 8)^2 - 8(0.3) + 2(1.5 + 3)$. Then apply the arithmetic operations to evaluate the expression: $(-4)^2 - (2.4) + 2(4.5) = 16 - 2.4 + 9 = 22.6$.

Biology

1. D

High specific heat value (A), strong polarity (B), and ability to dissolve many substances (C) are all characteristics of water. Very low adhesion (D) is not characteristic of water, which exhibits both adhesion (stickiness to other substances) and cohesion (stickiness to itself).

2. C

An individual with two different alleles for a specific gene is heterozygous for that gene. An individual with two of the same allele for a specific gene is homozygous (D) for that gene. Alleles themselves may be either dominant (A) or recessive (B).

3. B

Amino acids (B) are proteins. Fatty acids (A), steroids (C), and phospholipids (D) are all lipids.

4. C

Mitochondria create ATP, the energy used by the cell. The Golgi apparatus (A) collects and packages proteins for use in the cell. The endoplasmic reticulum (B) folds protein molecules and transports them to the Golgi apparatus. The nucleus (D) stores genetic material and controls gene replication during cell division.

5. A

The process of photosynthesis can be expressed as $6CO_2 + 6H_2O + \text{Light energy} \rightarrow C_6H_{12}O_6 + 6O_2$. Water (B), carbon dioxide (C), and photons (D) are raw materials that go into photosynthesis. The products are glucose (A) and oxygen.

Chemistry

1. C

8.323×10^5 is the same as $8.323 \times 100{,}000$, or $832{,}300$.

2. B

The Kelvin scale begins at absolute zero, or -273 Celsius. Therefore, 273K is equivalent to 0 degrees Celsius.

3. A

The nucleus of an atom contains protons and neutrons. Electrons orbit around the nucleus.

4. D

In the chemical reaction $C_3H_8 + 5\,O_2 \rightarrow 3\,CO_2 + 4\,H_2O$, the products are found to the right of the arrow. The products in this reaction are carbon dioxide (CO_2) and water (H_2O), choice (D). Propane (C_3H_8) and oxygen (O_2) (A) are the reactants, or starting substances, of this chemical reaction. Elemental carbon and hydrogen (B) are neither reactants nor products of the reaction, nor is elemental oxygen (C).

5. B

Decomposition (B) occurs when a compound breaks down into individual elements. In synthesis (A), elements combine to form a new product. In combustion (C), oxygen and a fuel compound react to produce energy. Single replacement (D) occurs when an active metal changes places with a metal in an existing compound.

Anatomy and Physiology

1. C

The transverse plane cuts horizontally through the middle of the torso. The frontal plane (A) cuts vertically through the torso from side to side, dividing the body into front and back. The sagittal plane (B) cuts vertically through the torso from front to back, dividing the body into left and right halves. The median plane (D) is another term for the sagittal plane.

2. D

The vertebral column includes lumbar (A), sacral (B), and thoracic (C) sections. The final section of vertebral column is cervical, not cranial (D).

3. B

The infundibulum is a stalk connecting the pituitary gland to the hypothalamus. The adrenal cortex (A) is the outermost layer of the adrenal gland. The adenohypophysis (C) is another term for the anterior pituitary, the frontal lobe of the pituitary gland. The neurohypophysis (D) is the posterior pituitary, or rear lobe of the pituitary gland.

4. C

The human sex organs are responsible for producing both sex cells (or gametes) and certain hormones.

5. C

The alveoli are the main location where gas exchange occurs in the lungs during respiration. The bronchi (A) are passages connecting the trachea to the bronchioles. The trachea (B) is the main passageway for air entering the lungs. The larynx (D) protects the trachea from intrusion of food and foreign objects, and it houses the vocal cords.

Physics

1. D

Average speed is equal to total distance divided by total time. The answer options give rates in meters per second, so the units in the question must be converted:

9.2 kilometers = 9.2 kilometers × (1,000 meters/kilometer) = 9,200 meters.

3 minutes = (3 minutes) × (60 seconds/minute) = 180 seconds. Then 3 minutes and 50 seconds = (180 seconds) + (50 seconds) = 230 seconds.

The train traveled 9,200 meters in 230 seconds. Therefore, the average speed was (9,200 meters) ÷ (230 seconds) = 40 meters per second (m/s).

2. A

Acceleration is calculated as the change in velocity divided by the change in time. The change in velocity is (8.2 meters per second) − (0.4 meters per second) = 7.8 meters per second. The change in time is 60 seconds. Therefore, the acceleration is (7.8 meters per second) ÷ (60 seconds) = $\frac{7.8}{60}$ meters per second squared, or 0.13 meters per second squared (m/s^2).

3. C

The newton, a unit of force, is expressed as kilogram-meters per second squared, or kg-m/s^2. Therefore, 14N is 14 kg-m/s^2.

4. A

Angular acceleration is calculated as the change in angular speed divided by the change in time. The change in angular speed is the final angular speed minus the initial angular speed. Here the change in angular speed is (15 revolutions per second) − (3 revolutions per second) = 12 revolutions per second. The change in time is the final time minus the initial time. Here, the change in time is (60 seconds) − (0 seconds) = 60 seconds.

If the change in angular speed is 12 revolutions per second and the change in time is 60 seconds, then the angular acceleration of the wheel is (12 revolutions per second) ÷ (60 seconds) = 0.2 revolutions per second squared (s^2).

5. B

Kinetic energy (expressed in joules when the mass is in kilograms and the velocity is in meters per second) is calculated as $\frac{1}{2}$mass × velocity^2. Substitute 600 kg for the mass and 5 $\frac{\text{meters}}{\text{second}}$ for the velocity into the formula Kinetic energy = $\frac{1}{2}$mass × velocity^2: Kinetic energy = $\frac{1}{2}$mass × velocity^2 = $\frac{1}{2}$ (600 kg)(5 m/s)^2 = $\frac{1}{2}$(600)(5^2) kg-m/s^2 = 300(25) J = 7,500 J.

Learning Resources

- Common Word Roots and Prefixes
- Frequently Misspelled Words
- Words Commonly Confused for One Another
- Math in a Nutshell

Common Word Roots and Prefixes

AB/ABS: off, away from, apart, down

abdicate: to renounce or relinquish a throne; abduct: to carry off or lead away

ANTE: before

antebellum: before the war (especially the American Civil War); antecedent: existing, being, or going before

BEL/BELL: war

belligerent: warlike, given to waging war; rebel: a person who resists authority, control, or tradition

BEN/BON: good

benefit: anything advantageous to a person or thing; bonus: something given over and above what is due

CAP/CIP/CEPT: to take, to get

anticipate: to realize beforehand, foretaste, or foresee; capture: to take by force or stratagem

CHRON: time

anachronism: an obsolete or archaic form; chronic: constant, habitual

CO/COL/COM/CON: with, together

coerce: to compel by force, intimidation, or authority; collaborate: to work with another, cooperate

DIC/DICT/DIT: to say, to tell, to use words

dictionary: a book containing a selection of the words of a language; interdict: to forbid, prohibit

DOG/DOX: opinion

dogma: a system of tenets, as of a church; orthodox: sound or correct in opinion or doctrine

DUC/DUCT: to lead

abduct: to carry off or lead away; conducive: contributive, helpful

E/EF/EX: out, out of, from, former

efface: to rub or wipe out; evade: to escape from, avoid; exclude: to shut out, leave out

FER: to bring; to carry; to bear

confer: to grant, bestow; offer: to present for acceptance, refusal, or consideration

FERV: to boil, to bubble

effervescent: with the quality of giving off bubbles of gas; fervor: passion

JOIN/JUNCT: to meet; to unite

adjoin: to be next to and joined with; junction: the act of joining, combining; junta: clique, usually military, that takes power after a coup d'état

LECT/LEG: to select, to choose

collect: to gather together or assemble; eclectic: selecting ideas, etc. from various sources; select: to choose with care

MAG/MAJ/MAX: big

magnanimous: generous in forgiving an insult or injury; magnate: a powerful or influential person

MON/MONIT: to remind, to warn

admonish: to counsel against something, to caution; monitor: one that admonishes, cautions, or reminds

NOV/NEO/NOU: new

innovate: to begin or introduce something new; neologism: a newly coined word, phrase, or expression

OB/OC/OF/OP: toward, to, against, over

obese: extremely fat, corpulent; obfuscate: to render indistinct or dim, to darken

PAN: all, everyone

pandemic: widespread, general, universal; panegyric: formal or elaborate praise at an assembly

PARA: next to, beside

parable: a short, allegorical story designed to illustrate a moral lesson or religious principle; paragon: a model of excellence

SACR/SANCT/SECR: sacred

sacrament: something regarded as possessing sacred character; secret: known by one or only a few

SENS/SENT: to feel, to be aware

dissent: to differ in opinion, esp. from the majority; insensate: without feeling or sensitivity

TEND/TENS/TENT/TENU: to stretch; to thin

attenuate: to weaken or reduce in force; contentious: quarrelsome, disagreeable, belligerent

VEN/VENT: to come or to move toward

adventitious: accidental; contravene: to come into conflict with

Frequently Misspelled Words

Absence: One *a*, two *e*'s.

Accommodate, accommodation: Two *c*'s, two *m*'s

Accompany: Two *c*'s.

All right: Two words. *Alright* is *NOT* all right.

A lot: Always two words, never one; do not confuse with *allot*.

Argument: No *e* after the *u*.

Calendar: *A*, *e*, then another *a*.

Campaign: Remember the *aig* combination.

Cannot: Usually spelled as a single word, except where the meaning is "able not to."

- CORRECT: One *cannot* ignore the importance of conformity.
- CORRECT: Anyone *can not* pay taxes, but the consequences may be serious.

Comparative, comparatively: Yes, *comparison* has an *i* after the *r*. These words don't.

Conscience: Spell it with *science*.

Correspondent, correspondence: No *dance*.

Definite: Spell it with *finite*, not *finate*.

Develop, development: No *e* after the *p*.

Embarrass: Two *r*'s, two *s*'s.

Every day (adv.): Two words with *every* modifying *day*. Note that there is also an adjective.

Everyday (adj.): Meaning *commonplace, usual.*

- ADVERB: We see this error *every day*.
- ADJECTIVE: Getting stuck behind an elephant in traffic is no longer an *everyday* occurrence in Katmandu.

Exaggerate: One *x*, two *g*'s.

Foreign: Think of the *reign* of a *foreign* king.

Grammar: No *e*.

Grateful: Spell it with *grate*.

Harass: One *r*, two *s*'s.

Independent, independence: No *dance*.

Indispensable: It's something you are not *able* to dispense with.

Judgment: No *e* on the end of *judge*.

Leisure: Like *pleasure* but with an *i* instead of *a*.

License: In alphabetical order: *c* then *s*, not *lisence*.

Maintenance: *Main*, then *ten*, then *ance* (reverse alphabetical order for your vowels preceding *n*).

Maneuver: Memorize the unusual *eu* combo.

No one: Two words. Don't be misled by *nobody, nothing, everyone, someone,* and *anyone*.

Noticeable: Notice that this one keeps the *e* when adding the suffix.

Occur, occurred, occurrence: Double the *r* when you add a suffix beginning with a vowel.

Parallel, unparalleled: Two *l*'s, then one.

Parenthesis (pl. parentheses): Likewise, many other words of Greek origin are spelled with *-is* in the singular and *-es* in the plural; among the more common are *analysis, diagnosis, prognosis, synthesis, thesis.*

Perseverance: Only two *r*'s—*sever*, not *server*. Remember that the *a* in the suffix keeps it from being all *e*'s.

Professor, professional: One *f*.

Pronunciation: Never mind *pronounce* and *pronouncement*: *pronunciation* has no *o* in the second syllable.

Questionnaire: Two *n*'s, one *r*.

Regardless: Not *irregardless*, an unacceptable yoking of *irrespective* and *regardless*.

Responsible, responsibility: While the French and Spanish cognates end in *-able*, it's *-ible* in English.

Separate: Look for *a rat* in *separate*.

Unanimous: *Un-* and then *-an-*.

Vacuum: One *c*, two *u*'s.

Words Commonly Confused for One Another

Accept or *except? Alter* or *altar? Discrete* or *discreet?* Even if you know the difference between these words, when you're under pressure and short on time, it's easy to get confused. So, here's a quick review of some of the most common troublemakers.

Accept (v.): To take or receive. The CEO accepted the treasurer's resignation.

Except (prep.): Leave out. The Town Council approved all elements of the proposal except the tax increase.

Adverse (adj.): Unfavorable. This plan would have an adverse impact on the environment.

Averse (adj.): Opposed or reluctant. I am averse to doing business with companies that don't treat their employees fairly.

Advice (n.): Recommendation as to what should be done. I would like your advice about how to handle this situation.

Advise (v.): To recommend what should be done. I will be happy to advise you.

Affect (v.): To have an impact or influence on. The expansion of Pyramid Shopping Mall will certainly affect traffic on the access roads.

Effect (n.): Result, impact. The proposal will have a deleterious effect on everyone's quality of life.
(v.): To cause, implement. The engineers were able to effect a change in the train's performance at high speeds.

Altar (n.): An elevated structure, typically intended for the performance of religious rituals. The court refused to allow the construction of an altar on public property.

Alter (v.): To change. It should be a simple matter to alter one's will.

Among (prep.): Used to compare three or more items or entities. We can choose from among dozens of styles.

Between (prep.): Used to compare two items or entities. We can choose between these two styles.

Assent (n.): Agreement; **(v.):** to agree. Peter has given his assent to the plan.

Assure (v.): To convince or guarantee. He has assured me that this is a safe investment.

Ensure (v.): To make certain. Please ensure that this is a safe investment.

Insure (v.): To guard against loss. There is no way to insure this investment.

Bazaar (n.): A market. I found these fantastic trinkets at the bazaar.

Bizarre (adj.): Very strange, weird. No one knew how to respond to such a bizarre question.

Cite (v.): To quote, to refer to. The article cited our annual report.

Sight (n.): Something seen or visible; the faculty of seeing. What an amazing sight!

Site (n.): Location; **(v.):** to place or locate. This is the perfect site for a new office.

Complement (n.): Something that completes; **(v.):** to go with or complete. This item really complements our product line.

Compliment (v.): To flatter; **(n.):** a flattering remark. That was a sincere compliment.

Continual (adj.): Repeated regularly and frequently. Alan's continual telephone calls finally wore Rosa down and she agreed to a meeting.

Continuous (adj.): Extended or prolonged without interruption. The continuous banging from the construction site gave me a severe headache.

Decent (adj.): Proper, acceptable. You can trust Lena to do what is decent.

Descent (n.): Downward movement. The rapid descent of the balloon frightened its riders.

Discrete (adj.): Separate, not connected. These are two discrete issues.

Discreet (adj.): Prudent, modest, having discretion; not allowing others to notice. I must be very discreet about looking for a new job while I am still employed here.

Disinterested (adj.): Impartial, objective. We need a disinterested person to act as an arbitrator in this dispute.

Uninterested (adj.): Not interested. Charles is uninterested, but he'll come along anyway.

Eminent (adj.): Outstanding, distinguished. The eminent Dr. Blackwell will teach a special seminar in medical ethics this fall.

Imminent (adj.): About to happen, impending. Warned of imminent layoffs, Loretta began looking for another job.

Incidence (uncountable noun: occurrence): Frequency. The incidence of multiple births is on the rise.

Incident (pl.: incidents) (countable noun: events, cases): An occurrence of an event or situation. She preferred to forget the whole incident.

Personal (adj.): Private or pertaining to the individual. Please mark the envelope "personal and confidential."

Personnel (n.): Employees. This year we had a 5% increase in personnel.

Precede (v.): To come before. The list of resources should precede the financial worksheet.

Proceed (v.): To go forward. Although Jules will be absent, we will proceed with the meeting as planned.

Principal (n.): Head of a school or organization, primary participant, main sum of money; **(adj.):** main, foremost, most important. Joshua is one of the principals of the company.

Principle (n.): A basic truth or law. I have always run my business based on the principle that honesty is the best policy.

Reign (v.): To exercise power; **(n.):** period in which a ruler exercised power or a condition prevailed. Under the reign of King Richard, order was restored.

Rein (n.): A means of restraint or guidance; **(v.)** to restrain, control. You need to rein in your intern, Carol—she's taking on much too much responsibility and doesn't seem to know what she's doing.

Than (conj.): Used to compare. I will be more successful this time because I am more experienced than before.

Then (adv.): I was very naïve back then.

Weather (n.): Climatic conditions, state of the atmosphere. The bad weather is going to keep people away from our grand opening.

Whether (conj.): Used to refer to a choice between alternatives. I am not sure whether I will attend the grand opening or not.

Math in a Nutshell

We've listed the 64 most important concepts that you'll need for the math on your nursing school entrance exam in this learning resource. Use this list to remind yourself of the key areas you'll need to know. Do three concepts a day, and you'll be ready in three weeks. If a concept continually causes you trouble, circle it and refer back to it when correcting your practice tests.

Number Properties

1. Number Categories

Integers are **whole numbers;** they include negative whole numbers and zero.

A **rational number** is a number that can be expressed as a **ratio of two integers. Irrational numbers** are real numbers—they have locations on the number line—but they **can't be expressed precisely as a fraction or decimal.** For the purposes of nursing exams, the most important **irrational numbers** are $\sqrt{2}$, $\sqrt{3}$, and π.

2. Adding/Subtracting Signed Numbers

To **add a positive and a negative,** first ignore the signs and find the positive difference between the number parts. Then attach the sign of the original number with the larger number part. For example, to add 23 and -34, first ignore the minus sign and find the positive difference between 23 and 34—that's 11. Then attach the sign of the number with the larger number part—in this case it's the minus sign from the -34. So, $23 + (-34) = -11$.

Make **subtraction** situations simpler by turning them into addition. For example, you can think of $-17 - (-21)$ as $-17 + (+21)$.

To **add or subtract a string of positives and negatives,** first turn everything into addition. Then combine the positives and negatives so that the string is reduced to the sum of a single positive number and a single negative number.

3. Multiplying/Dividing Signed Numbers

To multiply and/or divide positives and negatives, treat the number parts as usual and **attach a minus sign if there were originally an odd number of negatives.** For example, to multiply -2, -3, and -5, first multiply the number parts: $2 \times 3 \times 5 = 30$. Then go back and note that there were *three*—an *odd* number—negatives, so the product is negative: $(-2) \times (-3) \times (-5) = -30$.

4. PEMDAS

When performing multiple operations, remember to perform them in the right order: **PEMDAS,** which means **P**arentheses first, then **E**xponents, then **M**ultiplication and **D**ivision (left to right), and lastly **A**ddition and **S**ubtraction (left to right). In the expression $9 - 2 \times (5 - 3)^2 + 6 \div 3$, begin with the parentheses: $(5 - 3) = 2$. Then do the exponent: $2^2 = 4$. Now the expression is: $9 - 2 \times 4 + 6 \div 3$. Next do the multiplication and division to get $9 - 8 + 2$, which equals 3. If you have difficulty remembering PEMDAS, use this sentence to recall it: Please Excuse My Dear Aunt Sally.

5. Counting Consecutive Integers

To count consecutive integers, **subtract the smallest from the largest and add 1.** To count the integers from 13 through 31, subtract: $31 - 13 = 18$. Then add 1: $18 + 1 = 19$.

KAPLAN

Number Operations and Concepts

6. Exponential Growth

If r is the ratio between consecutive terms, a_1 is the first term, a_n is the nth term, and S_n is the sum of the first n terms, then $a_n = a_1 r^{n-1}$ and $S_n = \dfrac{a_1 - a_1 r^n}{1} - r$. (For example, in 1, 2, 4, 8, $r = 2$, $a_1 = 1$ and $a_4 = 8$, the fourth term.)

7. Union and Intersection of Sets

The things in a set are called elements or members. The union of Set A and Set B, sometimes expressed as $A \cup B$, is the set of elements that are in either or both of Set A and Set B. If Set $A = \{1, 2\}$ and Set $B = \{3, 4\}$, then $A \cup B = \{1, 2, 3, 4\}$. The intersection of Set A and Set B, sometimes expressed as $A \cap B$, is the set of elements common to both Set A and Set B. If Set $A = \{1, 2, 3\}$ and Set $B = \{3, 4, 5\}$, then $A \cap B = \{3\}$.

Divisibility

8. Factor/Multiple

The **factors** of integer n are the positive integers that divide into n with no remainder. The **multiples** of n are the integers that n divides into with no remainder. For example, 6 is a factor of 12, and 24 is a multiple of 12. 12 is both a factor and a multiple of itself, since $12 \times 1 = 12$ and $12 \div 1 = 12$.

9. Prime Factorization

To find the prime factorization of an integer, just keep breaking it up into factors until **all the factors are prime**. To find the prime factorization of 36, for example, you could begin by breaking it into 4×9: $36 = 4 \times 9 = 2 \times 2 \times 3 \times 3$.

10. Relative Primes

Relative primes are integers that have no common factor other than 1. To determine whether two integers are relative primes, break them both down to their prime factorizations. For example: $35 = 5 \times 7$, and $54 = 2 \times 3 \times 3 \times 3$. They have **no prime factors in common**, so 35 and 54 are relative primes.

11. Common Multiple

A common multiple is a number that is a multiple of two or more integers. You can always get a common multiple of two integers by **multiplying** them, but, unless the two numbers are relative primes, the product will not be the *least* common multiple. For example, to find a common multiple for 12 and 15, you could just multiply: $12 \times 15 = 180$.

To find the **least common multiple (LCM)**, check out the **multiples of the larger integer** until you find one that's **also a multiple of the smaller**. To find the LCM of 12 and 15, begin by taking the multiples of 15: 15 is not divisible by 12; 30 is not; nor is 45. But the next multiple of 15, 60, *is* divisible by 12, so it's the LCM.

12. Greatest Common Factor (GCF)

To find the greatest common factor, break down both integers into their prime factorizations and multiply all the **prime factors they have in common**. $36 = 2 \times 2 \times 3 \times 3$, and $48 = 2 \times 2 \times 2 \times 2 \times 3$. What they have in common is two 2s and one 3, so the GCF is $2 \times 2 \times 3 = 12$.

13. Even/Odd

To predict whether a sum, difference, or product will be even or odd, just **take simple numbers like 1 and 2 and see what happens.** There are rules—"odd times even is even," for example—but there's no need to memorize them. What happens with one set of numbers generally happens with all similar sets.

14. Multiples of 2 and 4

An integer is divisible by 2 (even) if the **last digit is even.** An integer is divisible by 4 if the **last two digits form a multiple of 4.** The last digit of 562 is 2, which is even, so 562 is a multiple of 2. The last two digits form 62, which is *not* divisible by 4, so 562 is not a multiple of 4. The integer 512, however, is divisible by four because the last two digits form 12, which is a multiple of 4.

15. Multiples of 3 and 9

An integer is divisible by 3 if the **sum of its digits is divisible by 3.** An integer is divisible by 9 if the **sum of its digits is divisible by 9.** The sum of the digits in 957 is 21, which is divisible by 3 but not by 9, so 957 is divisible by 3 but not by 9.

16. Multiples of 5 and 10

An integer is divisible by 5 if the **last digit is 5 or zero.** An integer is divisible by 10 if the **last digit is zero.** The last digit of 665 is 5, so 665 is a multiple of 5 but *not* a multiple of 10.

17. Remainders

The remainder is the **whole number left over after division.** 487 is 2 more than 485, which is a multiple of 5, so when 487 is divided by 5, the remainder will be 2.

Fractions and Decimals

18. Reducing Fractions

To reduce a fraction to its lowest terms, **factor out and cancel** all factors the numerator and denominator have in common.

$$\frac{28}{36} = \frac{4 \times 7}{4 \times 9} = \frac{7}{9}$$

19. Adding/Subtracting Fractions

To add or subtract fractions, first find a **common denominator,** then add or subtract the numerators.

$$\frac{2}{15} + \frac{3}{10} = \frac{4}{30} + \frac{9}{30} = \frac{4+9}{30} = \frac{13}{30}$$

20. Multiplying Fractions

To multiply fractions, **multiply** the numerators and **multiply** the denominators.

$$\frac{5}{7} \times \frac{3}{4} = \frac{5 \times 3}{7 \times 4} = \frac{15}{28}$$

21. Dividing Fractions

To divide fractions, **invert** the second one and **multiply.**

$$\frac{1}{2} \div \frac{3}{5} = \frac{1}{2} \times \frac{5}{3} = \frac{1 \times 5}{2 \times 3} = \frac{5}{6}$$

22. Mixed Numbers and Improper Fractions

To convert a mixed number to an improper fraction, **multiply** the whole number part by the denominator, then **add** the numerator. The result is the new numerator (over the same denominator). To convert $7\frac{1}{3}$, first multiply 7 by 3, then add 1 to get the new numerator of 22. Put that over the same denominator, 3, to get $\frac{22}{3}$.

To convert an improper fraction to a mixed number, divide the denominator into the numerator to get a **whole number quotient with a remainder.** The quotient becomes the whole number part of the mixed number, and the remainder becomes the new numerator—with the same denominator. For example, to convert $\frac{108}{5}$, first divide 5 into 108, which yields 21 with a remainder of 3. Therefore, $\frac{108}{5} = 21\frac{3}{5}$.

23. Reciprocal

To find the reciprocal of a fraction, **switch the numerator and the denominator.** The reciprocal of $\frac{3}{7}$ is $\frac{7}{3}$. The reciprocal of 5 is $\frac{1}{5}$. The product of reciprocals is 1.

24. Comparing Fractions

One way to compare fractions is to **re-express them with a common denominator.** $\frac{3}{4} = \frac{21}{28}$ and $\frac{5}{7} = \frac{20}{28}$. $\frac{21}{28}$ is greater than $\frac{20}{28}$, so $\frac{3}{4}$ is greater than $\frac{5}{7}$. Another method is to **convert them both to decimals.** $\frac{3}{4}$ converts to 0.75, and $\frac{5}{7}$ converts to approximately 0.714.

25. Converting Fractions and Decimals

To convert a fraction to a decimal, **divide the bottom into the top.** To convert $\frac{5}{8}$, divide 8 into 5, yielding 0.625.

To convert a decimal to a fraction, set the decimal over 1 and **multiply the numerator and denominator by 10** raised to the number of digits to the right of the decimal point.

To convert 0.625 to a fraction, you would multiply $\frac{0.625}{1}$ by $\frac{10^3}{10^3}$ or $\frac{1000}{1000}$. Then simplify: $\frac{625}{1000} = \frac{5 \times 125}{8 \times 125} = \frac{5}{8}$.

26. Repeating Decimal

To find a particular digit in a repeating decimal, note the **number of digits in the cluster that repeats.** If there are 2 digits in that cluster, then every second digit is the same. If there are 3 digits in that cluster, then every third digit is the same. And so on. For example, the decimal equivalent of $\frac{1}{27}$ is 0.037..., which is best written $0.\overline{037}$. There are 3 digits in the repeating cluster, so every third digit is the same: 7. To find the 50th digit, look for the multiple of 3 just less than 50—that's 48. The 48th digit is 7, and with the 49th digit the pattern repeats with zero. The 50th digit is 3.

27. Identifying the Parts and the Whole

The key to solving most fractions and percents story problems is to identify the part and the whole. Usually you'll find the **part** associated with the verb *is/are* and the **whole** associated with the word *of*. In the sentence, "Half of the boys are blonds," the whole is the boys ("*of* the boys"), and the part is the blonds ("*are* blonds").

Percents

28. Percent Formula

Whether you need to find the part, the whole, or the percent, use the same formula:

$$\text{Part} = \text{Percent} \times \text{Whole}$$

Example: What is 12% of 25?
Setup: Part = 0.12 × 25

Example: 15 is 3% of what number?
Setup: 15 = 0.03 × Whole

Example: 45 is what percent of 9?
Setup: 45 = Percent × 9

29. Percent Increase and Decrease

To increase a number by a percent, **add the percent to 100%,** convert to a decimal, and multiply. To increase 40 by 25%, add 25% to 100%, convert 125% to 1.25, and multiply by 40. 1.25 × 40 = 50.

30. Finding the Original Whole

To find the **original whole before a percent increase or decrease,** set up an equation. Think of the result of a 15% increase over *x* as 1.15*x*.

Example: After a 5% increase, the population was 59,346. What was the population before the increase?

Setup: 1.05*x* = 59,346

31. Combined Percent Increase and Decrease

To determine the combined effect of multiple percent increases and/or decreases, **start with 100 and see what happens.**

Example: A price went up 10% one year, and the new price went up 20% the next year. What was the combined percent increase?

Setup: First year: 100 + (10% of 100) = 110.
Second year: 110 + (20% of 110) = 132.
That's a combined 32% increase.

Ratios, Proportions, and Rates

32. Setting up a Ratio

To find a ratio, put the number associated with the word *of* **on top** and the quantity associated with the word *to* **on the bottom** and reduce. The ratio of 20 oranges to 12 apples is $\frac{20}{12}$, which reduces to $\frac{5}{3}$.

33. Part-to-Part Ratios and Part-to-Whole Ratios

If the parts add up to the whole, a part-to-part ratio can be turned into two part-to-whole ratios by putting **each number in the original ratio over the sum of the numbers.** If the ratio of males to females is 1 to 2, then the males-to-people ratio is $\frac{1}{1+2} = \frac{1}{3}$ and the females-to-people ratio is $\frac{2}{1+2} = \frac{2}{3}$. In other words, $\frac{2}{3}$ of all the people are female.

34. Solving a Proportion

To solve a proportion, **cross-multiply:**

$$\frac{x}{5} = \frac{3}{4}$$
$$4x = 3 \times 5$$
$$x = \frac{15}{4} = 3.75$$

35. Rate

To solve a rates problem, **use the units** to keep things straight.

Example: If snow is falling at the rate of 1 foot every 4 hours, how many inches of snow will fall in 7 hours?

Setup:
$$\frac{1 \text{ foot}}{4 \text{ hours}} = \frac{x \text{ inches}}{7 \text{ hours}}$$
$$\frac{12 \text{ inches}}{4 \text{ hours}} = \frac{x \text{ inches}}{7 \text{ hours}}$$
$$4x = 12 \times 7$$
$$x = 21$$

36. Average Rate

Average rate is *not* simply the average of the rates.

$$\text{Average } A \text{ per } B = \frac{\text{Total } A}{\text{Total } B}$$

$$\text{Average Speed} = \frac{\text{Total distance}}{\text{Total time}}$$

To find the average speed for 120 miles at 40 mph and 120 miles at 60 mph, **don't just average the two speeds.** First, figure out the total distance and the total time. The total distance is 120 + 120 = 240 miles. The times are 2 hours for the first leg and 3 hours for the second leg, or 5 hours total. The average speed, then, is $\frac{240}{5} = 48$ miles per hour.

Averages

37. Average Formula

To find the average of a set of numbers, **add them up and divide by the number of numbers.**

$$\text{Average} = \frac{\text{Sum of the Terms}}{\text{Number of Terms}}$$

To find the average of the 5 numbers 12, 15, 23, 40, and 40, first add them: 12 + 15 + 23 + 40 + 40 = 130. Then, divide the sum by 5: 130 ÷ 5 = 26.

Powers and Roots

38. Multiplying and Dividing Powers

To multiply powers with the same base, **add the exponents and keep the same base:**

$$x^3 \times x^4 = x^{3+4} = x^7$$

To divide powers with the same base, **subtract the exponents and keep the same base:**

$$y^{13} \div y^8 = y^{13-8} = y^5$$

39. Raising Powers to Powers

To raise a power to a power, **multiply the exponents:**

$$(x^3)^4 = x^{3 \times 4} = x^{12}$$

40. Simplifying Square Roots

To simplify a square root, factor out the perfect squares under the radical, unsquare them, and put the result in front.

$$\sqrt{12} = \sqrt{4 \times 3} = \sqrt{4} \times \sqrt{3} = 2\sqrt{3}$$

41. Adding and Subtracting Roots

You can add or subtract radical expressions **when the part under the radicals is the same:**

$$2\sqrt{3} + 3\sqrt{3} = 5\sqrt{3}$$

Don't try to add or subtract when the radical parts are different. There's not much you can do with an expression like:

$$3\sqrt{5} + 3\sqrt{7}$$

42. Multiplying and Dividing Roots

The product of square roots is equal to the **square root of the product:**

$$\sqrt{3} \times \sqrt{5} = \sqrt{3 \times 5} = \sqrt{15}$$

The quotient of square roots is equal to the **square root of the quotient:**

$$\frac{\sqrt{6}}{\sqrt{3}} = \sqrt{\frac{6}{3}} = \sqrt{2}$$

43. Negative Exponent and Rational Exponent

To find the value of a number raised to a negative exponent, simply rewrite the number, without the negative sign, as the bottom of a fraction with 1 as the numerator of the fraction: $3^{-2} = \frac{1}{3^2} = \frac{1}{9}$. If x is a positive number and a is a nonzero number, then $x^{\frac{1}{a}} = \sqrt[a]{x}$. So $4^{\frac{1}{2}} = \sqrt[2]{4} = 2$. If p and q are integers, then $x^{\frac{p}{q}} = \sqrt[q]{x^p}$. So $4^{\frac{3}{2}} = \sqrt[2]{4^3} = \sqrt{64} = 8$.

Algebraic Expressions

44. Evaluating an Expression

To evaluate an algebraic expression, **plug in** the given values for the unknowns and calculate according to **PEMDAS.** To find the value of $x^2 + 5x - 6$ when $x = -2$, plug in −2 for x: $(-2)^2 + 5(-2) - 6 = -12$.

45. Adding and Subtracting Monomials

To combine like terms, **keep the variable part unchanged while adding or subtracting the coefficients:**

$$2a + 3a = (2 + 3)a = 5a$$

46. Adding and Subtracting Polynomials

To add or subtract polynomials, **combine like terms.**

$$(3x^2 + 5x - 7) - (x^2 + 12) =$$
$$(3x^2 - x^2) + 5x + (-7 - 12) =$$
$$2x^2 + 5x - 19$$

47. Multiplying Monomials

To multiply monomials, **multiply the coefficients and the variables separately:**

$$2a \times 3a = (2 \times 3)(a \times a) = 6a^2$$

48. Multiplying Binomials: FOIL

To multiply binomials, use **FOIL.** To multiply $(x + 3)$ by $(x + 4)$, first multiply the First terms: $x \times x = x^2$. Next the Outer terms: $x \times 4 = 4x$. Then the Inner terms: $3 \times x = 3x$. And finally the Last terms: $3 \times 4 = 12$. Then add and combine like terms:

$$x^2 + 4x + 3x + 12 = x^2 + 7x + 12$$

49. Multiplying Other Polynomials

FOIL works only when you want to multiply two binomials. If you want to multiply polynomials with more than two terms, make sure you **multiply each term in the first polynomial by each term in the second.**

$$(x^2 + 3x + 4)(x + 5) =$$
$$x^2(x + 5) + 3x(x + 5) + 4(x + 5) =$$
$$x^3 + 5x^2 + 3x^2 + 15x + 4x + 20 =$$
$$x^3 + 8x^2 + 19x + 20$$

After multiplying two polynomials together, the number of terms in your expression before simplifying should equal the number of terms in one polynomial multiplied by the number of terms in the second. In the example, you should have $3 \times 2 = 6$ terms in the product before you simplify like terms.

Factoring Algebraic Expressions

50. Factoring out a Common Divisor

A factor common to all terms of a polynomial can be **factored out.** All three terms in the polynomial $3x^3 + 12x^2 - 6x$ contain a factor of $3x$. Pulling out the common factor yields $3x(x^2 + 4x - 2)$.

51. Factoring the Difference of Squares

One of the test makers' favorite factorables is the **difference of squares.**

$$a^2 - b^2 = (a - b)(a + b)$$

$x^2 - 9$, for example, factors to $(x - 3)(x + 3)$.

52. Factoring the Square of a Binomial

Recognize polynomials that are squares of binomials:

$$a^2 + 2ab + b^2 = (a + b)^2$$
$$a^2 - 2ab + b^2 = (a - b)^2$$

For example, $4x^2 + 12x + 9$ factors to $(2x + 3)^2$, and $n^2 - 10n + 25$ factors to $(n - 5)^2$.

53. Factoring Other Polynomials: FOIL in Reverse

To factor a quadratic expression, **think about what binomials you could use FOIL on to get that quadratic expression.** To factor $x^2 - 5x + 6$, think about what First terms will produce x^2, what Last terms will produce $+6$, and what Outer and Inner terms will produce $-5x$. Some common sense—and a little trial and error—lead you to $(x - 2)(x - 3)$.

54. Simplifying an Algebraic Fraction

Simplifying an algebraic fraction is a lot like simplifying a numerical fraction. The general idea is to **find factors common to the numerator and denominator and cancel them.** Thus, simplifying an algebraic fraction begins with factoring.

For example, to simplify $\dfrac{x^2 - x - 12}{x^2 - 9}$, first factor the numerator and denominator:

$$\frac{x^2 - x - 12}{x^2 - 9} = \frac{(x - 4)(x + 3)}{(x - 3)(x + 3)}$$

Canceling $x + 3$ from the numerator and denominator leaves you with $\dfrac{x - 4}{x - 3}$.

Solving Equations

55. Solving a Linear Equation

To solve an equation, do whatever is necessary to both sides to **isolate the variable.** To solve the equation $5x - 12 = -2x + 9$, first get all the x's on one side by adding $2x$ to both sides: $7x - 12 = 9$. Then add 12 to both sides: $7x = 21$. Then divide both sides by 7: $x = 3$.

56. Solving "In Terms Of"

To solve an equation for one variable **in terms of** another means to **isolate the one variable on one side of the equation,** leaving an expression containing the other variable on the other side of the equation. To solve the equation $3x - 10y = -5x + 6y$ for x in terms of y, isolate x:

$$3x - 10y = -5x + 6y$$
$$3x + 5x = 6y + 10y$$
$$8x = 16y$$
$$x = 2y$$

57. Translating from English into Algebra

To translate from English into algebra, look for the key words and systematically turn phrases into algebraic expressions and sentences into equations. Be careful about order, especially when subtraction is called for.

Example: The charge for a phone call is r cents for the first 3 minutes and s cents for each minute thereafter. What is the cost, in cents, of a phone call lasting exactly t minutes? ($t > 3$)

Setup: The charge begins with r, and then something more is added, depending on the length of the call. The amount added is s times the number of minutes past 3 minutes. If the total number of minutes is t, then the number of minutes past 3 is $t - 3$. So the charge is $r + s(t - 3)$.

58. Solving a Quadratic Equation

To solve a quadratic equation, put it in the "$ax^2 + bx + c = 0$" form, **factor** the left side (if you can), and set each factor equal to 0 separately to get the two solutions. To solve $x^2 + 12 = 7x$, first rewrite it as $x^2 - 7x + 12 = 0$. Then factor the left side:

$$(x - 3)(x - 4) = 0$$
$$x - 3 = 0 \text{ or } x - 4 = 0$$
$$x = 3 \text{ or } 4$$

59. Solving a System of Equations

You can solve for 2 variables only if you have 2 distinct equations. 2 forms of the same equation will not be adequate. **Combine the equations** in such a way that **one of the variables cancels out.** To solve the 2 equations $4x + 3y = 8$ and $x + y = 3$, multiply both sides of the second equation by -3 to get: $-3x - 3y = -9$. Now add the 2 equations; the $3y$ and the $-3y$ cancel out, leaving: $x = -1$. Plug that back into either one of the original equations and you'll find that $y = 4$.

60. Solving an Inequality

To solve an inequality, do whatever is necessary to both sides to **isolate the variable.** Just remember that when you **multiply or divide both sides by a negative number,** you must **reverse the sign.** To solve $-5x + 7 < -3$, subtract 7 from both sides to get: $-5x < -10$. Now divide both sides by -5, remembering to reverse the sign: $x > 2$.

61. Radical Equations

A radical equation contains at least one radical expression. Solve radical equations by using standard rules of algebra. If $5\sqrt{x} - 2 = 13$, then $5\sqrt{x} = 15$ and $\sqrt{x} = 3$, so $x = 9$.

Functions

62. Function Notation and Evaluation

Standard function notation is written $f(x)$ and read "f of x." To evaluate the function $f(x) = 2x + 3$ for $f(4)$, replace x with 4 and simplify: $f(4) = 2(4) + 3 = 11$.

63. Direct and Inverse Variation

In direct variation, $y = kx$, where k is a nonzero constant. In direct variation, the variable y changes directly as x does. If a unit of Currency A is worth 2 units of Currency B, then $A = 2B$. If the number of units of B were to double, the number of units of A would double, and so on for halving, tripling, etc. In inverse variation, $xy = k$, where x and y are variables and k is a constant. A famous inverse relationship is $rate \times time = distance$, where distance is constant. Imagine having to cover a distance of 24 miles. If you were to travel at 12 miles per hour, you'd need 2 hours. But if you were to halve your rate, you would have to double your time. This is just another way of saying that rate and time vary inversely.

64. Domain and Range of a Function

The domain of a function is the set of values for which the function is defined. For example, the domain of $f(x) = \dfrac{1}{1 - x^2}$ is all values of x except 1 and -1, because for those values the denominator has a value of 0 and is therefore undefined. The range of a function is the set of outputs or results of the function. For example, the range of $f(x) = x^2$ is all numbers greater than all or equal to zero, because x^2 cannot be negative.